PHOTOGRAPHY BY CLIFFORD L. FREEHE

ILLUSTRATIONS BY VIRGINIA E. BROOKS
(Excluding Chapter 12 and Appendix)

Second Edition

AN ATLAS OF PEDODONTICS

JOHN M. DAVIS, D.D.S., M.S.D.

Associate Professor of Pedodontics,
University of Washington School of Dentistry,
Seattle, Washington

DAVID B. LAW, B.S.D., D.D.S., M.S.

Professor of Pedodontics,
University of Washington School of Dentistry,
Seattle, Washington

THOMPSON M. LEWIS, D.D.S., M.S.D.

Professor of Pedodontics,
University of Washington School of Dentistry,
Seattle, Washington

1981

W.B. SAUNDERS COMPANY   Philadelphia   London   Toronto

W. B. Saunders Company: West Washington Square
                           Philadelphia, PA   19105

                           1 St. Anne's Road
                           Eastbourne, East Sussex BN21 3UN, England

                           1 Goldthorne Avenue
                           Toronto, Ontario M8Z 5T9, Canada

Library of Congress Cataloging in Publication Data

Davis, John M 1936–

An atlas of pedodontics.

First ed. (1969) by D. B. Law, T. M. Lewis, and J. M. Davis.

1. Pedodontics — Atlases.   I. Law, David B., 1914–
   joint author.   II. Lewis, Thompson M., 1924–
   joint author.   III. Davis, John M., 1936–   . Atlas of
   pedodontics.   IV. Title. [DNLM: 1. Pedodontics —
   Atlases. WU17 D262a]

RK55.C5L37 1980   617.6′45   79–64596

ISBN 0–7216–2977–6

Listed here are the latest translated editions of this book together
with the language of the translation and the publisher.

Japanese (*1st Edition*) — Igaku Shoin, Ltd., Tokyo, Japan

French (*1st Edition*) — Julian Prelat, Paris, France

Italian (*1st Edition*) — Scienza e Tecnica Dentistica Edizioni
                          Internazionali, Milan, Italy (Saccardin)

An Atlas of Pedodontics   ISBN   0-7216-2977-6

Last digit is the print number   9   8   7   6   5   4   3   2   1

TO
OUR WIVES

Patricia, Marian, and Betty Jean

CONTRIBUTORS

MARC W. ANDERSON, D.D.S., M.S.D.
Director of Dental Department, Children's Orthopedic Hospital and Medical Center, Seattle, Washington

Chapter 19: Sedation

MICHAEL R. FEY, D.D.S., M.S.D.
Assistant Professor, Departments of Pedodontics and Orthodontics, University of Washington School of Dentistry, Seattle, Washington

Co-author, Chapter 20: The Handicapped Child

KENNETH E. GLOVER, D.D.S., M.S.D.
Associate Professor, Division of Orthodontics, Faculty of Dentistry, University of Alberta, Edmonton, Alberta

Co-author, Chapter 4: Radiography

MARC R. JOONDEPH, D.D.S., M.S.D.
Assistant Professor, Department of Orthodontics, University of Washington School of Dentistry, Seattle, Washington

Chapter 14: Orthodontic Diagnosis

ROGER A. MEYER, D.D.S., M.D.
Diplomate, American Board of Oral and Maxillofacial Surgery; Associate Professor, Chairman, Department of Oral and Maxillofacial Surgery Emory University School of Dentistry, Atlanta, Georgia

Chapter 12: Pediatric Oral Surgery

vii

PATRICK K. TURLEY, D.D.S., M.S.D., M.Ed.
   Assistant Professor, Section of Orthodontics and Pediatric Dentistry, University of California School of Dentistry, Los Angeles, California
Co-author, Chapter 20: The Handicapped Child

BRYAN J. WILLIAMS, D.D.S., M.S.D., M.Ed.
   Assistant Professor, Departments of Pediatric Dentistry and Orthodontics, University of Detroit School of Dentistry, Detroit, Michigan
Co-author, Chapter 4: Radiography

PREFACE

The purpose of this book is to give the practicing dentist a photographic presentation of clinical pedodontics characterized by clarity and brevity. There are several fine textbooks on pedodontics but there is need for the pictorial type of reference which can supply immediate and practical assistance to the clinician, who in turn can pass this knowledge on to patients and their parents.

The field of pedodontics is so all-inclusive that it is impossible for any one book to portray everything that might be considered pertinent and worthwhile. Improvements in intra-oral photography, however, make it possible to show clinical material in a far more easily understood fashion than would be feasible with the printed word alone. A good example of this is the recognition and diagnosis of dental anomalies. The subject of patient management, on the other hand, does not lend itself to the photographic format of an Atlas and therefore has been presented in abbreviated form.

There are many different ways of accomplishing most clinical procedures in pedodontics; the authors, however, have presented their method of choice, fully cognizant that other techniques may be equally acceptable.

Time is the most precious factor in the life of the precise, conscientious, and understanding dentist. It is hoped that this Atlas will provide a readily accessible source of information that will be frequently used.

JOHN M. DAVIS

DAVID B. LAW

THOMPSON M. LEWIS

ACKNOWLEDGMENTS

The authors wish to express their appreciation to Clifford Freehe, R.B.P. It was his high standard of dental photography that originally inspired this text. Our thanks also to David Andrews and Jim Clark for many hours of photographic preparation.

Virginia Brooks, scientific illustrator for the Health Sciences at the University of Washington, is to be highly commended for her excellent illustrations. We are also grateful for the illustrations prepared by Dr. Gerald Harper for Chapter 12. We wish to thank as well Trese Rand, medical illustrator at Children's Orthopedic Hospital and Medical Center in Seattle, for the illustrations in the appendix.

We are indebted to the clinicians and educators from whom we have borrowed special material. They have been acknowledged individually in the appropriate legends. Of vital importance to this text have been the contributions of the Pedodontic Faculty and Graduate Pedodontic students at the University of Washington.

To Nancy Felts go our heartfelt thanks for her patience in typing this text.

Saving the best till last, we thank our wives for their understanding and support.

CONTENTS

Chapter 15

Chapter 16

Chapter 17

Chapter 18

Chapter 19
by Marc W. Anderson

Chapter 20
by Michael R. Fey and Patrick K. Turley

AN ATLAS OF PEDODONTICS

GROWTH AND DEVELOPMENT

Chapter 1 _____

A thorough understanding of the fundamental principles of growth and development of the facial complex is essential in the practice of pedodontics. Without a knowledge of the manner in which teeth calcify and erupt, it would be difficult to differentiate between a hypoplastic condition induced by local factors and an inherited syndrome. Normal stages in the development of the dentition can be mistaken for malocclusion by the untrained observer. It is not within the scope of this book to treat the subject of growth and development in all its ramifications. Rather, the purpose is to focus attention on some of the key areas in which the clinician who treats children should be knowledge-able. It is the responsibility of the practitioner to give accurate answers to the questions frequently asked by parents concerning tooth position, spacing, labial frenum, and the effect of traumatic injuries, to mention only a few. More exhaustive information, if needed, can readily be obtained from textbooks on orthodontics and pedodontics.

Figure 1–1 Maxillary growth sites. The primary *centers* of growth contributing to the downward and forward direction of the maxilla are the following:

A. Growth at the spheno-occipital and sphenoethmoidal junctions.

B. Growth of the nasal cartilaginous septum.

The following sutures are considered secondary or accommodating growth *sites* for the primary centers of growth:

A. Frontomaxillary suture.
B. Zygomaticomaxillary suture.
C. Zygomaticotemporal suture.
D. Pyramidal process of palatal bone.
E. Alveolar process.

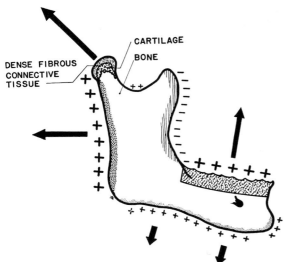

Figure 1–2 Mandibular growth sites. Growth in the condyle increases the anterior-posterior (downward and forward pattern of growth) dimension of the mandible. Anterior-posterior dimension of the mandible is also increased by resorption of bone on the anterior border of the ramus and apposition of bone on the posterior border of the ramus. Appositional growth of alveolar bone increases the superior-inferior dimension of the mandible. (From Graber, T. M.: *Orthodontics*, 3rd ed., W. B. Saunders Co., Philadelphia, 1972, p. 61.)

Figure 1–3 Tracing of superimposed films of head showing the normal downward and forward facial growth pattern — ages 6 months, 3 years, and 8 years.

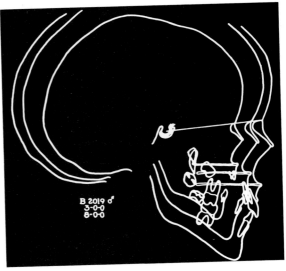

TABLE 1-1   MODIFICATION OF THE TABLE "CHRONOLOGY OF THE HUMAN DENTITION" (LOGAN AND KRONFELD, SLIGHTLY MODIFIED BY MCCALL AND SCHOUR), SUGGESTED BY LUNT AND LAW,[1,2] FOR THE CALCIFICATION AND ERUPTION OF THE PRIMARY DENTITION[*]

DECIDUOUS TOOTH	HARD TISSUE FORMATION BEGINS (FERTILIZATION AGE IN UTERO, WEEKS)		AMOUNT OF ENAMEL FORMED AT BIRTH	ENAMEL COMPLETED (MONTHS AFTER BIRTH)	ERUPTION (MEAN AGE IN MONTHS, ±1 SD)	ROOT COMPLETED (YEARS)
Maxillary						
Central incisor	14	(13–16)	Five sixths	1½	10 (8–12)	1½
Lateral incisor	16	(14⅔–16½)	Two thirds	2½	11 (9–13)	2
Canine	17	(15–18)	One third	9	19 (16–22)	3¼
First molar	15½	(14½–17)	Cusps united; occlusal completely calcified plus one-half to three-fourths crown height	6	16 (13–19) boys (14–18) girls	2½
Second molar	19	(16–23½)	Cusps united; occlusal incompletely calcified; calcified tissue covers one-fifth to one-fourth crown height	11	29 (25–33)	3
Mandibular						
Central incisor	14	(13–16)	Three fifths	2½	8 (6–10)	1½
Lateral incisor	16	(14⅔–16½)	Three fifths	3	13 (10–16)	1½
Canine	17	(16–18)	One third	9	20 (17–23)	3¼
First molar	15½	(14½–17)	Cusps united; occlusal completely calcified	5½	16 (14–18)	2¼
Second molar	18	(17–19½)	Cusps united; occlusal incompletely calcified	10	27 (23–31) boys (24–30) girls	3

[*]Critical points of difference in deciduous dentition—new tables versus Logan and Kronfeld's—include the following:
1. The calcification of deciduous teeth is initiated in incisors and canines from only one center.
2. The sequence of calcification is central, first molar, lateral, cuspid, and second molars.
3. Deciduous teeth calcify in a range of time rather than at fixed points in time. Therefore fixed values for times of initial calcification should be replaced with ranges and mathematical means.
4. Times of initial calcifications should be 2 to 6 weeks earlier than specified in the old "chronology."
  Points of difference in eruption include the following:
1. Two months or more later than in Logan and Kronfeld's table.
2. Much variation in sequence and time of eruption.
3. No sex differences.
4. In the maxilla, the lateral incisor, first molar, and cuspid erupt earlier than their counterparts in the mandible.

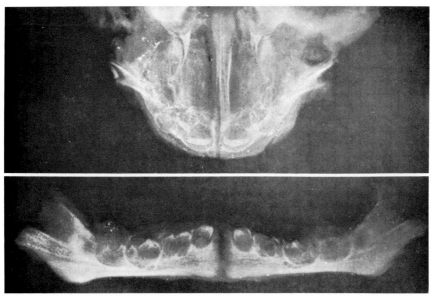

Figure 1–4 Eight-month fetus (wet specimen). Note areas of dental calcification in the mandibular incisors, cuspids, and first primary molars, as well as in the maxillary central and lateral incisors and first primary molars. There is only slight calcification in the maxillary cuspids and cusp tips of the second primary molars. (From McCall, J. O., and Wald, S. S.: *Clinical Dental Roentgenology*, 4th ed., W. B. Saunders Co., Philadelphia, 1957, p. 153.)

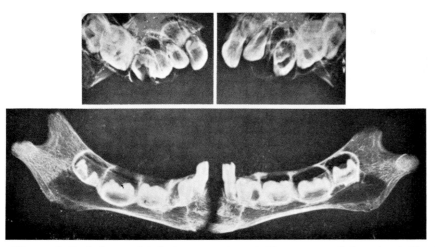

Figure 1–5 Infant at birth (wet specimen). Note areas of dental calcification similar to those shown in Figure 1–4. Maxillary calcification is slightly less advanced. (From McCall, J. O., and Wald, S. S.: *Clinical Dental Roentgenology*, 4th ed., W. B. Saunders Co., Philadelphia, 1957, p. 154.)

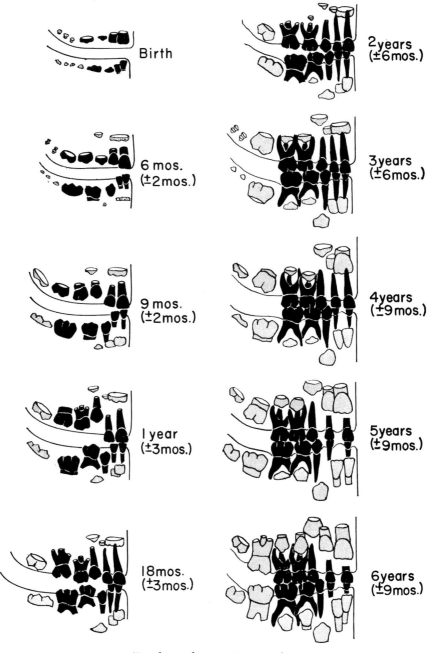

Birth

6 mos.
(±2mos.)

9 mos.
(±2mos.)

1 year
(±3mos.)

18mos.
(±3mos.)

2years
(±6mos.)

3years
(±6mos.)

4years
(±9mos.)

5years
(±9mos.)

6years
(±9mos.)

(See legend opposite page.)

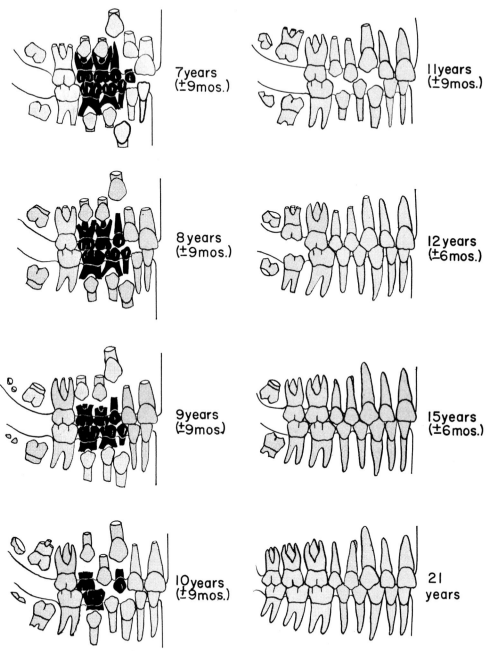

7years
(±9mos.)

8years
(±9mos.)

9years
(±9mos.)

10years
(±9mos.)

11years
(±9mos.)

12years
(±6mos.)

15years
(±6mos.)

21
years

Figure 1–6 Development of human dentition. (Modified from Schour and Massler. *In* Graber, T. M.: *Orthodontics,* 3rd ed., W. B. Saunders Co., Philadelphia, 1972, pp. 90 and 91.)

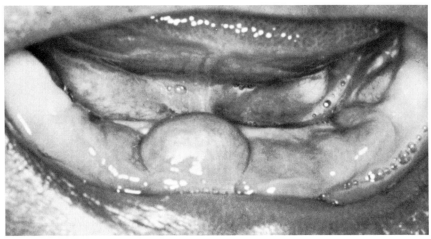

Figure 1–7 Eruption cyst in newborn infant. Note primary incisor visible through cyst. (Courtesy Dr. James R. Hooley.)

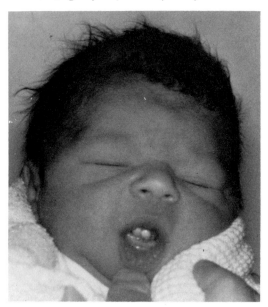

Figure 1–8 Male child, 1 day old. Mandibular right and left primary central incisors erupted at birth (natal tooth). Natal teeth are present in oral cavity at birth. Neonatal teeth erupt within first 30 days after birth. Most natal and neonatal teeth are normal primary central incisors and should be left in the mouth.

Figure 1–9 Natal mandibular primary central incisors in this 4-year-old girl were extracted the first week after birth. Note the position of the mandibular primary lateral incisors and cuspids in relation to the maxillary primary lateral incisors and cuspids. A possible loss in mandibular arch length may occur.

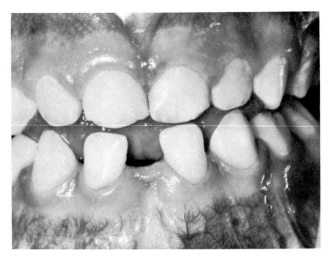

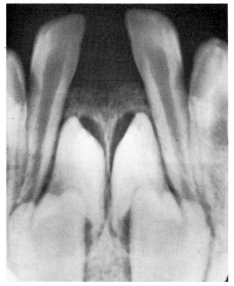

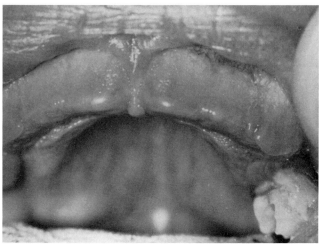

Figure 1–10 Radiograph of patient seen in Figure 1–9, showing space closure. Extraction of natal or neonatal teeth should be avoided if possible.

Figure 1–11 An 8-day-old male with a natal maxillary left primary molar and an epithelial cyst in the area of the maxillary right primary molars.

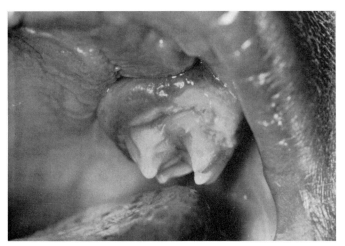

Figure 1–12 Close-up view of the natal maxillary left primary molar illustrated in Figure 1–11.

Figure 1–13 Close-up view of the epithelial cyst in the maxillary right primary molar area seen in Figure 1–11. According to Hooley, pea-sized cysts may form over one or more of the first primary molars. These cysts are shed during the first 2 months of life.

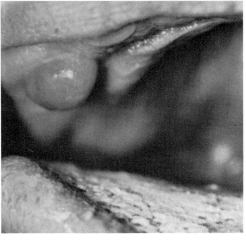

9

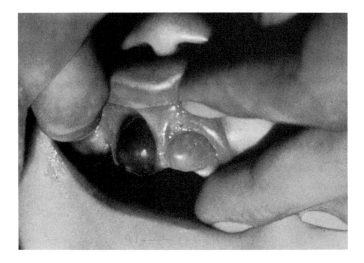

Figure 1-14 Eruption hematoma in the area of the maxillary right primary central incisor on a 7-month-old infant. This is nonpathologic and may occur prior to the eruption of some teeth. No treatment is indicated unless child is extremely irritable. Lancing of tissue should be avoided. Gentle rubbing with a teething ring may be helpful.

Figure 1-15 Slight eruption hematoma prior to the eruption of the maxillary left primary first molar in a 14-month-old child.

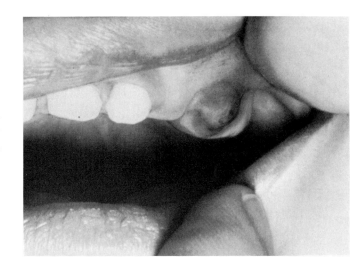

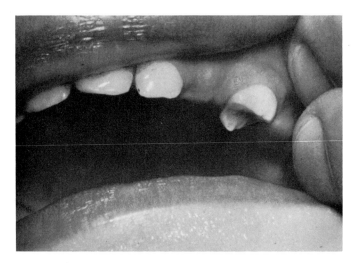

Figure 1-16 Same patient as seen in Figure 1-15 after eruption of the maxillary left primary first molar. Note the normal sequence of eruption of the first primary molar before the primary cuspid.

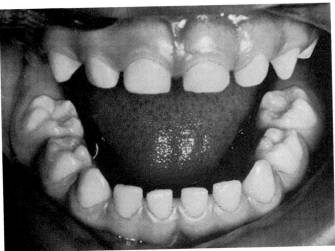

Figure 1–17 A 4-year-old child with normal healthy teeth and supporting tissues. Note the desirable spacing of the anterior teeth in the primary dentition.

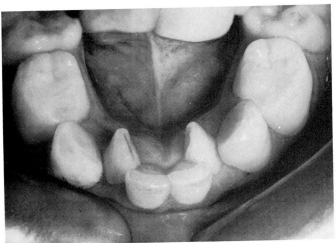

Figure 1–18 A 4-year-old child with abnormal crowding of the primary dentition. Most children with primary anterior teeth that are in contact or crowded will eventually require orthodontic care.

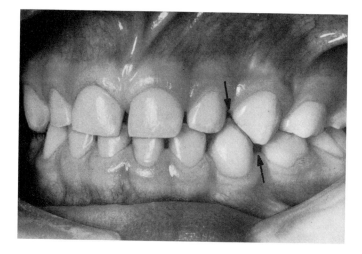

Figure 1–19 Normal dentition of a preschool child, showing maxillary primate space between lateral and cuspid incisors and mandibular primate space between the cuspid incisor and the first primary molar.

Figure 1–20 Step relationship of distal surfaces of maxillary and mandibular primary second molars and its effect on the occlusion of the first permanent molars. Note the permanent molars erupting into normal occlusion. (From Hitchcock, P. H. *In* Finn, S. B.: *Clinical Pedodontics,* 4th ed., W. B. Saunders Co., Philadelphia, 1973, p. 323.)

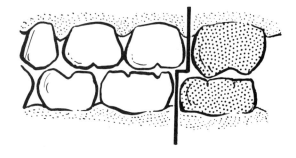

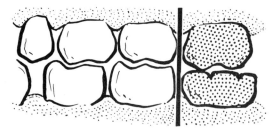

Figure 1–21 Flat plane relationship of distal surfaces of maxillary and mandibular primary second molar and its effect on the occlusion of the first permanent molar. Note the end-to-end occlusion of the permanent molars. (From Hitchcock, P. H. *In* Finn, S. B.: *Clinical Pedodontics*, 4th ed., W. B. Saunders Co., Philadelphia, 1973, p. 323.)

Figure 1–22 Five-year-old child with occlusal wear due to bruxism. Bruxism is common in the primary dentition, resulting in varying degrees of occlusal wear.

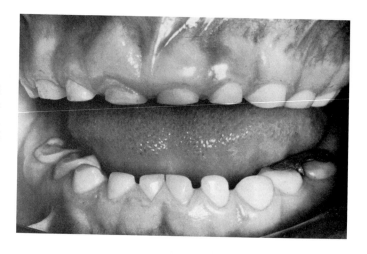

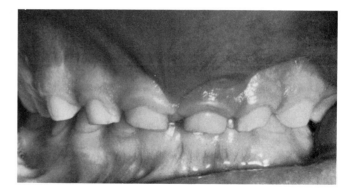

Figure 1–23 Five-year-old child with a deep overbite in the primary dentition.

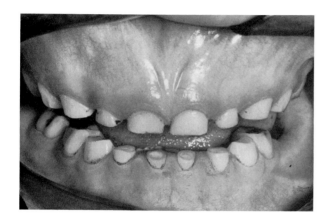

Figure 1–24 Six-year-old child with extreme incisal wear of the mandibular primary incisors. Note the erupting mandibular right permanent central incisor. Bilateral extraction of the primary central incisors is indicated.

Figure 1–25 Six-year-old child with mandibular left permanent central incisor erupting lingually. Since neither of the mandibular *primary* central incisors was loose and ready to be naturally exfoliated, the dentist extracted them, allowing the permanent incisor to erupt into normal position. After the primary incisor or incisors are exfoliated or extracted, the action of the tongue usually moves the permanent incisor labially into a normal labiolingual position.

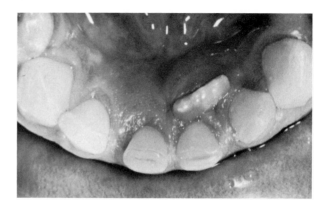

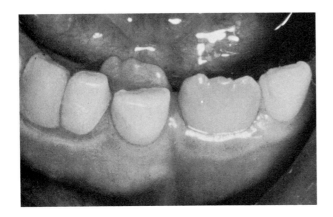

Figure 1–26 A 6½-year-old child with a lingually erupting mandibular right permanent central incisor. Immediate treatment consists of extraction of the mandibular right primary central incisor.

Figure 1–27 A 7-year-old child with extreme crowding of primary and permanent teeth in the mandibular arch (same child as shown in Figure 1–18). A complete orthodontic evaluation should be done at this time prior to any treatment.

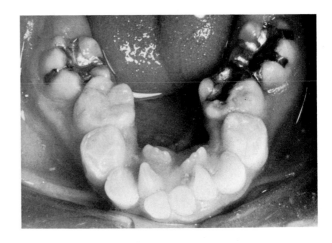

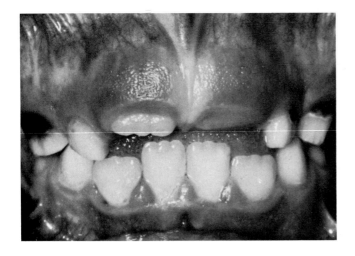

Figure 1–28 A 7½-year-old child with normal beginning of mixed dentition. Note swollen gingivae around erupted mandibular teeth and bulging tissues over erupting maxillary permanent central incisors.

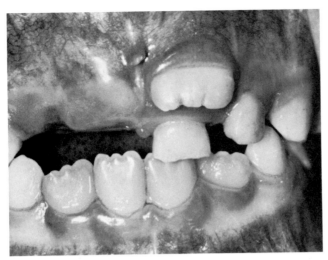

Figure 1–29 A 7½-year-old child with a maxillary left permanent central incisor erupting labially. Maxillary permanent central incisors often erupt labial to the *primary* central incisor. The maxillary primary central incisor should be extracted to provide room for the permanent incisor. Pressure from the lip will usually move the permanent incisor lingually into better alignment.

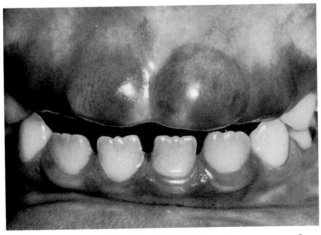

Figure 1–30 An 8-year-old child with delayed eruption of maxillary permanent central incisors. Treatment consists of removing tissue from the incisal one third of the labial and lingual crowns.

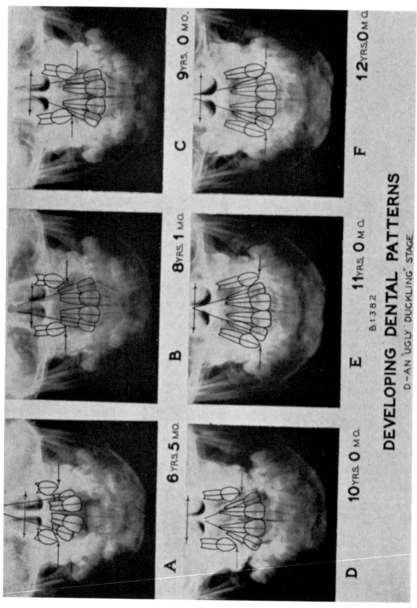

Figure 1-31 Normal developmental pattern of maxillary permanent teeth in children between 6 and 12 years of age. The central diastema and distally flaring lateral incisors are usually self-correcting with the eruption of maxillary permanent cuspids. (From Broadbent, H. B.: The face of the normal child. Angle Orthodontist 7:183–208, Oct., 1937.)

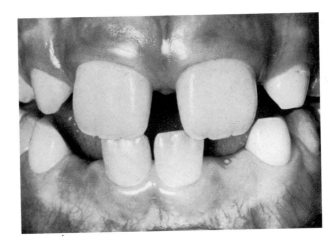

Figure 1–32 A 7½-year-old child. Note diastema between the maxillary permanent central incisors. Radiographs are indicated to determine the presence or absence of maxillary permanent lateral incisors.

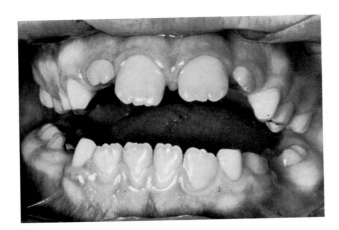

Figure 1–33 An 8-year-old child. Note eruption of maxillary permanent lateral incisors. Frenectomy is usually not considered until permanent cuspids have erupted. Mamelons on incisal edges of teeth are very prominent but will become less noticeable as wear occurs.

Figure 1–34 A 9-year-old patient. Maxillary and mandibular central and lateral incisors are well erupted, but primary cuspids are still present. Interdental spaces usually close with the eruption of permanent cuspids.

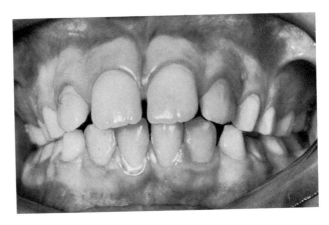

REFERENCES

1. Lunt, R. C., and Law, D. B.: A review of the chronology of calcification of deciduous teeth. J.A.D.A. 89:599, Sept., 1974.
2. Lunt, R. C., and Law, D. B.: A review of the chronology of eruption of deciduous teeth. J.A.D.A. 89:872–879, Oct., 1974.

ORAL DIAGNOSIS

Chapter 2 _____

A good diagnostician evaluates all aspects of a child's appearance and behavior before arriving at any conclusions concerning his or her oral condition. From the moment a youngster walks into the office for the first time until the termination of his appointment, a great deal of pertinent information can be elicited by the alert clinician. The gait and stance of the child may be an indication of medical problems, as may be complexion, hair, and other physical features. It is important to get into the habit of always noting these obvious physical characteristics before narrowing down to the area of particular interest to the dentist, which is the oral cavity. Such evaluation is not necessarily time consuming if the observer is perceptive.

Some kind of health questionnaire or past medical and dental history should be completed in writing by the parent prior to the child's introduction to the dentist. The nature of the questions on this form will reflect the individual dentist's ideas and concepts of diagnosis. Good examples of adequate health questionnaires are the Cornell Medical Index and the Minnesota Multiphasic Personality Inventory. The health questionnaire should provide basic information such as the child's name, nickname, age, weight, and place of birth, in addition to the chief complaint and past medical and dental history. Using this type of form as a guide, the dentist can then complete his or her own case history in conference with the parent, securing additional facts as indicated by the answers previously supplied.

The clinical examination of the child patient should begin with a survey of the head and neck (see Chapter 12) and should continue with a detailed inspection of the soft and hard tissues of the mouth, including a radiographic survey. When this is completed, the need will be established for special tests, diet surveys, medical reports, or consultation with specialists. A systematic approach to the examination of soft and hard tissues is essential. A good order of sequence is to inspect the lips, externally and internally, the buccal mucosa and mucobuccal fold, the hard palate, the pharyngeal area, the sublingual area, the tongue, and the gingivae. An evaluation of the occlusion should be performed next, noting both the position of teeth in contact and the path of closure. The individual condition of each tooth may then be verified with respect to color, mobility, caries, and other abnormalities. All information should be accurately recorded on the patient's chart and later augmented by careful examination of the radiographs. Regardless of the dentist's individual preference for a particular type of radiographic survey, there should be sufficient exposures to include periapical areas as well as the customary interproximal areas. In treating children, it is particularly important to make an early determination of missing teeth, supernumeraries, and similar abnormalities, which will be missed if only bitewing radiographs are obtained.

The dentist who sees children should have as his goal the ability to make an accurate diagnosis of every case that he treats. To meet this challenge, he will have to keep abreast of the professional literature, use all known methods of examination, and above all maintain close relationships with allied specialists who can cooperate with him on his referrals.

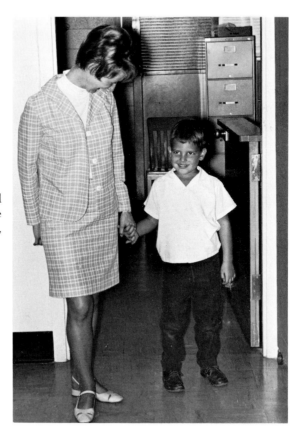

Figure 2–1 Child and mother walking into office. Note the child's gait, stature, dress, and speech.

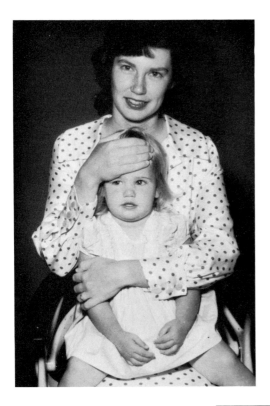

Figure 2–2 Young child seated on mother's lap for dental examination. Note the position of mother's arms and hands to stabilize the child during the examination. This approach may be used on the very young child who feels more secure when seated in the mother's lap.

Figure 2–3 Fingers being examined. Look for abnormalities of shape that may be an indication of an oral habit, a systemic disease, or other condition.

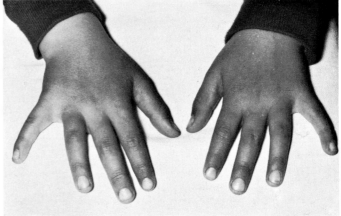

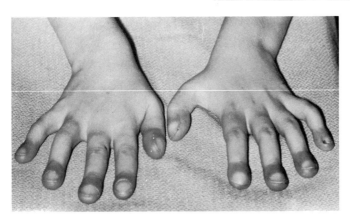

Figure 2–4 Fingers of a child with a congenital heart defect. Note clubbing of the ends of the fingers.

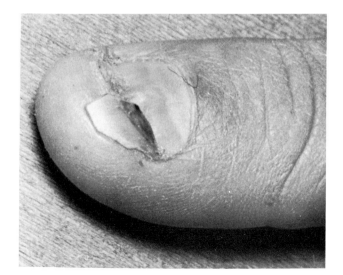

Figure 2–5 Thumb of a child with sucking habit.

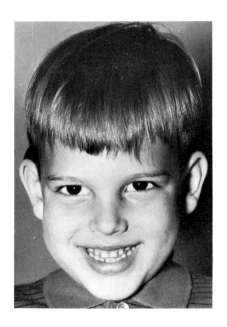

Figure 2–6. Anterior view of the head. Examine the skin, eyes, nose, and lips, and check for facial asymmetry.

Figure 2–7 Lateral view of the head. Observe the shape of the head and the nose. Note the quality and distribution of hair.

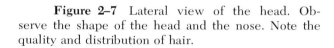

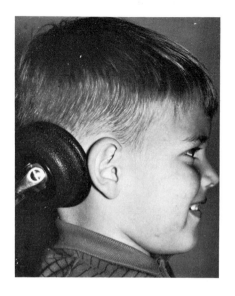

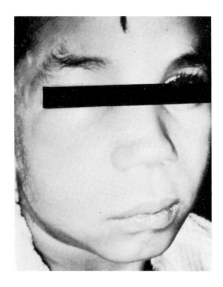

Figure 2–8 Severe swelling of the right side of the face extending from the lower border of the mandible to the orbital region as a result of a periapical abscess of the maxillary right primary second molar.

Figure 2–9 Bulbous area on the lower right side of the lip associated with a lip-sucking habit.

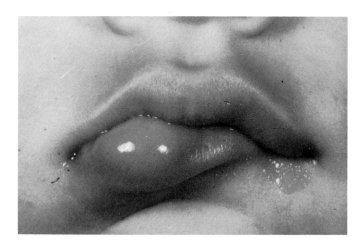

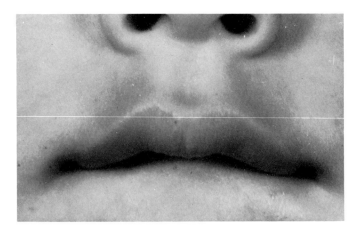

Figure 2–10 Child sucking on lip (same child as shown in Figure 2–9).

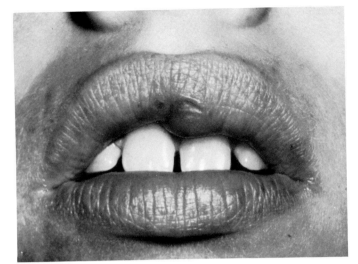

Figure 2–11 An 8½-year-old child with a history of falling and biting the upper lip.

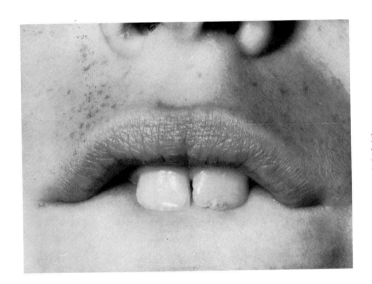

Figure 2–12 Typical appearance of mouth in a child with lip-biting and lip-sucking habits.

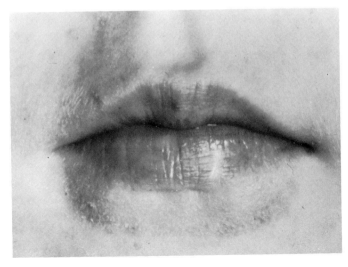

Figure 2–13 Patient with chapped lower lip (see Figure 2–14).

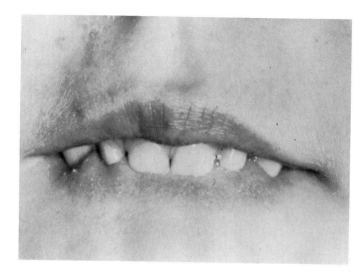

Figure 2–14 Patient with chronic lip-sucking and lip-chewing habits.

Figure 2–15 Dryness of the commissure of the lips on the right side. May be caused by a licking habit.

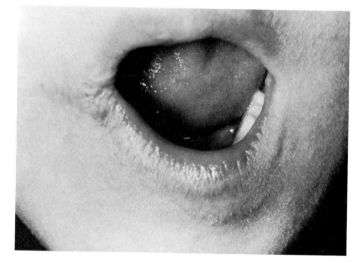

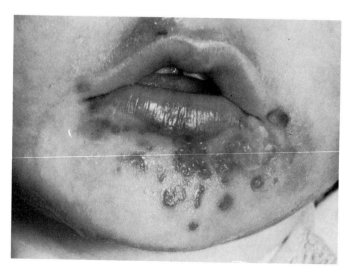

Figure 2–16 Primary herpetic gingivostomatitis on the lower face. This is a very painful condition, and the patient usually does not wish to eat or drink. Treatment consists mainly of preventing dehydration and secondary infection. Hospitalization may be necessary if dehydration does occur. The lesions heal within 7 to 14 days without causing scars.

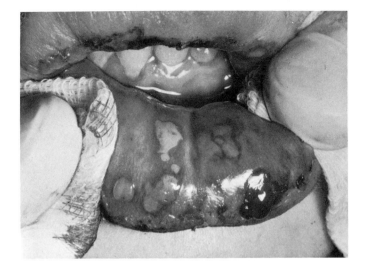

Figure 2–17 Primary herpetic gingivostomatitis of the lower lip and oral mucosa. Same patient as presented in Figure 2–16.

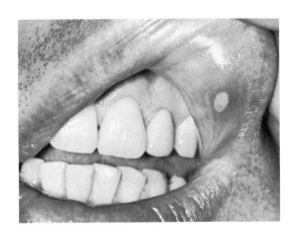

Figure 2–18 Canker sore (recurrent aphthous ulcer) of the oral mucosa of the upper lip. Treatment is palliative; these lesions heal within 7 to 14 days and cause no scars.

Figure 2–19 Severe infection of forefinger from contact with herpetic lesions in the mouth. Rubber gloves should be used in oral examination when such lesions are present.

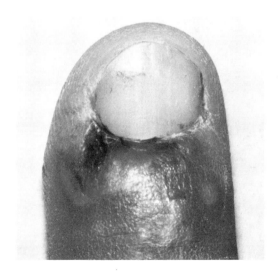

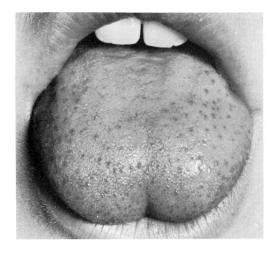

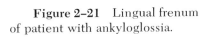

Figure 2–20 Mobility of tongue inhibited because of ankyloglossia.

Figure 2–21 Lingual frenum of patient with ankyloglossia.

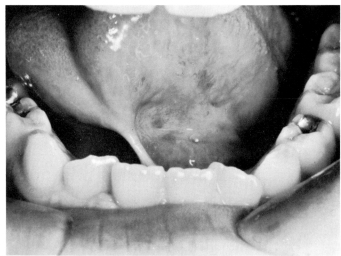

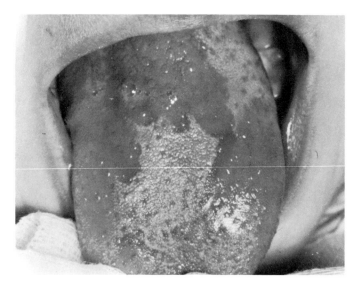

Figure 2–22 Geographic tongue. These lesions usually disappear spontaneously; however, recurrences are not uncommon. Always inspect the superior, inferior, and lateral surfaces of the tongue.

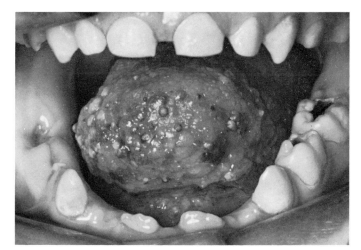

Figure 2-23 Cavernous hemangioma of the tongue in a young child.

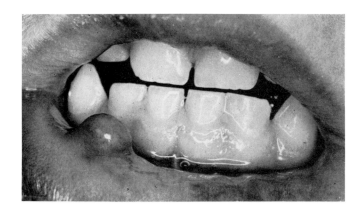

Figure 2-24 Mucocele caused by retention of mucin in the tissue following injury to the lip. (From Kerr, D. A., and Ash, M. M.: *Oral Pathology*, 2nd ed., Lea & Febiger, Philadelphia, 1965, p. 121.)

Figure 2-25 Inspection of the floor of the mouth. Note capillary hemangioma on the inferior surface of the tongue next to the lingual frenum.

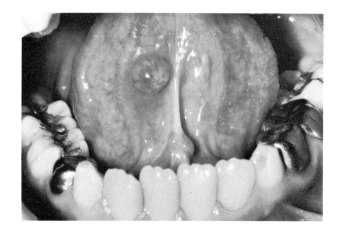

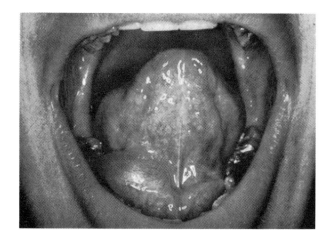

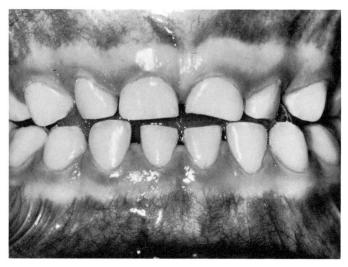

Figure 2–26 Ranula in the floor of the mouth. (From Krueger, G. O.: *Oral Surgery,* 2nd ed., C. V. Mosby Co., St. Louis, 1961, p. 271.)

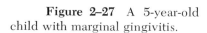

Figure 2–27 A 5-year-old child with marginal gingivitis.

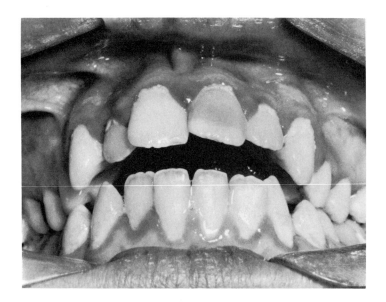

Figure 2–28 Teen-ager with gingivitis caused by accumulation of debris and materia alba around the teeth. Patient practiced poor oral hygiene. Gingival hemorrhage occurs easily on contact. Treatment consists of thorough prophylaxis followed by home care.

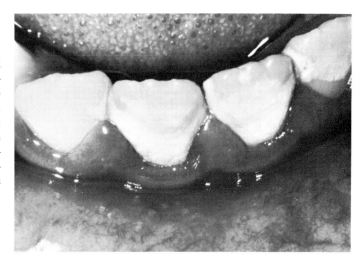

Figure 2–29 A 7-year-old child with heavy deposits of calculus on the labial surfaces of the mandibular permanent incisors. Note gingivitis. Calculus is the most common cause of gingivitis and must be removed. It is unusual for heavy deposits of calculus to develop in children less than 12 years of age.

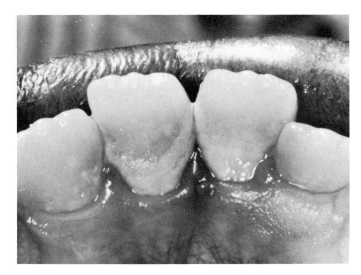

Figure 2–30 An 8-year-old child with calculus on the lingual surfaces of the mandibular permanent incisors. This is usually the first site of calculus accumulation.

Figure 2–31 Necrotizing ulcerative gingivitis. It is seldom seen in children less than 10 years of age. Interdental papillae often have a crater, with areas of sloughing tissue over the red, edematous gingiva. Initial treatment is prophylaxis to remove the local irritants, followed by diligent home care of the involved area. Antibiotics are used only to treat secondary infections. (Courtesy Department of Oral Biology, School of Dentistry, University of Washington.)

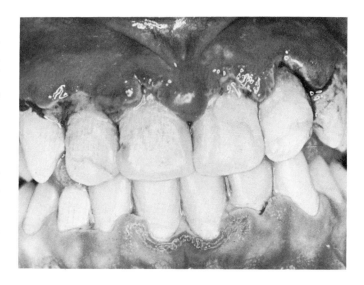

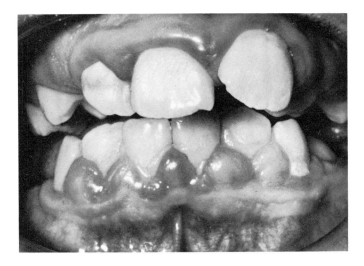

Figure 2–32 Pubertal gingivitis. Tissues are soft and bleed easily. The condition is associated with a hormonal imbalance during puberty and normally disappears when the hormonal balance is restored. The importance of good oral hygiene should be stressed to teenagers.

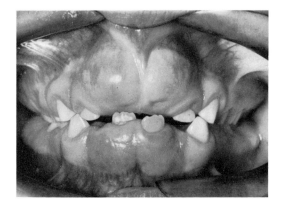

Figure 2–33 Idiopathic gingival fibromatosis (hereditary gingival fibromatosis). This is a familial defect similar in appearance to diphenylhydantoin (Dilantin) hyperplasia; however, it occurs in individuals with no history of having received diphenylhydantoin therapy. Although gingivoplasty improves the condition, the overgrowth of connective tissue tends to recur.

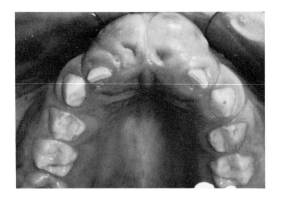

Figure 2–34 Idiopathic gingival fibromatosis of the maxillary arch (same patient as seen in Figure 2–33).

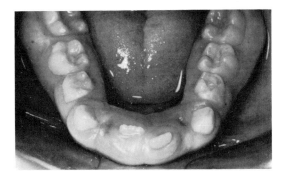

Figure 2–35 Idiopathic gingival fibromatosis of the mandibular arch (same patient as seen in Figures 2–33 and 2–34).

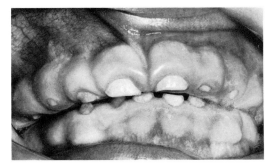

Figure 2–36 Idiopathic fibromatosis in a preschool child.

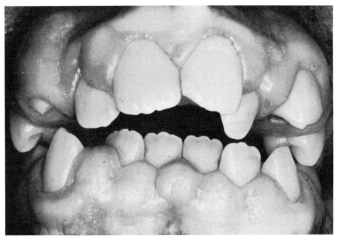

Figure 2–37 Diphenylhydantoin (Dilantin) hyperplasia in a teenager. Gingivoplasty is the treatment of choice; however, following removal of the tissue the gingiva will become hyperplastic once again if the patient continues to ingest diphenylhydantoin. *Careful* oral hygiene will retard this tendency (see Figure 2–38).

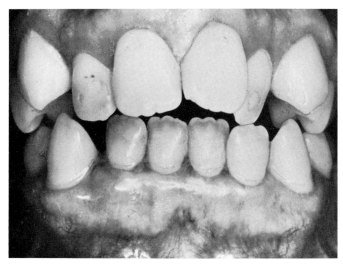

Figure 2–38 Teenager with diphenylhydantoin (Dilantin) hyperplasia following gingivoplasty (same patient as seen in Figure 2–37).

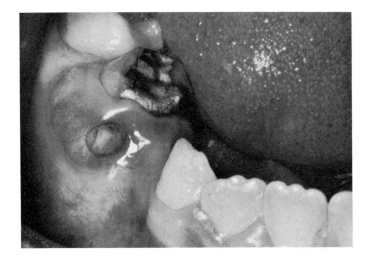

Figure 2–39 Periapical abscess of mandibular right primary second molar. In many cases this condition is not painful and consequently may be present for a long time. The tooth was extracted.

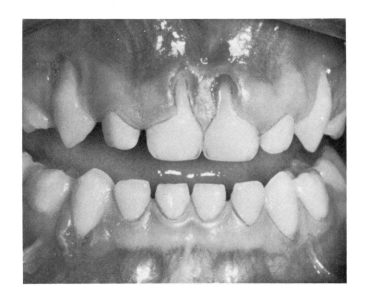

Figure 2–40 Localized gingival recession resulting from a habit of picking at the tissue with the fingernail. Note tissue around maxillary primary central incisors and cuspids and the mandibular right primary cuspid.

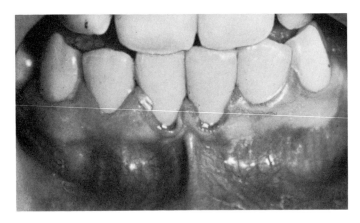

Figure 2–41 Loss of integrity (stripping) of gingival margin around the mandibular permanent central incisors. Numerous factors compound this periodontal problem—e.g., occlusal trauma, area of food impaction, frenum attachment, and encroachment of the alveolar mucosa. Periodontal treatment is definitely indicated, otherwise stripping will continue.

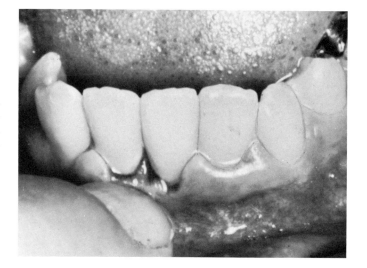

Figure 2–42 Patient has a habit of picking at the labial gingiva with a fingernail. A careful history is required to determine the true cause of this habit.

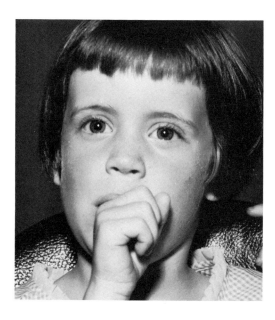

Figure 2–43 A 5-year-old child with an anterior open bite caused by a finger-sucking habit.

Figure 2–44 An anterior open bite caused by a finger-sucking habit in a pre-school child.

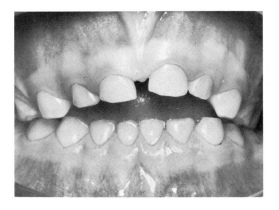

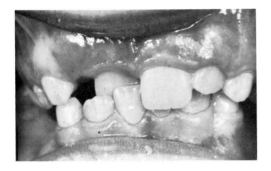

Figure 2–45 An 8-year-old child with an anterior crossbite.

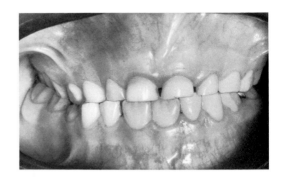

Figure 2–46 A 6½-year-old child with a posterior crossbite.

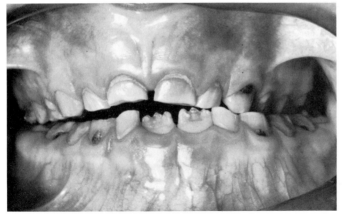

Figure 2–47 Tetracycline staining of primary dentition in a 6-year-old child. Before the dentist examines the teeth for caries and prepares radiographs, he should check the color, shape, structure, size, and number of teeth. (See Chapter 3, Anomalies of the Dentition.)

Figure 2–48 A 5½-year-old child with the habit of bruxism. Note extreme abrasion of the primary incisors.

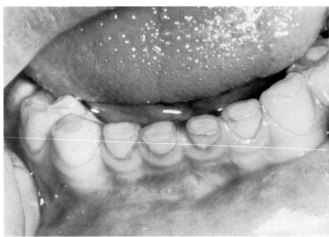

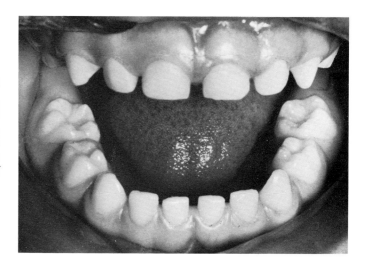

Figure 2–49 A 5-year-old child with a favorable dentition, ready to be examined for dental caries. A good set of radiographs, adequate light and air, dental floss, and a sharp explorer are necessary to determine areas of caries.

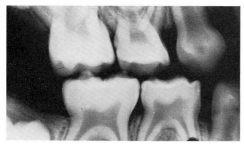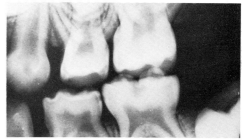

Figure 2–50 Patient J. D., bitewings of a 4-year-old child showing areas of initial caries on the proximal surfaces of maxillary and mandibular primary molars. Parent disregarded advice of the dentist to restore the involved teeth, and chose to postpone treatment. See Figure 2–51 for bitewings of same child 12 months later.

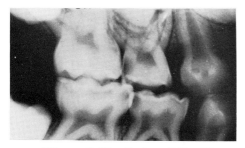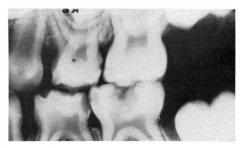

Figure 2–51 Patient J.D., 12 months after first examination. Note the extent of the carious involvement of the mandibular left primary second molar. This series of bitewings illustrates well the rapid progress of dental caries in the primary dentition and points out the need for early restoration.

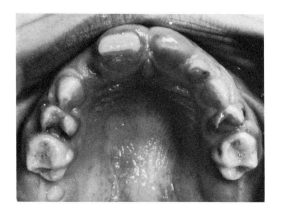

Figure 2–52 Loss of arch length caused by extensive caries of the disto-occlusal surfaces of the maxillary right and left primary first molars. Note how the primary second molars have drifted mesially. If the primary first molars had been restored to natural contour, this would not have occurred.

Figure 2–53 Radiographs showing mesial migration of maxillary right and left second primary molars into carious area of the primary first molars. Note the reduced space in which the bicuspids may erupt.

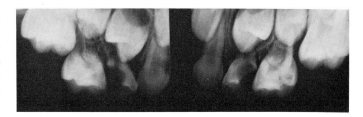

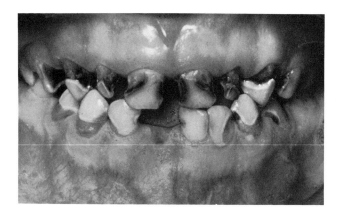

Figure 2–54 Rampant caries in a 5-year-old child.

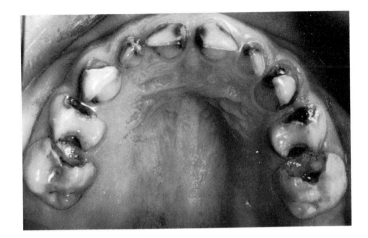

Figure 2–55 Maxillary arch (same patient as seen in Figure 2–54).

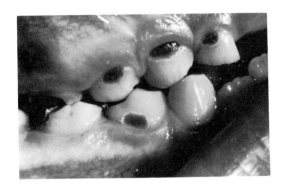

Figure 2–56 Gingival caries in a 7½-year-old child.

Figure 2–57 Caries of an occlusal pit in a mandibular primary second molar. Lesions like this may be overlooked clinically because of the small size of the external opening. Although there are no other areas of caries, the condition has progressed until it now involves a pulp horn. When inspecting radiographs, it is important to look at all susceptible surfaces and not just the involved proximal surfaces.

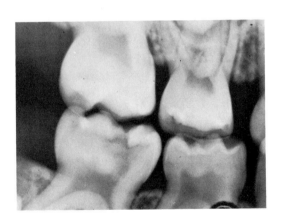

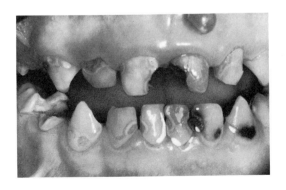

Figure 2–58 Rampant caries of the primary dentition. Note the fistula over the maxillary left central incisor.

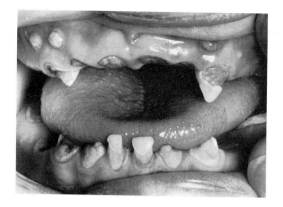

Figure 2–59 Rampant caries of the primary dentition. Teeth were extracted, and dentures were made for this child.

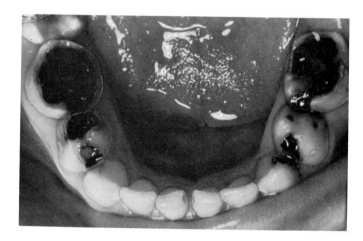

Figure 2–60 A 6-year-old child with arrested caries of the primary molars. There were no pulpal exposures (the dentin was stained and hard), and the teeth were restored with stainless steel crowns.

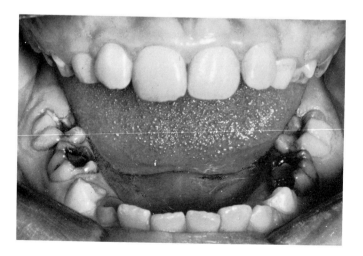

Figure 2–61 A 10-year-old child with extensive occlusal caries of the mandibular permanent first molars. These teeth are often lost because of the rapid progress of occlusal caries. Early restoration is important.

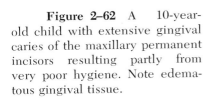

Figure 2-62 A 10-year-old child with extensive gingival caries of the maxillary permanent incisors resulting partly from very poor hygiene. Note edematous gingival tissue.

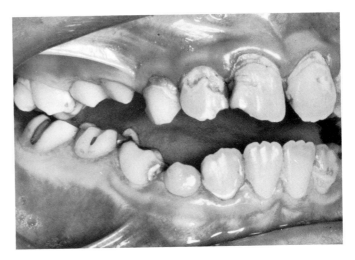

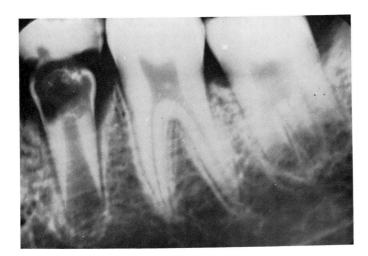

Figure 2-63 Idiopathic internal resorption of a mandibular second bicuspid. These teeth may be saved if early treatment is initiated. (See Figure 2-64 for illustration of treatment of a case of idiopathic internal resorption.)

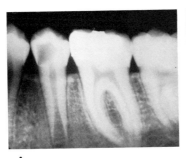

A

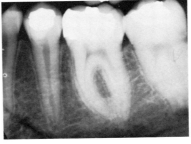

B

Figure 2-64 Idiopathic internal resorption of a mandibular second bicuspid. A, Preoperative radiograph. B, Postoperative radiograph following pulpotomy done with calcium hydroxide paste in the area of internal resorption. The tooth was then restored with zinc phosphate cement base and an amalgam restoration. Note continued root development.

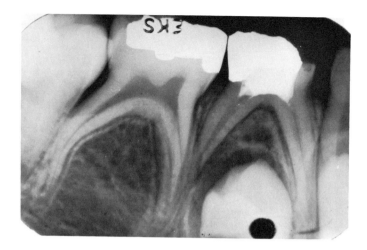

Figure 2–65 Periapical radiograph of the mandibular primary first molar following pulpotomy done with formocresol (see Figures 2–66 and 2–67).

Figure 2–66 Bitewing radiograph taken 12 months after pulpotomy with formocresol. Note the radiolucent area under the mandibular primary first molar (indicative of a pulpotomy failure). The dentist then took a periapical radiograph of the involved area (see Figure 2–67).

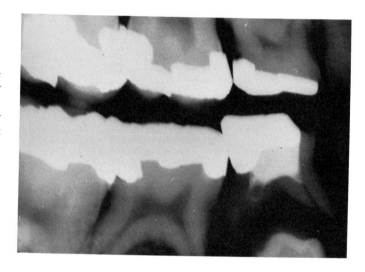

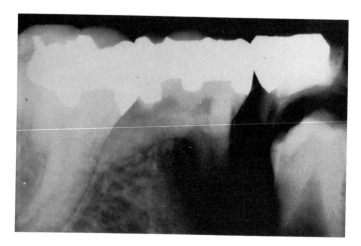

Figure 2–67 Periapical view of the involved area. The mandibular first and second primary molars were extracted, and the pathologist diagnosed the condition as a dentigerous cyst. This case illustrates the necessity for taking adequate radiographs.

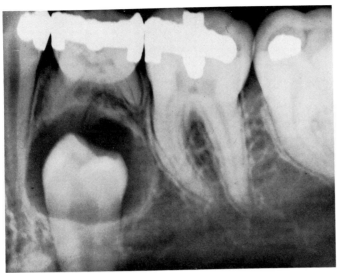

Figure 2–68 A questionable radiolucent area around a mandibular second bicuspid. Early establishment of a diagnosis and treatment are important to prevent further damage. The pathologist diagnosed this condition as a dentigerous cyst.

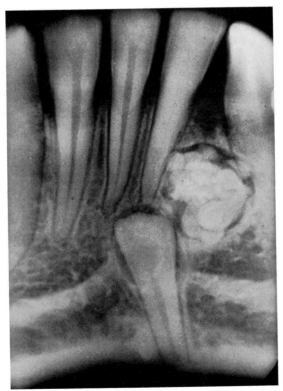

Figure 2–69 An odontoma that obstructed eruption of the mandibular lateral incisor.

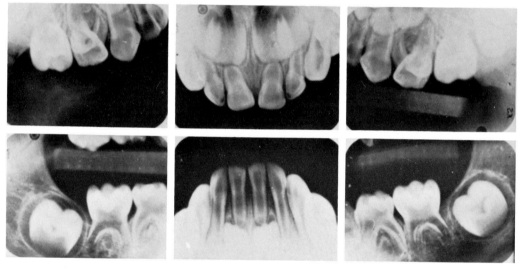

Figure 2–70   Radiographs of a 3-year-old boy with vitamin D–resistant rickets. Note the large size of pulp chambers. This type of case requires prophylactic placement of steel crowns to prevent enamel wear and subsequent dentin exposure and pulpal abscess. (Courtesy Dr. William Tracy, University of Oregon Dental School.)

ANOMALIES OF THE DENTITION

Chapter 3 _____

A majority of the bizarre and unusual anomalies of human teeth become evident during the childhood years. In these cases, the dentist who treats the family is usually called on first to make the diagnosis and perform whatever immediate treatment may be required. Too often hereditary conditions are incorrectly diagnosed and dismissed as the result of "fever" or "faulty nutrition." Parents may thus feel unnecessarily guilty about circumstances over which they have no control whatsoever. It is a source of satisfaction to the practitioner to be able to pinpoint the nature of a particular anomaly, and it is the purpose of this chapter to enable him or her to do so.

A classification of anomalies of the dentition is of value to the clinician seeking information useful in making a diagnosis. The six chief categories listed below are further subdivided in the section just preceding their detailed descriptions.

    I. Anomalies of number of teeth
    II. Anomalies of shape of teeth
   III. Anomalies of color of teeth
   IV. Anomalies of structure and texture of teeth
    V. Anomalies of eruption and exfoliation of teeth
   VI. Anomalies of position of teeth

Anomalies of Number of Teeth

Supernumerary teeth result from aberrations in the initiation or proliferation period of the life cycle of the tooth. The best available evidence points to genetic factors as being responsible for this anomaly. Several large-scale studies have been reported on the incidence of supernumerary teeth in children, and although there is some variation in data, there is agreement that the anomaly is much more prevalent in the permanent dentition than in the primary. Published reports on the prevalence of supernumeraries in the primary dentition range from a low figure of 0.3 per cent[7] to a high figure of 1.8 per cent.[5] The majority of these teeth are located in the maxillary or mandibular incisor region and are of normal shape. No reliable evidence exists for prevalence of supernumerary teeth in the primary dentition in one sex over the other.

The incidence of supernumerary teeth in the permanent dentition in children under 14 years of age has been reported by different investigators as ranging from 2 to 3 per cent. Grahnen[7] in a study of Swedish children reported a figure of 3.1 per cent, Castaldi[4] in a similar study of Canadian children reported 3.1 per cent, and Clayton[5] in a group of American children found an incidence of 2.7 per cent. It is of interest that both Castaldi and Clayton found a significantly higher number of supernumeraries in boys than in girls. The majority of these teeth are located in the maxillary incisor region (mesiodens), with a smaller percentage in the bicuspid region, and are generally conical or of unusual shape. An observation of importance to the diagnostician is that in cleidocranial dysostosis, a familial and dominant hereditary syndrome involving missing clavicles, there are usually a number of supernumerary teeth.

Teeth that are congenitally or developmentally missing cause many problems for the practicing dentist. Early recognition depends upon careful clinical examination and adequate radiographic surveys. As with supernumeraries, missing teeth represent a fault or aberration in either the initiation or proliferation stage of the life cycle of the tooth. There is ample evidence in the literature that the chief causative factor is hereditary, and there are well-documented reports of pedigrees through several generations. In rare instances, bone disease, tumors, or radiation may result in the lack of tooth formation.

Missing teeth occur less frequently in the primary than in the permanent dentitions. Since the primary tooth bud gives rise to the anlage of the succedaneous tooth, it follows that the absence of the primary tooth should mean the absence of the permanent tooth also. This is not always the case, however. Studies of the incidence of missing primary teeth in different population groups show considerable variation, but in all instances primary teeth are missing less frequently than are permanent teeth. Menczer[8] reported 0.09 per cent missing primary teeth in a group of American preschool children, whereas Grahnen[7] reported 0.4 per cent in a comparable group of Swedish children. Both investigators found the maxillary primary lateral incisor most commonly missing.

In the permanent dentition, the incidence of hypodontia, exclusive of third molars, was found to be 3.8 per cent in the Evanston[1] dental caries study. The group studied comprised over 13,000 children aged 12 to 14 years. In Grahnen's comparable survey[7] of 1006 Swedish school children aged 11 to 14 years, the incidence of missing teeth was 6.1 per cent. In all studies in which radiographs have been employed, there is agreement that in children the most commonly missing tooth is the mandibular second bicuspid, followed by the maxillary lateral incisor, and finally by the maxillary second bicuspid. On the basis of family studies, Grahnen[6] feels that the so-called peg lateral is actually a modified manifestation of hypodontia.

Certain characteristic syndromes have long been observed to be associated with multiple missing teeth. In hereditary anhidrotic ectodermal dysplasia there is usually oligodontia or anodontia. This condition chiefly affects males. It has been classified as a sex-linked recessive trait. In Down's syndrome (mongolism), Brown and Cunningham[3] reported that as many as 43 per cent of affected children exhibited missing teeth, usually the maxillary lateral incisors.

The clinical management of cases involving missing teeth can be decided only on an individual basis. In some instances no treatment may be indicated, whereas in others orthodontic correction plus prostheses may be required.

I. ANOMALIES OF NUMBER

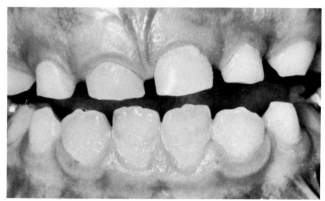

Figure 3–1   Intraoral view of a 7-year-old child with a supernumerary tooth in the area of the developing maxillary right permanent central incisor. At this age, the anomaly will be detected only by radiographic survey.

I. ANOMALIES OF NUMBER *Continued*

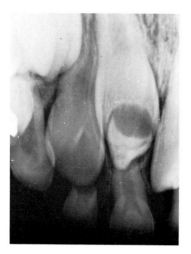

Figure 3–2 Radiograph of the patient seen in Figure 3–1. Note supernumerary tooth in area of right permanent central incisor. If supernumerary teeth are not extracted, they usually cause eruption to be delayed or deflection in the normal path of eruption of the neighboring developing permanent tooth or teeth.

Figure 3–3 Supernumerary mandibular primary incisor.

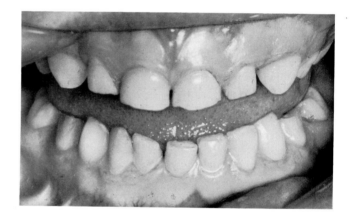

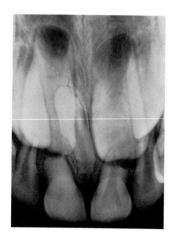

Figure 3–4 Midline supernumerary (mesiodens) in a 5-year-old child. Extraction of the mesiodens is the treatment of choice.

I. ANOMALIES OF NUMBER *Continued*

Figure 3–5 Two supernumerary teeth in area of maxillary permanent central incisor in an 8½-year-old child. Note how the supernumeraries caused delayed eruption of the permanent central incisors. Both maxillary permanent lateral incisions have erupted. Immediate extraction of the supernumeraries is indicated.

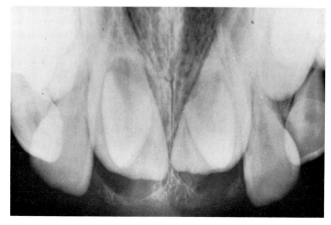

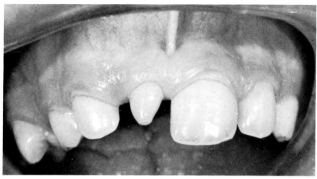

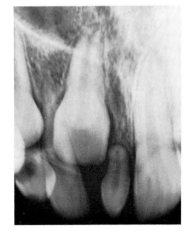

Figure 3–6 Erupted midline supernumerary (mesiodens).

Figure 3–7 Midline supernumerary (mesiodens). Radiograph of the patient seen in Figure 3–6. Note that the eruption of maxillary right permanent central incisor is retarded. Immediate extraction of the supernumerary is necessary for the incisor to erupt. Even then, it is likely that the incisor will erupt in a poor position. Minor orthodontic treatment is frequently necessary to align a permanent incisor whose eruption has been retarded because of a supernumerary tooth.

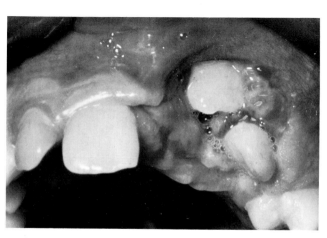

Figure 3–8 An erupting permanent maxillary left central incisor following removal of a supernumerary tooth in the area. Eruption is frequently slow in these cases.

I. ANOMALIES OF NUMBER *Continued*

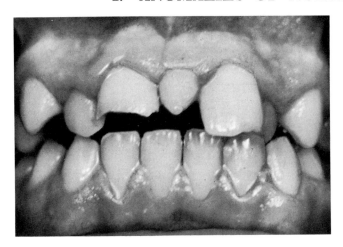

Figure 3–9 Midline supernumerary (mesiodens). Note crowding in area of maxillary permanent lateral incisors. The supernumerary must be extracted.

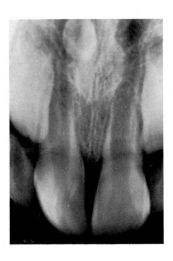

Figure 3–10 Midline supernumerary (mesiodens). Note that the maxillary right permanent central incisor has rotated. It was most likely deflected from its normal path of eruption by the mesiodens. The mesiodens should be extracted.

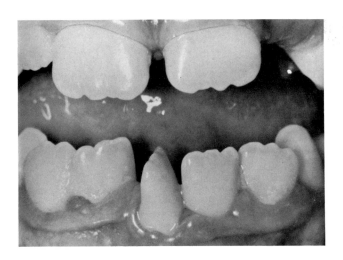

Figure 3–11 Midline supernumerary (mesiodens) of the mandibular arch. Mesiodentes usually occur in the maxillary arch. Note the crowding of the mandibular permanent incisors. Extraction of the mesiodens is the treatment of choice.

Figure 3–12 Developing supernumerary teeth in area of mandibular cuspid and bicuspid. Extraction of supernumeraries is the treatment of choice.

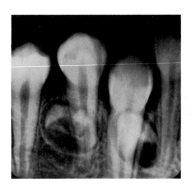

I. ANOMALIES OF NUMBER *Continued*

Figure 3–13 A 9-year-old girl with cleidocranial dysostosis. Note how the patient can closely approximate the right and left shoulders (a diagnostic sign). These individuals usually have supernumerary teeth, and the eruption of their permanent dentition is retarded.

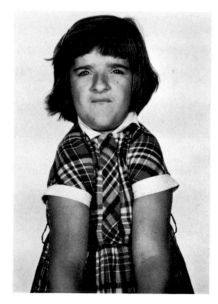

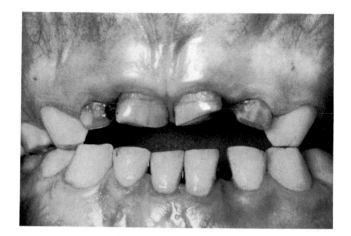

Figure 3–14 Intraoral view of the 9-year-old girl shown in Figure 3–13. Note that the eruption of maxillary and mandibular incisors is retarded.

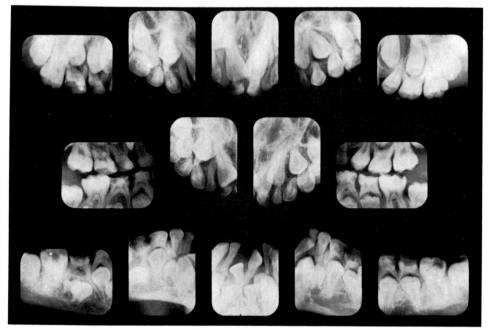

Figure 3–15 Full-mouth radiographs of a 9-year-old girl with cleidocranial dysostosis. Note that the eruption of permanent teeth is retarded, and there are supernumeraries in the upper and lower left quadrants.

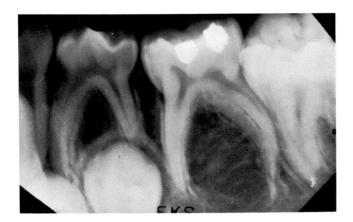

Figure 3–16 Mandibular second bicuspid is missing. Next to the third molar, this tooth is the one most frequently missing in the human dentition.

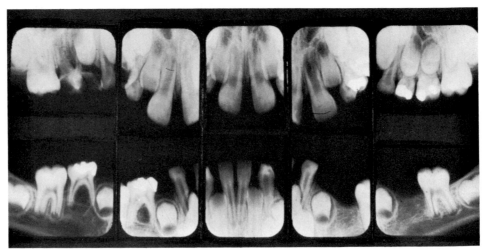

Figure 3–17 Full-mouth radiographs of a 7-year-old boy in whom the mandibular second bicuspids and the maxillary right second bicuspid are missing.

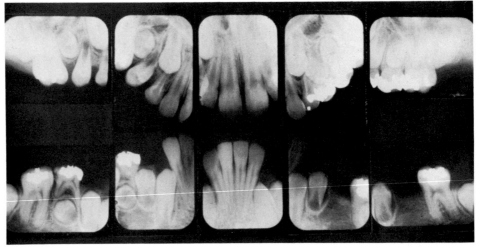

Figure 3–18 Same boy as seen in Figure 3–17, 2 years later. Note the development of right maxillary and mandibular second bicuspids. During the preschool years it is unwise to prognosticate about the failure of development of the bicuspids.

I. ANOMALIES OF NUMBER *Continued*

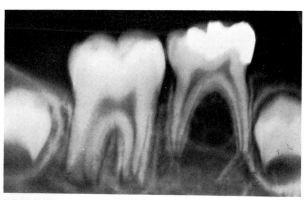

Figure 3–19 Periapical view of mandibular right bicuspid area in boy shown in Figure 3–17. It appears that the second bicuspid is missing.

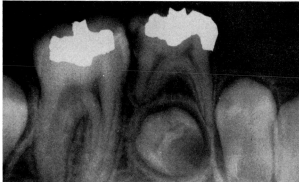

Figure 3–20 Same area as seen in Figure 13–19, 2 years later. Note the development of second bicuspid crown.

Figure 3–21 Same patient as seen in Figures 3–19 and 3–20. Periapical view of maxillary right bicuspid. Second bicuspid apparently is missing.

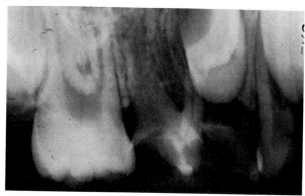

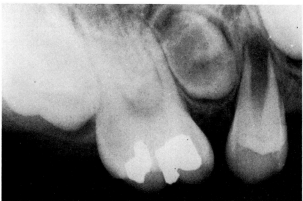

Figure 3–22 Same area seen in Figure 13–21, 2 years later. Note the development of second bicuspid crown.

I.   ANOMALIES OF NUMBER *Continued*

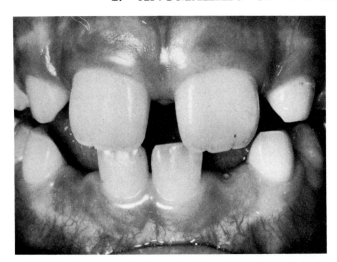

Figure 3–23 A 7½-year-old child in whom maxillary permanent lateral incisors were developmentally missing. Next to the third molars and mandibular second bicuspids, these permanent teeth are the ones most often developmentally missing.

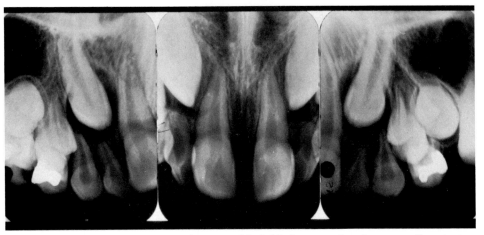

Figure 3–24   Radiograph of 9-year-old child showing developmentally missing maxillary permanent lateral incisors.

Figure 3–25 Extraoral view of a child in whom maxillary permanent lateral incisors are developmentally missing. The wide diastema is often an indication that lateral incisors are missing.

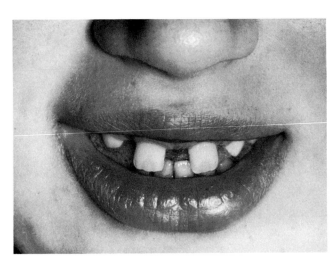

I.   ANOMALIES OF NUMBER *Continued*

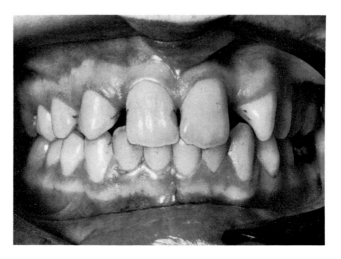

Figure 3–26 Adult with developmentally missing maxillary lateral incisors.

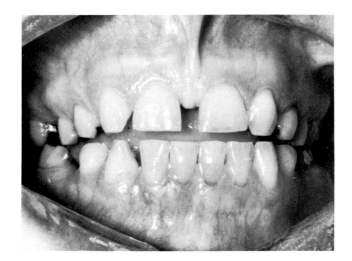

Figure 3–27 Adult with developmentally missing maxillary lateral incisors. Note how maxillary cuspids have been recontoured (incisal edges) to more closely resemble lateral incisors for esthetic improvement.

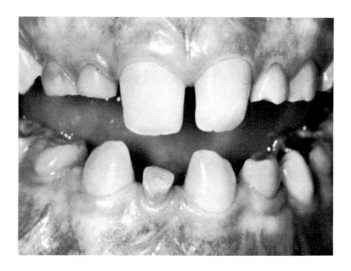

Figure 3–28 Child with some missing permanent incisors. There is no history of hereditary ectodermal dysplasia.

I. ANOMALIES OF NUMBER *Continued*

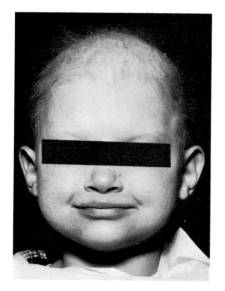

Figure 3–29 Facial view of boy with hereditary anhidrotic ectodermal dysplasia. This condition is a sex-linked recessive trait that mainly affects males. It is characterized by a lack of sweat glands, sparse hair, dry skin, and the absence of teeth.

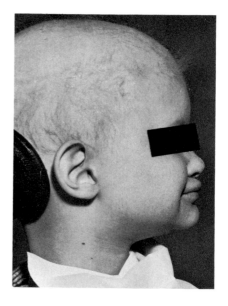

Figure 3–30 Same boy as shown in Figure 3–29. Note saddle nose, prominent lips, sparse hair, and lack of eyebrows — all typical of ectodermal dysplasia.

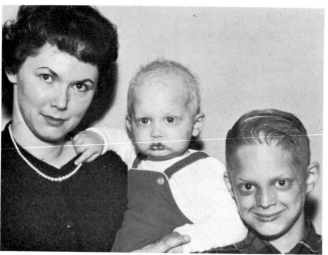

Figure 3–31 Two male children in family have ectodermal dysplasia. Mother shows no manifestations of this condition. Older boy has normal hair distribution.

I.   ANOMALIES OF NUMBER *Continued*

Figure 3–32 Boy aged 3 years with anhidrotic ectodermal dysplasia. Conical teeth are characteristic and usually require modification for reasons of appearance.

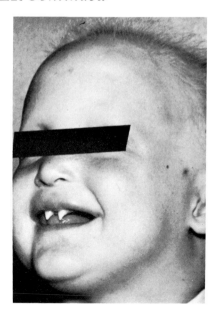

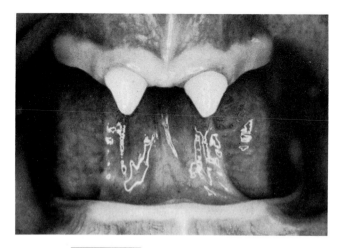

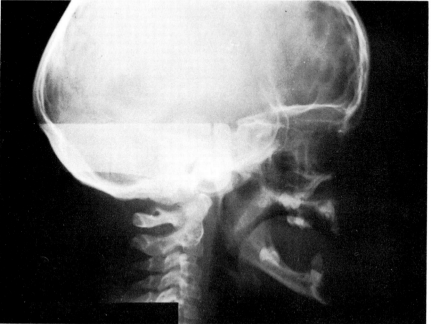

Figure 3–33 Same child as seen in Figure 3–32. The lack of alveolar bone development is due to the absence of teeth.

Figure 3–34 Cephalometric radiograph of a child with ectodermal dysplasia showing lack of tooth development. Although alveolar bone is deficient in these cases, basal bone or skeletal bone development proceeds normally.

I. ANOMALIES OF NUMBER *Continued*

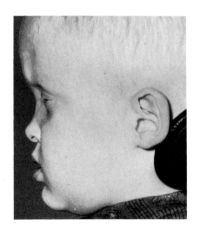

Figure 3–35 Four-year old boy with anhidrotic ectodermal dysplasia. Note characteristic facial appearance in profile.

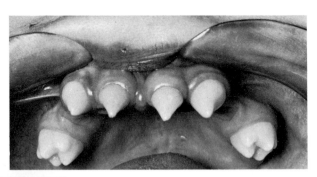

Figure 3–36 Maxillary arch of boy shown in Figure 3–35. Note conical shape of primary incisors — a typical finding. Alveolar bone development is lacking because of the absence of permanent teeth.

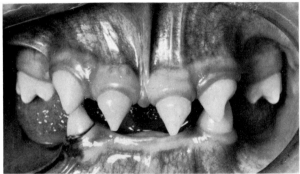

Figure 3–37 Anterior intraoral view of boy seen in Figure 3–35. Note lack of ridge in area posterior to lower canines. (See Chapter 15 for a description of the prosthetic treatment of this patient.)

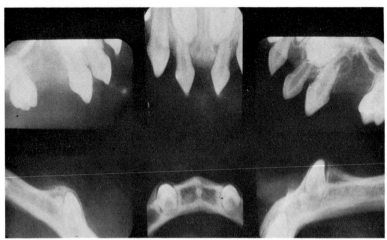

Figure 3–38 Radiographs of boy seen in Figure 3–35. Note the lack of primary as well as permanent teeth. This patient was fitted with a lower denture and upper partial denture after the upper teeth were modified (see Chapter 15).

Anomalies of Shape of Teeth

Variations in crown and root configuration of teeth may be of a hereditary nature or may result from disease or trauma. Frequently these anomalies are limited to one or two teeth. In making a diagnosis, the radiograph is a necessity, and in most cases the patient's history will also be of value. Few studies have been reported on the incidence of these conditions. Grahnen[7] in a survey of 1006 children aged 11 to 14 years, found that 1.7 per cent exhibited peg lateral incisors in the upper arch. He found fused or geminated teeth in 0.5 per cent of a group of 3- to 5-year-old children. Clayton[5] reported that 0.47 per cent of a group of children aged 3 to 12 years had geminated or fused teeth, a figure that compares closely with Grahnen's. The occurrence of fused or geminated teeth in the permanent dentition is much less common than in the primary dentition. A classification of anomalies of shape of teeth is of value in reaching a diagnosis.

CLASSIFICATION

  A. Gemination
  B. Fusion
  C. Dilaceration
  D. Concrescence
  E. Hutchinson's incisor*
  F. Mulberry molar*
  G. Peg lateral
  H. Exaggerated cingulum
  I. Supernumerary cusps
  J. Claw-shaped incisors
  K. Taurodontism
  L. Dens-in-dente
  M. Macrodontia
  N. Microdontia†
  O. Hypoplastic defects and generalized malformations resulting from trauma, exanthematous disease, and genetic syndromes.‡

---

*Associated disease complex, congenital syphilis.
†Associated genetic syndrome, primordial dwarfism.
‡See the section on Anomalies of Structure and Texture in this chapter as well as Chapter 16, Trauma to Primary Teeth, and Chapter 17, Trauma to Permanent Teeth.

II. ANOMALIES OF SHAPE

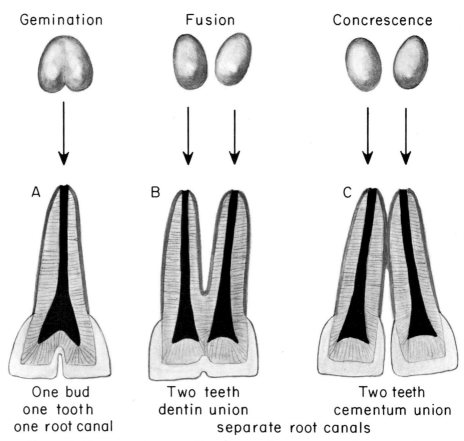

Figure 3–39 Diagrammatic illustration of gemination, fusion, and concrescence. (Modified from Tannenbaum, K. A., and Alling, E. E.: Anomalous tooth development: case report of gemination and twinning. Oral Surg. Oral Med. Oral Path. *16*:883–887, July, 1963).

II. ANOMALIES OF SHAPE *Continued*

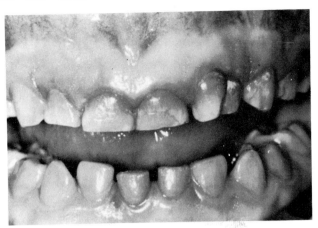

Figure 3–40 Gemination of a maxillary left primary lateral incisor.

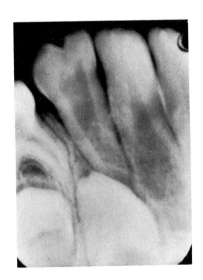

Figure 3–41 Radiograph of geminated mandibular primary cuspid.

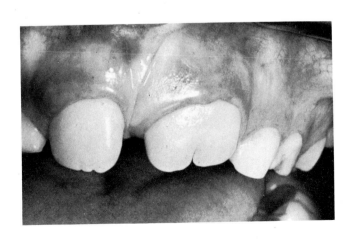

Figure 3–42 Gemination of the maxillary left permanent central incisor.

II. ANOMALIES OF SHAPE *Continued*

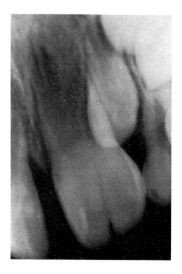

Figure 3–43 Radiograph of the geminated left permanent maxillary central incisor shown in Figure 3–42. Note the presence of one pulp chamber and pulp canal.

Figure 3–44 Fusion of the mandibular primary right cuspid and lateral incisor.

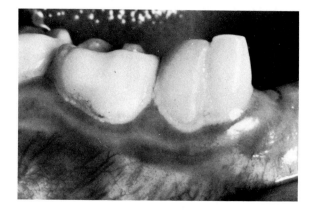

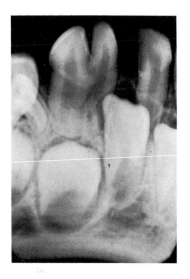

Figure 3–45 Radiograph of fused mandibular right cuspid and lateral incisor. Note the presence of separate pulp chambers and pulp canals.

II. ANOMALIES OF SHAPE *Continued*

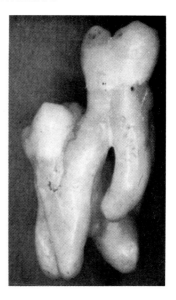

Figure 3–46 Concrescence. Fusion of molar roots by cementum. (From Kerr, D. A., and Ash, M. M., *Oral Pathology*, 2nd ed., Lea & Febiger, Philadelphia, 1965, p. 55).

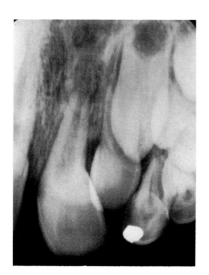

Figure 3–47 Dilaceration of the maxillary left permanent central incisor.

Figure 3–48 Dilaceration of the mandibular right permanent central incisor.

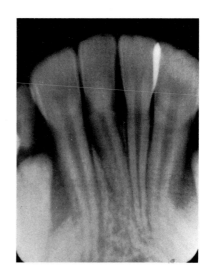

II. ANOMALIES OF SHAPE *Continued*

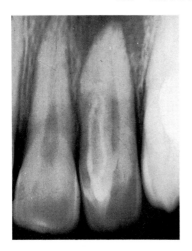

Figure 3-49 Dens-in-dente of the maxillary left permanent central incisor.

Figure 3-50 Peg-shaped maxillary right permanent lateral incisor.

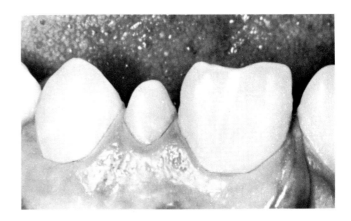

Figure 3-51 Radiograph of peg-shaped lateral incisor illustrated in Figure 3-50.

Figure 3-52 Maxillary central incisors with exaggerated cingula.

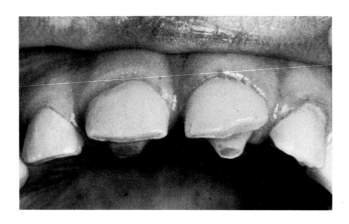

II. ANOMALIES OF SHAPE *Continued*

Figure 3–53 Hutchinson's incisors. These may be the end result of congenital syphilis. (From Kerr, D. A., and Ash, M. M.: *Oral Pathology*, 2nd ed., Lea & Febiger, Philadelphia, 1965, p. 52.)

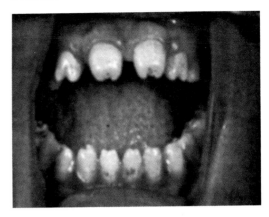

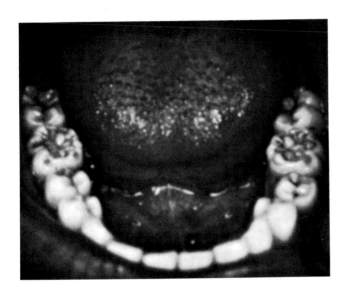

Figure 3–54 Mulberry molars. Typical shape associated with congenital syphilis (From Colby, R. A., Kerr, D. A., and Robinson, H. B. G.: *Color Atlas of Oral Pathology*, 2nd ed., J. B. Lippincott Co., Philadelphia, 1961, p. 48.)

Figure 3–55 Taurodontism of a mandibular left first primary molar. Note the unusual root configuration, in which there is an increased height of the pulp chamber and less constriction at the cementoenamel junction. Taurodontism may be associated with Klinefelter's syndrome. (Courtesy Dr. Lloyd B. Austin.)

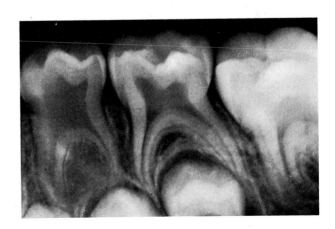

Anomalies of Color of Teeth

Often the first evidence of variation from normal in the human dentition is an observable difference in the color of the teeth. Some of these variations are apparent only to the trained eye, others are so obvious that they are a cause of great concern to parent and child alike. In recent years, the widespread use of tetracycline has added a new category of intrinsic discoloration of teeth, emphasizing again the role of the dentition as a permanent record of the life cycle of the individual.

Although a series of color photographs of dental anomalies would be instructive, it should be pointed out that color is never a reliable diagnostic criterion in itself. Clinical examination, patient history, and radiographs are always essential in making a final diagnosis. The first consideration is whether the color or stain in a particular case is intrinsic or extrinsic. Prophylaxis utilizing pumice should be done to remove green stains or yellow pigmentation caused by vitamin syrups or tobacco. If the color is intrinsic it will be necessary to consider its distribution and the patient's history, place of residence, early illnesses, and family background.

CLASSIFICATION

1. Yellow teeth: tetracycline staining, pigmentation due to premature birth, amelogenesis imperfecta.
2. Brown teeth: tetracycline staining, amelogenesis imperfecta, dentinogenesis imperfecta, pigmentation due to premature birth, cystic fibrosis, porphyria.
3. Blue to blue-green teeth: erythroblastosis fetalis.
4. White or cream-colored opaque teeth: amelogenesis imperfecta.
5. Teeth with specific white areas: fluorosis, snow-capped teeth, idiopathic opacities.
6. Reddish-brown teeth: porphyria.
7. Gray-brown teeth: dentinogenesis imperfecta.
8. Miscellaneous discolorations due to extrinsic staining from foods, drugs, tobacco, or other agents.

Note: Examples of amelogenesis imperfecta and dentinogenesis imperfecta will be found in the next section under Anomalies of Structure and Texture of Teeth.

III. ANOMALIES OF COLOR

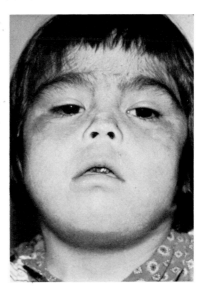

Figure 3–56 Full-face view of 6-year-old girl with hereditary porphyria, a rare metabolic error resulting in failure of the conversion of porphyrins. Urine is a burgundy color, and there is discoloration of teeth and bones. (Figures 3–57 and 3–59 are illustrations of same patient.)

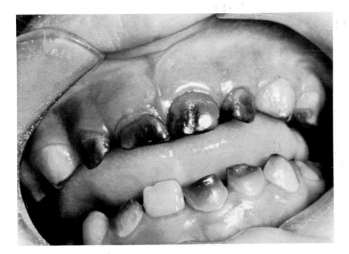

Figure 3–57 Intraoral view. Note discolored primary incisors, which are reddish-brown and fluoresce under ultraviolet light. These features are characteristic of tissues containing porphyrins. See Figure 3–59 for illustration of permanent teeth of same patient.

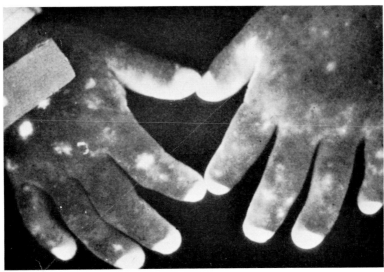

Figure 3–58 Note fluorescence of skin and fingernails under ultraviolet light.

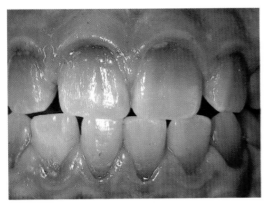

Figure 3–59 Hereditary porphyria. Same patient as seen in Figure 3–56 at 14 years of age. Brown pigmentation is more pronounced on posterior teeth.

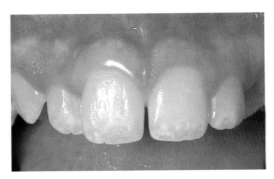

Figure 3–60 Mild fluorosis. Tips of cusps of first permanent molars are also affected.

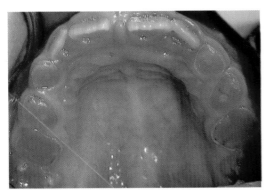

Figure 3–61 Dentinogenesis imperfecta. Characteristic brown color of teeth may be partly due to extrinsic staining of exposed dentin.

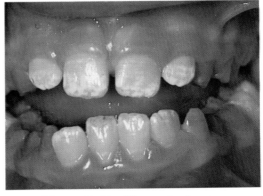

Figure 3–62 Fluorosis due to excess prescription fluoride. See Table 5–1 for correct administration of fluoride at different age levels.

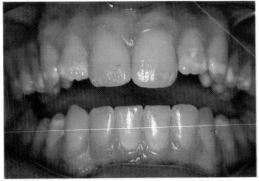

Figure 3–63 Hereditary snow-capped teeth. Not to be confused with fluorosis. This rare enamel anomaly is usually more pronounced in maxillary than in mandibular teeth.

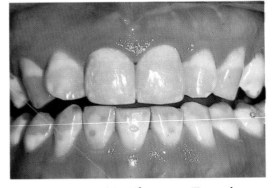

Figure 3–64 Fluorosis. Typical mottling with brownish areas. Patient grew up in area containing 4 ppm. fluoride in the water supply.

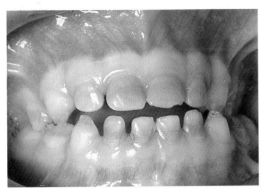

Figure 3–65 Tetracycline pigmentation of primary teeth.

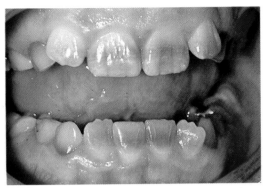

Figure 3–66 Tetracycline pigmentation in permanent teeth. Color is grayer than in Figure 3–65.

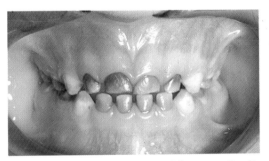

Figure 3–67 Erythroblastosis fetalis (hemolytic disease of the newborn). Primary teeth that are undergoing calcification up to the time of birth exhibit characteristic blue-green color because of absorption of bile pigments by dentin.

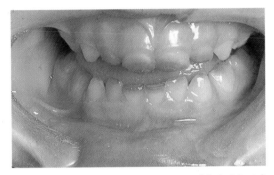

Figure 3–68 A five-year-old child with yellow-brown staining and hypoplasia as a result of jaundice associated with premature birth.

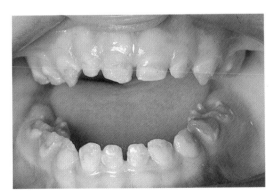

Figure 3–69 X-linked recessive hypomaturation of enamel. Primary teeth show brown pigmentation and some hypoplasia.

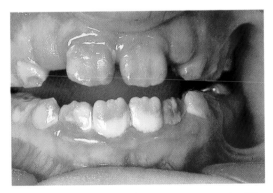

Figure 3–70 Same patient as in Figure 3–69 with erupted anterior permanent incisors. Mottled appearance is typical, along with reduced hardness of enamel.

Anomalies of Structure and Texture of Teeth

Included in this category are the hereditary syndromes, such as amelogenesis imperfecta and dentinogenesis imperfecta, as well as the miscellaneous factors that may affect enamel or dentin formation. It should be pointed out that there are conflicting reports in the literature concerning the genetic analysis of these syndromes; consequently, in order to make a diagnosis all aspects of the anomaly should be considered.

CLASSIFICATION

  I. Hereditary syndromes.
  A. Enamel (amelogenesis imperfecta).
   1. Hereditary enamel hypoplasia (four subdivisions).
   2. Hereditary enamel hypocalcification (three subdivisions).
  B. Dentin.
   1. Dentinogenesis imperfecta.
   2. Dentin dysplasia, radicular.
   3. Dentin dysplasia, coronal.
   4. Shell teeth.
 II. Other manifestations of anomalous structure and texture.
  A. Fluorosis.
  B. Porphyria.
  C. Hypophosphatasia.
  D. Hypoplasia due to febrile disease.
  E. Hypoplasia due to trauma.
  F. Hypoplasia due to radiation.
  G. Hypoplasia due to vitamin deficiency.
  H. Hypoplasia due to hypothyroidism.
   I. Hypoplasia due to pseudohypoparathyroidism.
   J. Hypoplasia due to vitamin D–resistant rickets.
  K. Hypoplasia due to premature birth and neonatal factors.

TABLE 3-1 TYPICAL PEDIGREE OF A FAMILY WITH DENTINOGENESIS IMPERFECTA

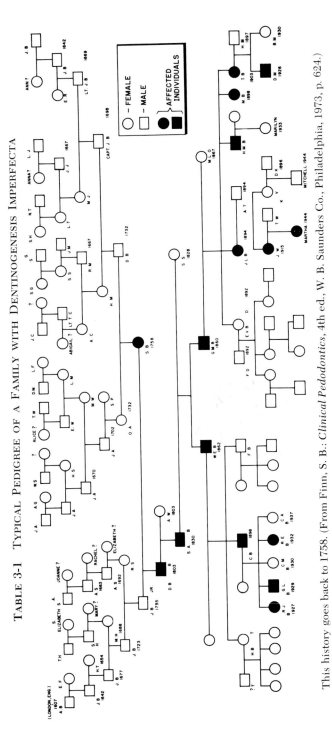

This history goes back to 1758. (From Finn, S. B.: *Clinical Pedodontics*, 4th ed., W. B. Saunders Co., Philadelphia, 1973, p. 624.)

TABLE 3-2 HEREDITARY ANOMALIES OF ENAMEL (AMELOGENESIS IMPERFECTA*)

	HEREDITARY ENAMEL HYPOPLASIA (FAULT OF APPOSITION-MATRIX FORMATION)				HEREDITARY ENAMEL HYPOCALCIFICATION† (FAULT OF CALCIFICATION-MATURATION)		
	Type 1	*Type 2*	*Type 3*	*Type 4*	*Type 1*	*Type 2*	*Type 3*
	Enamel thin but hard; smooth and glossy	Enamel hard but pitted on external surface	Enamel hard but vertically grooved and wrinkled on external surface (Witkop)	Local areas of hypoplasia, lines, or pits not related to febrile cause	Enamel soft and cheesy; can be easily removed by an instrument	Enamel dull, easily chipped; cuts readily with rotating instrument	Local areas of hypocalcification usually limited to incisal and occlusal "snow-capped" teeth
Color	Glossy yellow to orange-brown	Normal	Normal	Brown in hypoplastic areas only	Yellow to gray-brown	Dull paper white to creamy white	White tips on incisors, cuspids, and bicuspids
Radiographic appearance	Enamel of normal density but reduced in thickness (one quarter to one half normal thickness)	Mottled	Mottled	Radiolucency in areas of defects; no other variation	Enamel of same density as dentin but of normal thickness; crowns and roots otherwise normal	Enamel of normal thickness but of same density as dentin; may be a thin layer of normal enamel along dentoenamel junction	Not distinguishable
Genetic characteristics	Autosomal dominant	Unknown	Sex-linked dominant	Autosomal dominant	Autosomal dominant; occurs 1:1 in siblings	Autosomal dominant	Unreported but definitely familial; should be differentiated from mild fluorosis
Histological characteristics	Above normal organic substances in demineralized sections; stage of life cycle-apposition (matrix formation)	Not reported	Not reported	Not reported	Lack of calcification of matrix in ground sections; stage of life cycle calcification	Areas of deficient mineralization may be seen	Unreported

*Overall incidence reported by Witkop, 1:14,000–16,000[10]

†Another variant designated as X-linked recessive hypomaturation is illustrated in Figures 3–69 and 3–70. Primary teeth are yellow in color. Permanent teeth usually are mottled yellow-brown to white. Lack of radiographic contrast between enamel and dentin is characteristic, and enamel is relatively soft.

TABLE 3-3 HEREDITARY ANOMALIES OF DENTIN

	INCIDENCE	STAGE AFFECTED IN LIFE CYCLE OF TOOTH	COLOR	RADIOGRAPHIC CHARACTERISTICS	HISTOLOGICAL CHARACTERISTICS	GENETIC CHARACTERISTICS	MISCELLANEOUS
Dentinogenesis imperfecta (hereditary opalescent dentin)	1 in 8000	Histodifferentiation	Blue-gray to brown	Pulp chambers and root canals obliterated in mature teeth; crowns appear more bulbous; enamel (when not abraded) appears of normal thickness and density; roots often appear foreshortened	Dentoenamel junction smooth and unscalloped; reduced number of odontoblasts; dentinal tubules disorganized and may contain pulpal inclusions; interglobular dentin may be abundant; chemical analysis of dentin shows it to be high in water and organic content compared with normal dentin	Simple, dominant, nonsex-linked	Teeth abrade rapidly; caries infrequent; may be associated with blue sclera; may be associated with osteogenesis imperfecta
Dentin dysplasia type I radicular	Very rare; 1 in 96,000	Probably histodifferentiation	Normal	Obliteration of pulp chambers and root canals; lack of root formation; large radiolucent areas around roots	No reduction in number of odontoblasts; presence of large collagenous masses interspersed among tubules is characteristic	Autosomal dominant	No tendency to abrade
Dentin dysplasia type II coronal thistle tube teeth	Rare	Probably histodifferentiation	Deciduous, amber; permanent, normal	Primary teeth normal; thistle-shaped pulp chambers in permanent teeth	Radicular dentin atubular and amorphous	Autosomal dominant	Roots appear normal in both dentitions
Shell teeth	Extremely rare	Probably histodifferentiation	Normal	Normal enamel layer with thin layer of dentin and enormous pulp chamber	No odontoblasts; thin layer of irregular dentin; coarse collagen bundles	Unreported	May be a variant of dentinogenesis imperfecta; only case reported by Rushton[9]

IV. ANOMALIES OF STRUCTURE AND TEXTURE

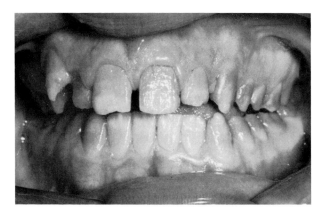

Figure 3–71 Hereditary enamel hypoplasia of the smooth, hard type in a 14-year-old boy. The enamel is about one fourth of the usual thickness and has a glossy orange-brown color.

Figure 3–72 Same boy as seen in Figure 3–71, at an earlier age. Radiograph of molar region. Note the thin enamel covering of the crowns and the lack of bell shape. Pulp chamber and dentin are normal.

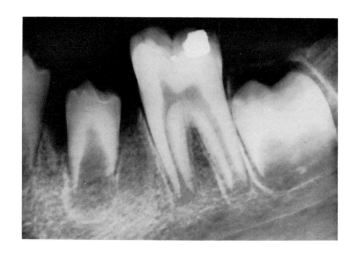

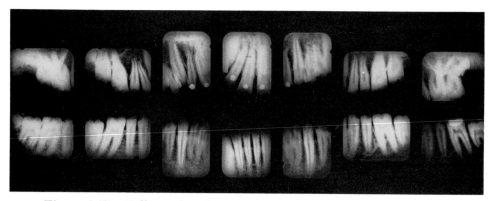

Figure 3–73 Full-mouth radiograph, same patient as illustrated in Figure 3–71. Teeth appear elongated and lacking in contour because of lack of enamel. Treatment consists of providing adequate coverage as teeth abrade.

IV. ANOMALIES OF STRUCTURE AND TEXTURE *Continued*

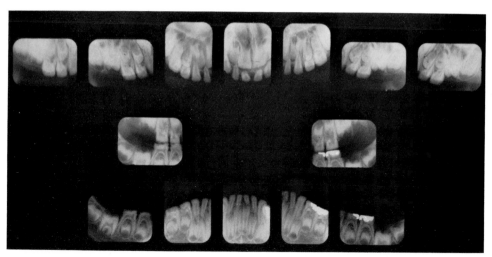

Figure 3–74   Figures 3–74 to 3–76 are full-mouth radiographs illustrating the delay in eruption of permanent teeth in a case of hereditary enamel hypoplasia. Note that the primary dentition exhibits the characteristic thin layer of enamel.

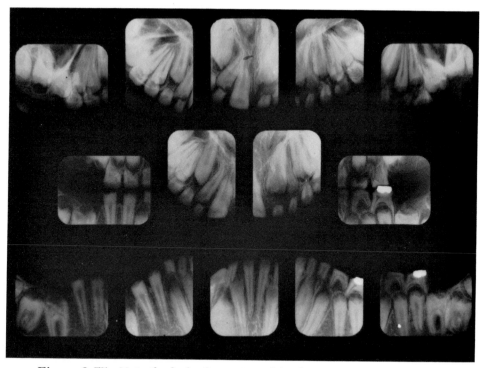

Figure 3–75   Note the lack of eruption of the first permanent molars as well as upper incisors in this 12-year-old patient.

IV. ANOMALIES OF STRUCTURE AND TEXTURE *Continued*

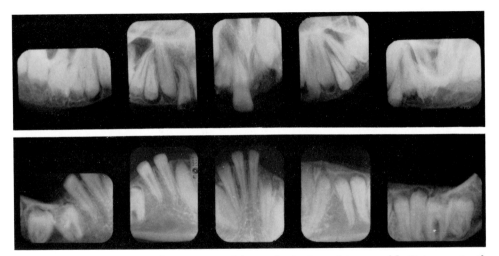

Figure 3–76 Hereditary enamel hypoplasia in a 14-year-old. Primary teeth were extracted to aid the eruption of permanent teeth, but no response is evident at this time. (See Figures 3–74 and 3–75.)

IV. ANOMALIES OF STRUCTURE AND TEXTURE *Continued*

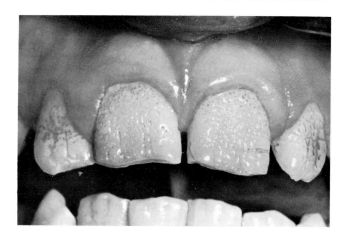

Figure 3–77 Hereditary enamel hypoplasia of the hard, pitted type. The enamel is lacking in thickness and is pitted and corrugated.

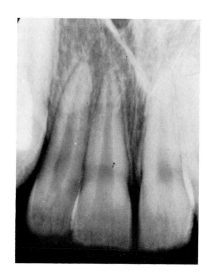

Figure 3–78 Radiograph of maxillary incisors of patient seen in Figure 3–77. Pitted areas appear radiolucent.

Figure 3–79 Another example of hereditary enamel hypoplasia of the hard, pitted type. The color of these teeth is usually close to normal.

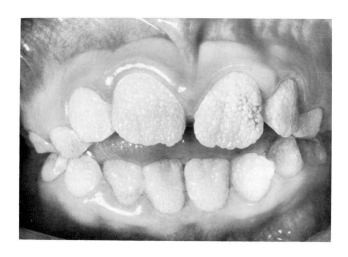

IV. ANOMALIES OF STRUCTURE AND TEXTURE *Continued*

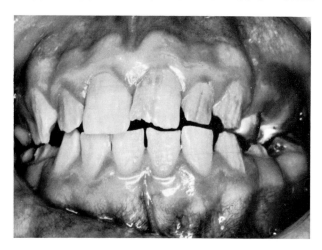

Figure 3–80 Hereditary enamel hypoplasia with vertical grooving. Enamel layer is lacking in thickness.

Figure 3–81 Hereditary enamel hypoplasia with horizontal wrinkling and grooving.

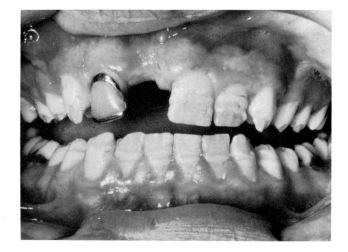

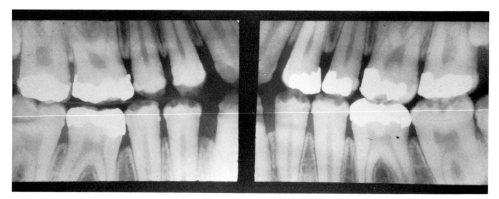

Figure 3–82 Radiographs of patient illustrated in Figure 3–81. Note crinkling and corrugation of crowns of all teeth.

IV. ANOMALIES OF STRUCTURE AND TEXTURE *Continued*

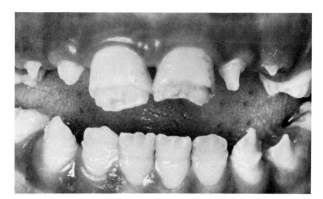

Figure 3–83 Intraoral view of girl with atypical hereditary enamel hypoplasia. The enamel is hard and glossy.

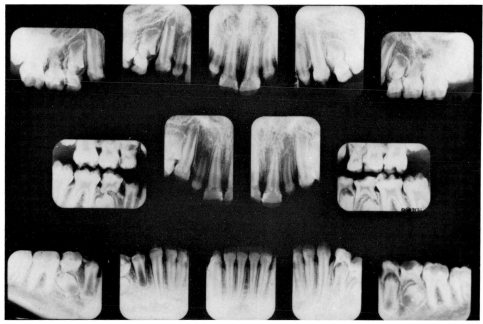

Figure 3–84 Full-mouth radiographs of girl seen in Figure 3–83, showing extent of hypoplasia in all teeth. Pulp canals and dentin appear normal.

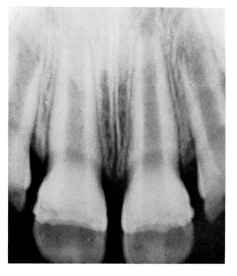

Figure 3–85 Radiographs of maxillary central incisors of girl illustrated in Figure 3–83. Note thin enamel and normal root canals.

IV. ANOMALIES OF STRUCTURE AND TEXTURE *Continued*

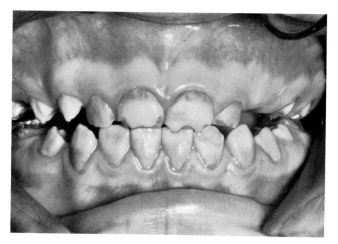

Figure 3–86 Hereditary enamel hypocalcification in an 11-year-old boy. The enamel on these teeth is soft and cheesy and can be dislodged with an explorer point. These cases require full coverage to prevent wear and loss of contour.

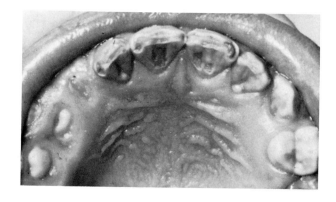

Figure 3–87 Same child as seen in Figure 3–86. Radiographs of these cases show normal pulp chamber morphology, but the enamel is lacking in normal radiopacity.

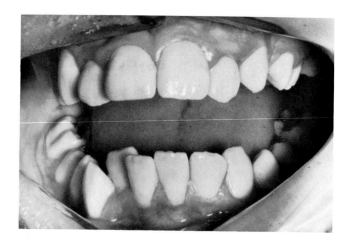

Figure 3–88 Hereditary enamel hypocalcification. In this type the enamel is dull and lusterless and is easily chipped.

IV. ANOMALIES OF STRUCTURE AND TEXTURE *Continued*

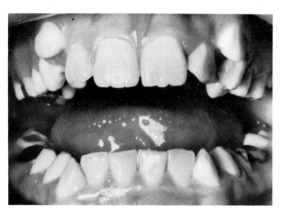

Figure 3–89 Another child exhibiting hereditary enamel hypocalcification. In this case the teeth have a creamy café-au-lait color and are easily abraded.

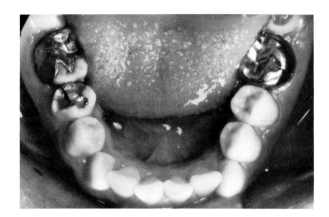

Figure 3-90 Intraoral view of patient illustrated in Figure 3–89. Note chipped enamel around amalgam restoration on the second bicuspid.

Figure 3–91 Radiograph, right side, in patient illustrated in Figure 3–89. The enamel and the dentin appear to be of equal density. Note the radiopaque line at the dentoenamel junction, particularly on the bicuspids, indicating a zone of more highly calcified enamel.

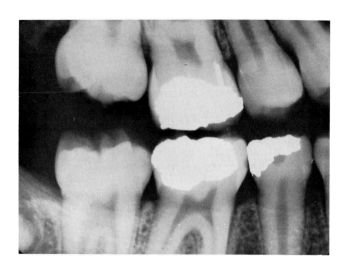

IV. ANOMALIES OF STRUCTURE AND TEXTURE *Continued*

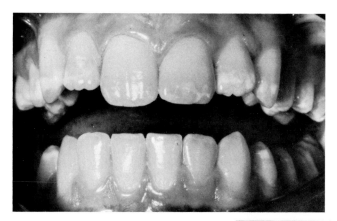

Figure 3–92   Snow-capped teeth, a typical form of hereditary enamel hypocalcification in which there are specific areas near the incisal and occlusal surfaces having a white ground-glass appearance.

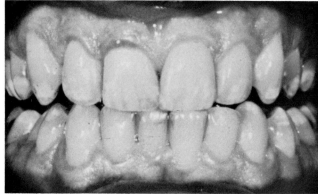

Figure 3–93   Snow-capped teeth. The white areas in this case are most prominent on the cuspids and bicuspids. Note that these markings do not conform to defects related to a febrile disease at a specific age.

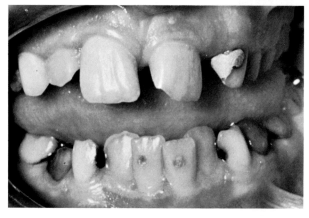

Figure 3–94   Defective enamel on two lower incisors, related to trauma. When child was 2 years of age he suffered a fall, which caused intrusion of the mandibular primary incisors. This type of hypoplasia is obviously not hereditary.

Figure 3–95   Local hypoplasia on a maxillary incisor in a boy with a history of a facial injury in infancy.

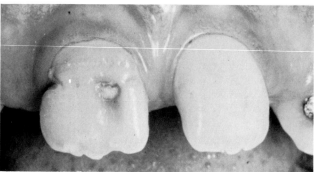

IV. ANOMALIES OF STRUCTURE AND TEXTURE *Continued*

Figure 3–96 Typical enamel hypoplasia related to a history of febrile disease. This child suffered a severe attack of pneumonia at age 8 months. Note that the maxillary lateral incisors are unaffected. This is because these teeth usually do not begin to calcify before 10 to 12 months of age.

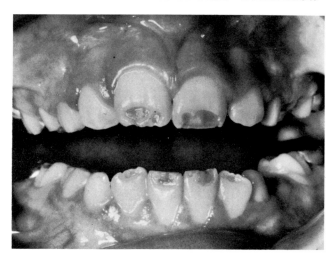

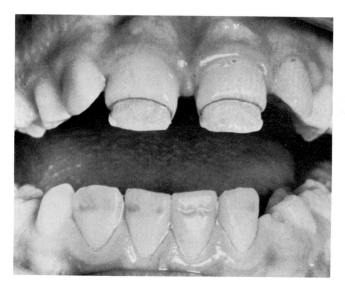

Figure 3–97 Local enamel hypoplasia related to a history of virus infection in infancy. Note that the maxillary laterals are normal, indicating that the disease probably terminated prior to age 10 months.

Figure 3–98 Close-up of mandibular molar region in patient shown in Figure 3–97. Note lack of enamel formation on occlusal of first permanent molar. The second primary molar appears unaffected.

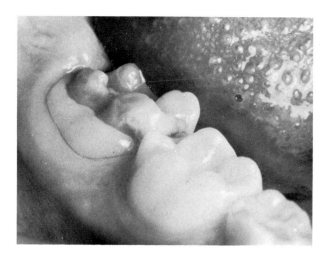

IV. ANOMALIES OF STRUCTURE AND TEXTURE *Continued*

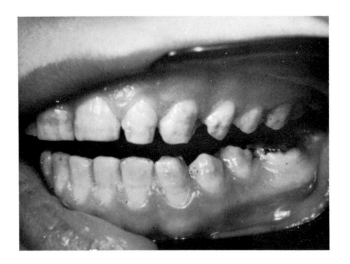

Figure 3–99 Fluorosis or mottled enamel. The effect of high concentrations of fluoride ion is to induce defective calcification in some areas. These in turn undergo distinctive staining giving a characteristic appearance.

Figure 3–100 Enamel hypoplasia in the primary dentition related to maternal disturbances during pregnancy. The areas affected are those that have calcified in the prenatal period.

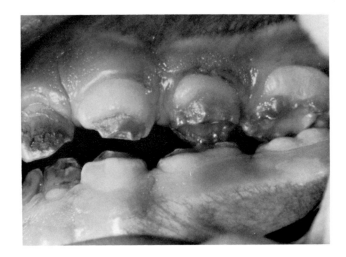

IV. ANOMALIES OF STRUCTURE AND TEXTURE *Continued*

Figure 3–101 Dentino-genesis imperfecta in a 5-year-old girl. An autosomal dominant trait, it is found in the ratio of 1:1 in siblings. Teeth are blue-gray or brown and abrade rapidly. (For a discussion of treatment, see Chapter 15, Prosthodontics.)

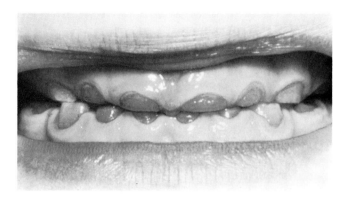

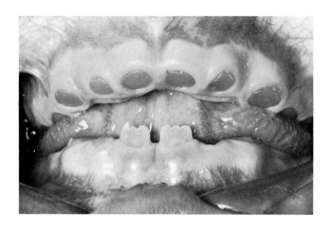

Figure 3–102 Same girl as seen in Figure 3–101. Lower permanent incisors have erupted, and maxillary primary teeth are abraded to a marked extent.

Figure 3–103 Maxillary arch showing extreme abrasion of primary crowns. Frequently these teeth become abscessed as a result of exposure of pulpal horns caused by wear. Full coverage is the treatment of choice.

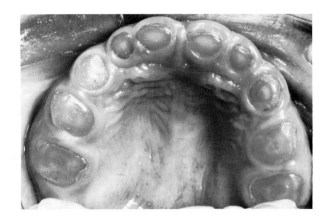

IV. ANOMALIES OF STRUCTURE AND TEXTURE *Continued*

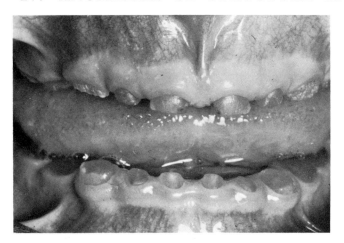

Figure 3–104 Dentinogenesis imperfecta in the primary dentition. Children with this condition may have psychological problems because of their appearance.

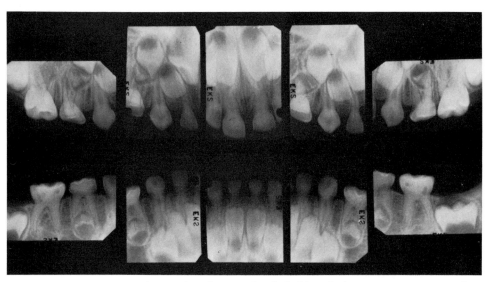

Figure 3–105 Radiographs of a preschool child with dentinogenesis imperfecta. Note obliteration of the pulp chambers with secondary dentin, a characteristic finding. Crowns generally appear more bulbous than usual.

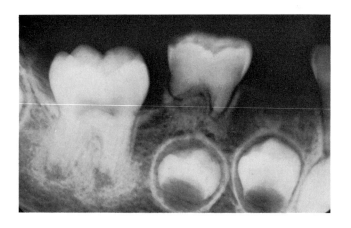

Figure 3–106 Radiograph of an 8-year-old child with dentinogenesis imperfecta. Note that the pulp chamber of the newly erupted permanent molar is not yet completely obliterated, as is the case with the adjacent primary molar.

IV. ANOMALIES OF STRUCTURE AND TEXTURE *Continued*

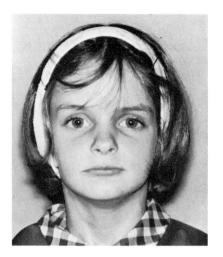

Figure 3–107 Eight-year-old girl with dentinogenesis imperfecta. Note the bite closure because of excessive loss of tooth substance from abrasion.

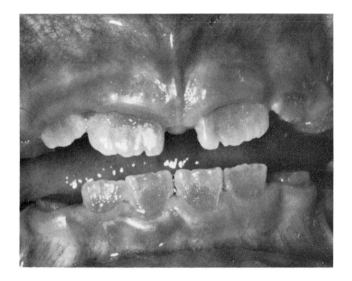

Figure 3–108 Anterior view of teeth of girl seen in Figure 3–107. The teeth have a brownish-gray color. Defects of enamel are sometimes associated with this condition, but the primary defect is one of the dentin.

Figure 3–109 Intraoral view of girl seen in Figure 3–107. Note complete abrasion of posterior teeth.

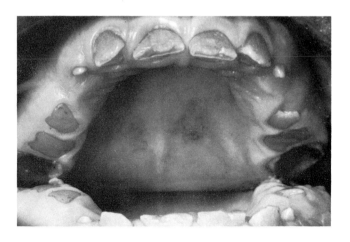

IV. ANOMALIES OF STRUCTURE AND TEXTURE *Continued*

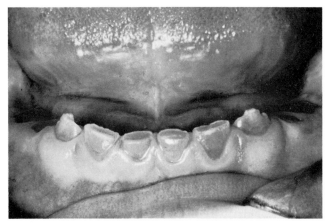

Figure 3–110 Same patient as seen in Figure 3–109. It is often advisable to provide coverage for permanent teeth as soon as they erupt.

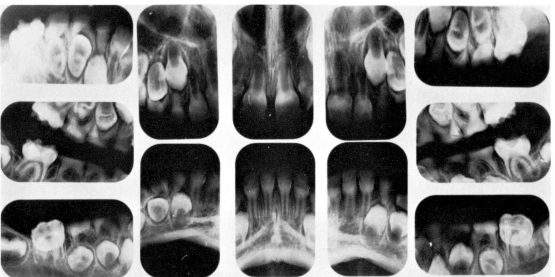

Figure 3–111 Radiographs of 8-year-old girl with dentinogenesis imperfecta. Pulp chambers of primary teeth are completely obliterated. Newly erupted permanent teeth have not as yet undergone significant abrasion and should be crowned.

Figure 3–112 An unusual case of dentinogenesis imperfecta in which the primary teeth exhibit the typical color and abrasion pattern but the erupting permanent teeth are normal in appearance.

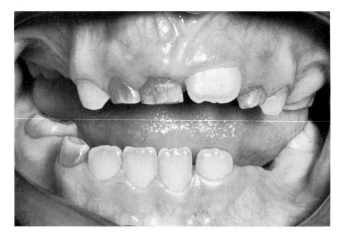

IV. ANOMALIES OF STRUCTURE AND TEXTURE *Continued*

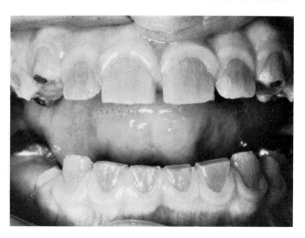

Figure 3–113 A 14-year-old girl with dentinogenesis imperfecta. (See Chapter 15, Prosthodontics, for a discussion of the treatment of this patient.)

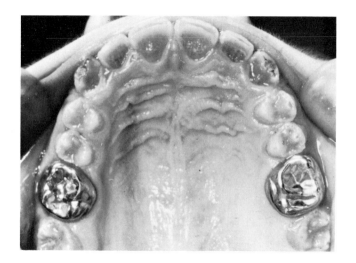

Figure 3–114 Same girl as seen in Figure 3–113. First permanent molars were crowned shortly after eruption to prevent abrasion.

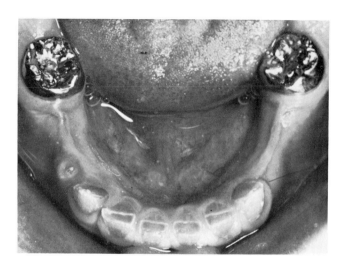

Figure 3–115 Lower arch of girl shown in Figure 3–113. Note wear on lower incisors.

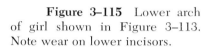

IV. ANOMALIES OF STRUCTURE AND TEXTURE *Continued*

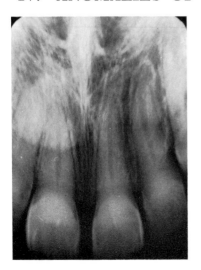

Figure 3–116 Radiographs of anterior teeth of girl with dentinogenesis imperfecta. Note obliteration of pulp chambers with secondary dentin.

Figure 3–117 Typical radiographic appearance in a case of dentinogenesis imperfecta. Pulp chambers and root canals are obliterated.

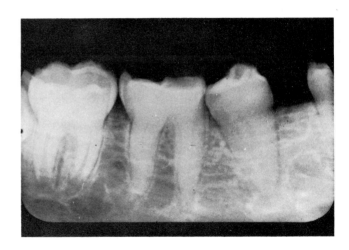

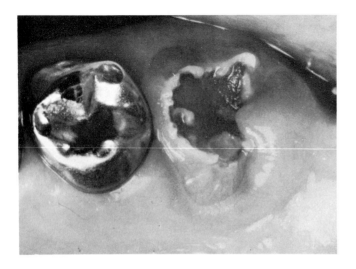

Figure 3–118 Intraoral view of erupting first permanent molar in a child with combined enamel and dentin defect. The dentin is similar to that found in dentinogenesis imperfecta. This anomaly has been variously designated as dysplasia of enamel and dentin and as odontogenesis imperfecta.

IV. ANOMALIES OF STRUCTURE AND TEXTURE *Continued*

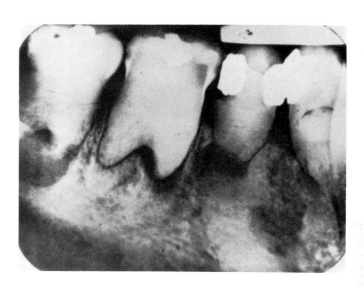

Figure 3–119 Dentinal dysplasia (also termed "rootless teeth"). This anomaly is comparatively rare and is characterized by crowns of normal color, but with pulp chambers obliterated and roots lacking in normal length. Radiolucent areas may be present around these roots. (From Rushton, M. A.: Anomalies of human dentin. Ann. Roy. Coll. Surg. *16:*94, 1955.)

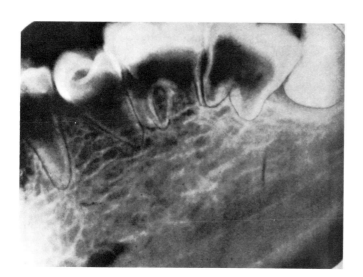

Figure 3–120 Shell teeth — a rare anomaly of dentin that has been described by Rushton. There is a thin layer of dentin surrounding the enormous pulp cavities. Roots are comparatively short. (From Rushton, M. A.: A new form of dentinal dysplasia: shell teeth. Oral Surg. Oral Med. Oral Path. 7:543–549, May, 1954.)

Anomalies of Eruption and Exfoliation

The age at which eruption and exfoliation of teeth occur varies widely. Many clinicians feel that there is a familial pattern of early or late eruption. A dramatic example of early eruption is the neonatal tooth, which is found occasionally in newborns. This has been reported to occur in 0.03 per cent of births (1 in 3000), usually in the lower incisor area.[2]

Local or systemic factors can influence eruption or exfoliation of teeth. In the case of premature loss of primary teeth resulting from caries, the effect on eruption of the succedaneous tooth depends on the age at which the extraction takes place. If it occurs during the preschool period, eruption of the underlying tooth is usually somewhat retarded. If it occurs during the mixed dentition period and there is extensive bone pathology, eruption of the permanent tooth is accelerated. A frequent cause of retarded eruption of permanent teeth is the presence of embedded supernumerary teeth or ankylosed primary teeth.

Retarded eruption is also associated with such conditions as cleidocranial dysostosis, hypothyroidism, and hypopituitarism. Conversely, precocious exfoliation may occur along with hypophosphatasia, acrodynia, and a form of reticular endotheliosis, such as Hand-Schüller-Christian disease.

Anomalies of Position of Teeth

In this classification there might properly be included all deviations from normal position — this would embrace all disharmonies of occlusion. For simplification, this section is limited to illustrations of deviations in tooth position due to ectopic eruption, ankylosis, and impaction.

V. ANOMALIES OF ERUPTION AND EXFOLIATION

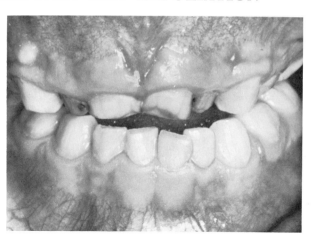

Figure 3–121 Delayed eruption of permanent teeth in an 8-year-old girl with cleidocranial dysostosis. In this hereditary condition the clavicles are absent, there are supernumerary teeth, and tooth eruption is delayed. (See also Figure 3–15.)

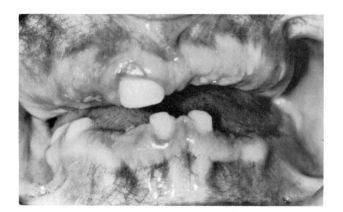

Figure   3–122 Intraoral view of 14-year-old girl with amelogenesis imperfecta (enamel hypoplasia type). Delayed eruption is sometimes associated with this anomaly.

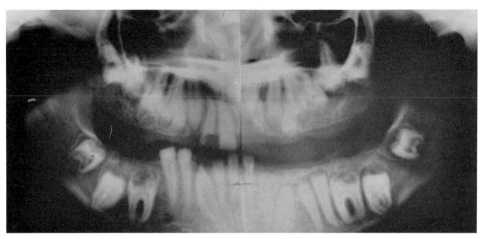

Figure 3–123 Radiographs of girl shown in Figure 3–122. Note multiple unerupted teeth.

V. ANOMALIES OF ERUPTION AND EXFOLIATION *Continued*

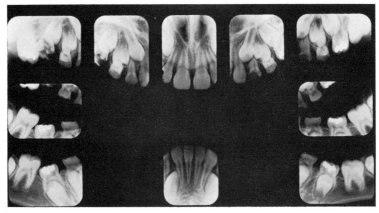

Figure 3–124 Radiographs of a 9-year-old girl with delayed eruption of all posterior permanent teeth. Some primary molars are ankylosed. There is no contact of teeth in the molar region, which might indicate the lack of vertical bone growth.

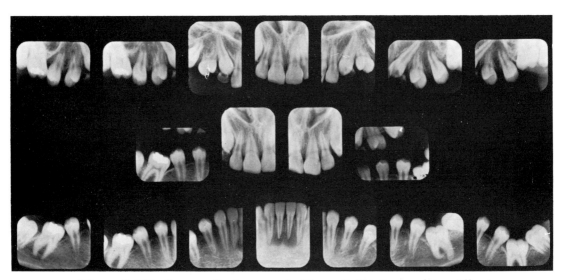

Figure 3–125 Same patient as seen in Figure 3–124, 2 years later. All primary teeth were extracted, but there is only limited eruption of posterior teeth. No other associated abnormalities were found.

V. ANOMALIES OF ERUPTION AND EXFOLIATION *Continued*

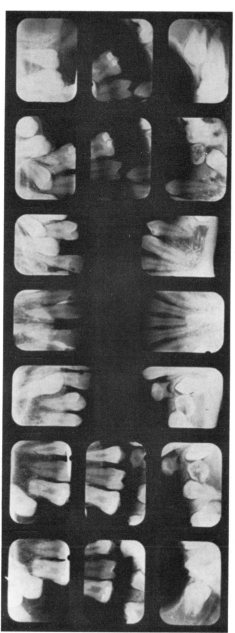

Figure 3–126 Delayed eruption in a 16-year-old boy with a history of hypothyroidism.

V. ANOMALIES OF ERUPTION AND EXFOLIATION *Continued*

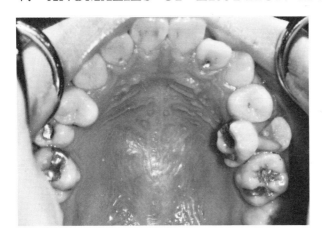

Figure 3–127 Delayed exfoliation of maxillary left primary second molar resulting from failure of resorption of lingual root.

Figure 3–128 Precocious exfoliation of primary dentition in a 3-year-old boy with hypophosphatasia. This condition is transmitted as an autosomal recessive trait and is characterized by a deficiency of alkaline phosphatase. Because of the absence of cementum, the tooth is deprived of its normal periodontal attachment.

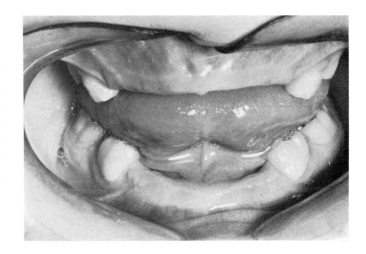

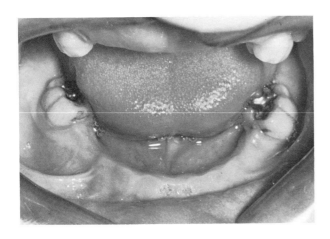

Figure 3–129 Same boy as shown in Figure 3–128, 1 year later. More teeth have loosened and been exfoliated. As this boy grew older, normal cementum developed around the permanent teeth, and the periodontal attachment was normal.

VI. ANOMALIES OF POSITION

Figure 3–130 Anterior crossbite. Before treatment is started, radiographs should be obtained to ascertain the presence or absence of supernumeraries. There must be adequate room for the lingually locked tooth to move forward.

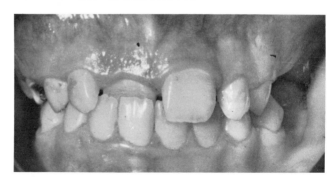

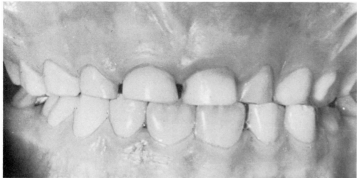

Figure 3–131 Posterior crossbite in the primary dentition. This condition can easily be overlooked. (See Chapter 14 concerning correction of anterior and posterior crossbites.) Note deviation of midline.

Figure 3–132 Labial eruption of maxillary permanent central incisor. Primary central incisors should be extracted. Some children exhibit over-retention of all primary teeth.

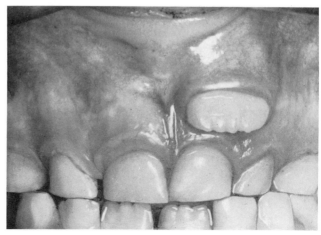

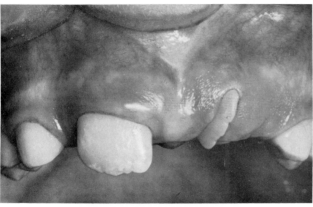

Figure 3–133 Permanent central incisor in abnormal position because of presence of a supernumerary tooth (mesiodens).

VI. ANOMALIES OF POSITION *Continued*

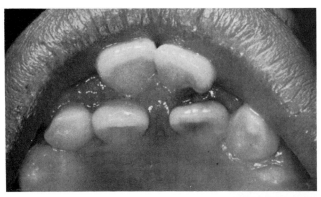

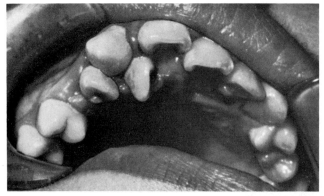

Figure 3–134 Extreme crowding in maxillary arch with lingual position of permanent lateral incisors. Orthodontic consultation should be sought.

Figure 3–135 Maxillary incisors crowded out of normal position because of the presence of a supernumerary tooth.

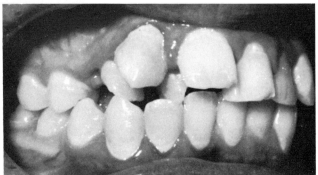

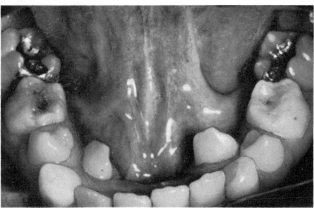

Figure 3–136 Occlusal view of patient shown in Figure 3–135. Extraction of the supernumerary tooth is indicated, followed by orthodontic treatment.

Figure 3–137 Ectopic eruption of mandibular permanent cuspids. Primary cuspids should be extracted and, if necessary, permanent cuspids repositioned.

VI.   ANOMALIES OF POSITION *Continued*

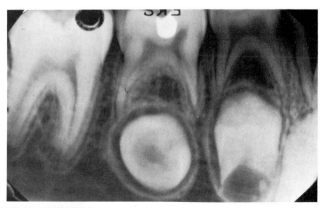

Figure 3–138 Rotated mandibular second bicuspid.

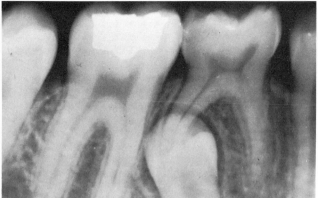

Figure 3–139 Over-retained second primary molar forces second bicuspid into distal position. The primary tooth should be extracted, the bone over the bicuspid removed, and the space maintained by a suitable appliance until the tooth erupts.

Figure 3–140 Ankylosed second primary molar has forced the second bicuspid to tip distally. The primary molar should be extracted and the space maintained until the permanent tooth erupts.

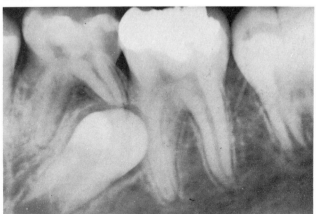

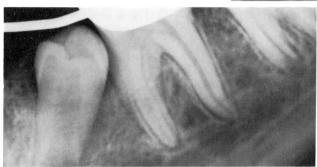

Figure 3–141 Same patient as in Figure 3–140, 3 months after extraction of the primary molar. The bicuspid is now upright and is erupting.

VI. ANOMALIES OF POSITION *Continued*

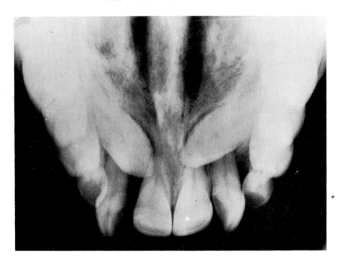

Figure 3–142 Permanent cuspids lying horizontally in the palate. Treatment of these cases should be done with the cooperation of the oral surgeon and the orthodontist.

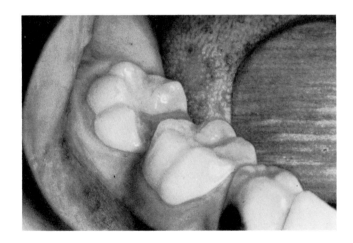

Figure 3–143 Ectopic eruption of mandibular first permanent molar. This is more commonly seen in the maxillary arch.

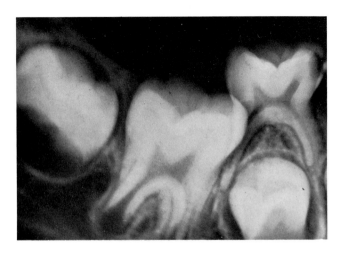

Figure 3–144 Radiograph of patient shown in Figure 3–143.

VI. ANOMALIES OF POSITION *Continued*

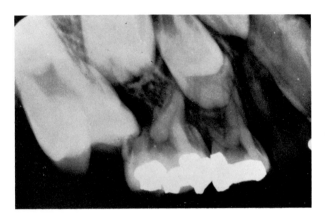

Figure 3–145 Ectopic eruption of maxillary first permanent molar. In a case as acute as this one, the primary second molar should be extracted, and the patient should wear a corrective headgear to reposition the permanent molar.

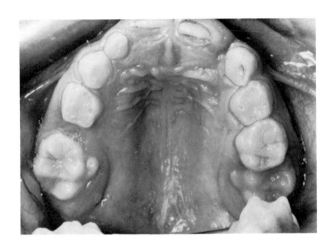

Figure 3–146 Maxillary occlusal view showing space loss created by an erupted ectopic first permanent molar that has not been treated. Note similar condition in opposite quadrant. Sometimes early intervention will prevent loss of second primary molar.

Figure 3–147 Bitewing radiograph illustrating a common situation: maxillary first permanent molar began to erupt ectopically, resorption took place, and the tooth assumed its proper position in the arch. Note the resorbed area on the distal root of the primary molar. Some ectopic eruptions are self correcting.

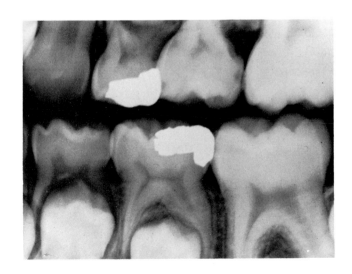

VI. ANOMALIES OF POSITION *Continued*

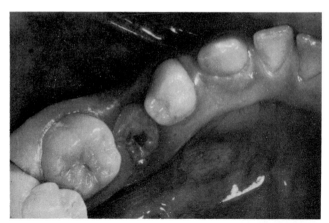

Figure 3–148 Ankylosis of a second primary molar. Growth of alveolar bone into lacunae on the root surface prevents normal vertical movement. The tooth should be extracted and the space maintained.

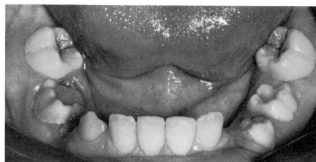

Figure 3–149 Ankylosis of mandibular primary molars. Loss of arch length can occur if ankylosed teeth fail to maintain proper position.

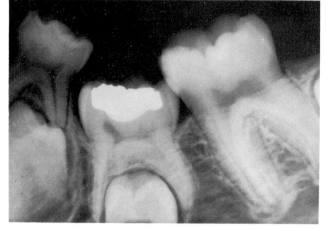

Figure 3–150 Radiograph of ankylosed primary second molar showing failure of tooth to maintain proper arch length. Extraction of the primary molar is indicated, followed by the use of a suitable appliance to reposition the tipped first permanent molar.

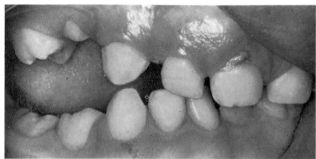

Figure 3–151 Ankylosis of all maxillary and mandibular primary molars on the right side resulting in loss of masticatory function in this area.

VI. ANOMALIES OF POSITION *Continued*

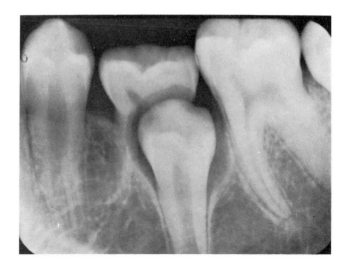

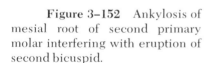

Figure 3–152 Ankylosis of mesial root of second primary molar interfering with eruption of second bicuspid.

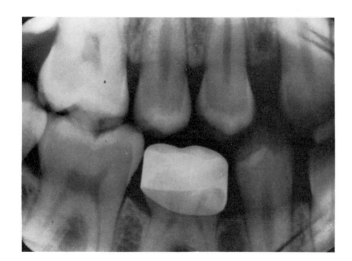

Figure 3–153 Use of a stainless steel crown to increase the height of an ankylosed molar and maintain arch length. This is advisable when the bicuspid is developmentally missing.

Figure 3–154 A cast gold crown can be constructed on an ankylosed primary molar, as shown here, to maintain arch length and occlusion. It is advisable to defer this type of restoration until vertical growth is attained, usually at 14 to 15 years of age.

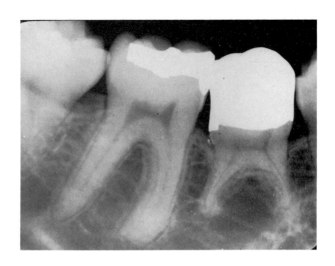

VI. ANOMALIES OF POSITION *Continued*

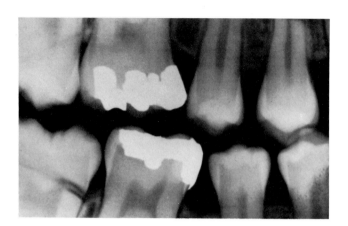

Figure 3–155 Permanent teeth seldom become ankylosed during the childhood years. This maxillary first permanent molar became ankylosed when the child was 12 years old and was well below the line of occlusion by age 14, necessitating restorative treatment.

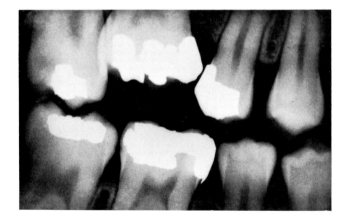

Figure 3–156 Same patient as seen in Figure 3–155, 2 years later. The extent of vertical bone growth that occurred during this period is indicated by the discrepancy in the line of occlusion and the occlusal relationship of the ankylosed tooth.

VI. ANOMALIES OF POSITION *Continued*

Figure 3–157 Periapical radiograph of ankylosed permanent molar shown in Figure 3–156. The exact areas of ankylosis cannot be detected.

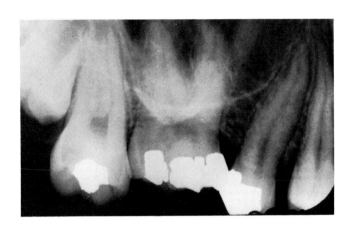

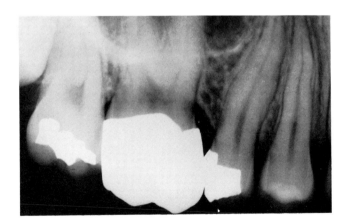

Figure 3–158 Treatment of ankylosed permanent molar by construction of full cast gold crown, which has restored proper occlusion.

REFERENCES

1. Blayney, J. R., and Hill, I. A.: Fluorine and dental caries. In Congenitally Missing Teeth. Special issue, J.A.D.A. 74:298–299, Jan., 1967.
2. Bodenhoff, J.: Dentitio connatalis et neonatalis. Odont. Tidskrift. 67:645–695, 1959.
3. Brown, H. R., and Cunningham, U. M.: Some dental manifestations in mongolism. Oral Surgery 14:664–676, 1961.
4. Castaldi, C. R., et al.: Incidence of congenital anomalies in permanent teeth of a group of Canadian children aged 6–9. J. Canad. Dent. Assoc. 32:154–159, March, 1966.
5. Clayton, J. M.: Congenital dental anomalies occurring in 3557 children. J. Dent. Child. 23:206–208, 1956.
6. Grahnen, H.: Hypodontia in the permanent dentition. Odont. Revy. 7:Suppl. 3, 1956.
7. Grahnen, H., and Granath, L.: Numerical variations in the primary dentition and their correlation with the permanent dentition. Odont. Revy. 4:348–357, 1961.
8. Menezer, L. F.: Anomalies of the primary dentition. J. Dent. Child. 22:57, 1955.
9. Rushton, M.: A new form of dentinal dysplasia: shell teeth. Oral Surg. Oral Med. Oral Path. 7:543–549, May, 1954.
10. Witkop, C. J., Jr.: Genetics and dentistry. Eugenics Qtrly. 5:15–21, 1959.
11. Chaudry, A. P., et al.: Hereditary enamel dysplasia. J. Pediatr. 54:776–785, 1959.
12. Schimmelpfennig, C. B., and McDonald, R. E.: Enamel and dentin aplasia, report of a case. Oral Surg. 6:1444–1449, 1953.

RADIOGRAPHY

Chapter 4 _____

KENNETH E. GLOVER
and
BRYAN J. WILLIAMS

An adequate radiographic survey is essential to complement the clinical examination of the pedodontic patient. The combination of these two procedures permits a diagnosis and treatment plan to be formulated on a sound data base. Radiographs of young children present challenges not usually associated with those of adults. The child's tolerance of the film packet as well as his or her attention span and patience are factors that may make radiographic surveys difficult. Some practitioners feel it easier to forgo the real or imagined challenge and base their treatment plan on clinical judgment alone. Failure to obtain adequate radiographs presents risks to both the patient and dentist by increasing the possibility of future management problems. Until adequate radiographs are available, it is best to postpone a comprehensive diagnosis and treatment plan.

Children are naturally curious and generally eager to please. These attributes can be used to advantage by an empathetic practitioner or radiographic technician to help introduce the child to radiography. Cooperation, as evidenced by a desire to help, can be utilized to obtain the necessary radiographs.

The initial introduction of the child to the radiographic procedure often determines subsequent cooperation. Terms such as "camera," "elephant's trunk," and "nose," are sometimes used to describe the x-ray tube head to young children. Some tube heads have even been characterized (Fig. 4–1). The child can examine the film packet with his or her fingers as the practitioner explains, simply and sincerely, that it contains film "like in a camera." The use of soft, vinyl-wrapped packets with gently rolled edges can minimize any discomfort. Prior to the film packet being placed in the mouth, the child's head position and the tube head angulation should be such that the time the patient has to tolerate the pack is minimized. If the child's attention is fixed on some object in the room, it will help minimize the "drift" of the head as the operator leaves the room to activate the timer.

Praise for the child who masters the techniques involved in obtaining a radiographic survey will generally enhance the desire to be of further assistance. The survey should begin with the easiest view (the maxillary anterior occlusal view) to demonstrate the technique and to gain the child's confidence.

Handicapped children present special problems, since in many cases they are unable to cooperate. In such instances, it is desirable to use the assistance of someone who is not regularly exposed to x-rays to help with the positioning and stabilization. This individual should be protected from radiation exposure by means of a lead apron and lead gloves (see Figures 4–2 and 4–3).

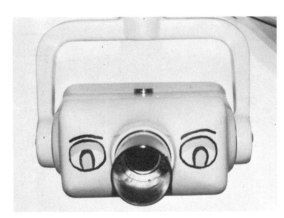

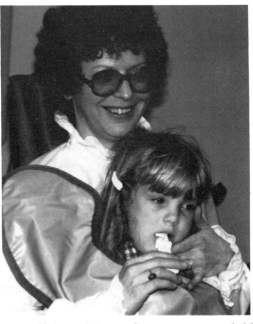

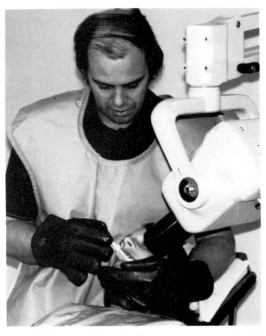

Figure 4–1 Characterized x-ray tube head.

Figure 4–2 Mother assisting child with film packet. A single lead apron protects both child and adult.

Figure 4–3 Father assisting child with film packet. The father is wearing lead gloves, and both the father and the daughter are wearing protective lead aprons. Holding the child's head against the parent's body helps to control undesirable movements.

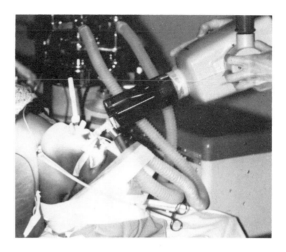

Figure 4–4 Obtaining radiographs in the operating room. When the patient is under general anesthesia, one means of holding the film in the proper position is with surgical tubing to support the mandible and occlude the teeth.

Radiographic Surveys

Individual discretion should be used in both the frequency of radiographic surveys and the number of films taken per survey. Even though there are suggested film surveys for different stages of development, it may not be practical — or desirable — to attempt all views in the survey at any one time. A combination of extraoral and selected intraoral radiographs may be a better alternative to traditional full mouth surveys in some patients (see Figure 4–5).

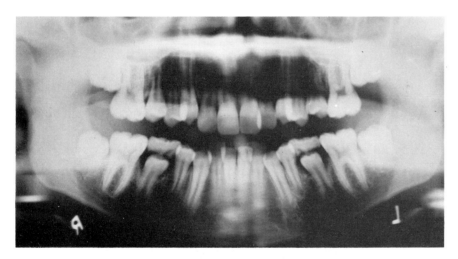

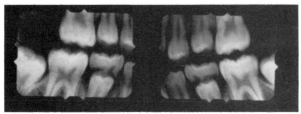

Figure 4–5 Panoramic film and bitewing radiographs. See Table 4–1 for comparative radiation dosages.

I. INTRAORAL RADIOGRAPHY

Intraoral radiographs are a necessity in caries detection and in the assessment of periodontal problems, as well as in the determination of tooth size for arch length analysis. The universal considerations in taking dental radiographs are as follows:

1. The child's body must be protected from radiation by means of a lead apron.

2. The horizontal plane as determined by the eyes should be parallel to the floor.

3. The film should closely approximate the tissue being examined.

4. In periapical views, the film should not project more than ¼ inch beyond the occlusal surface of the teeth.

5. The use of suggested preset angulations of the tube head will assist in obtaining diagnostically acceptable radiographs.

Figures 4–6 to 4–8 show suggested intraoral full mouth surveys for the primary, mixed, and young permanent dentition.

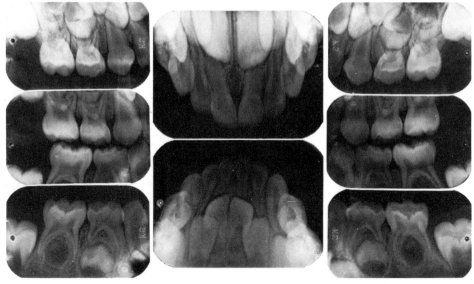

Figure 4–6 PRIMARY DENTITION. This survey should be performed prior to the eruption of any permanent teeth. (Courtesy of Dr. David B. Kennedy.)

I. INTRAORAL RADIOGRAPHY *Continued*

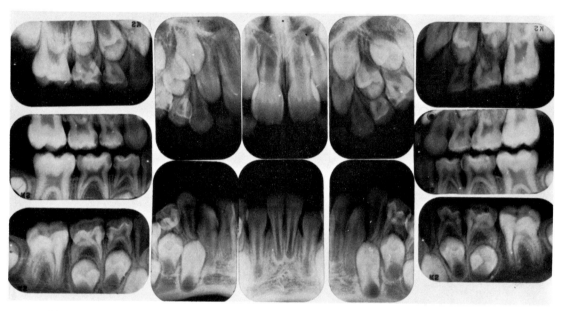

Figure 4–7 MIXED DENTITION. Adult-sized films are preferred for the posterior exposures. This survey is useful in determining the orthodontic spatial requirement.

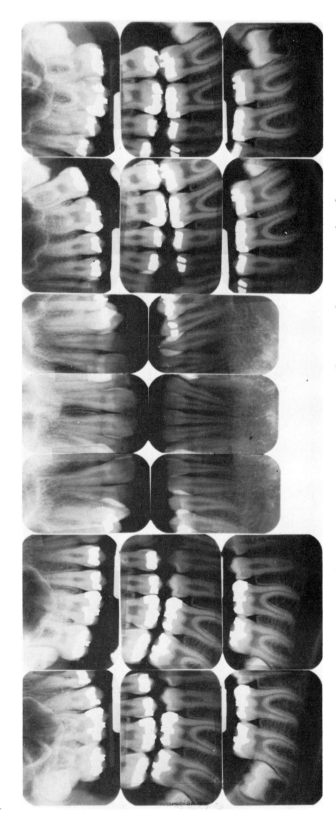

Figure 4–8 YOUNG PERMANENT. Evaluations of interproximal and occlusal relationships as well as periodontal status are visualized best from this survey.

I. INTRAORAL RADIOGRAPHY *Continued*

Figure 4–9 *Maxillary Occlusal View (+60°).* The film is placed between the maxillary and mandibular incisors and is held flat on the occlusal plane with a *gentle* biting pressure. The center of the film coincides with the midline of the incisors. In children, *after* eruption of the permanent central incisors, the film should be placed with its long axis in an anteroposterior direction.

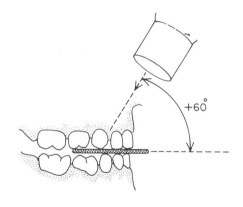

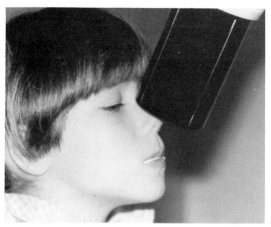

Figure 4–10 Angulation of cone in relation to patient and film for maxillary occlusal exposure.

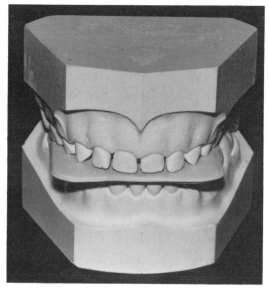

Figure 4–11 Placement of film for maxillary occlusal exposure.

Figure 4–12 Resulting radiograph of maxillary occlusal exposure.

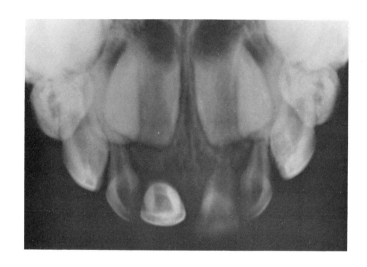

I. INTRAORAL RADIOGRAPHY *Continued*

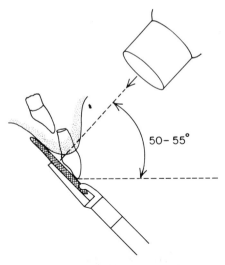

50-55°

Figure 4–13 *Maxillary Anterior Periapical View (+50 to 55°).* A film holder may be used for this view. The long axis of the film should be parallel to the incisors.

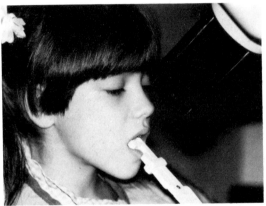

Figure 4–14 Angulation of cone in relation to patient and film for exposure of maxillary central and lateral incisors.

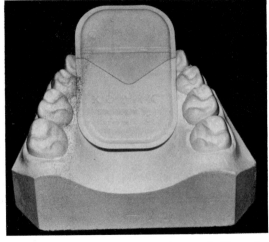

Figure 4–15 Placement of film for exposure of maxillary central and lateral incisors.

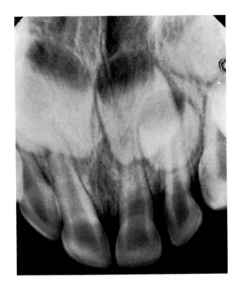

Figure 4–16 Resulting radiograph of maxillary central and lateral incisors.

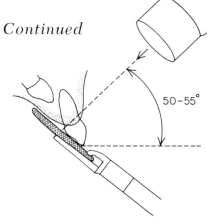

Figure 4–17 *Maxillary Canine (+50 to 55°).* A film holder may be used for this view. The long axis of the film should be placed parallel to the long axis of the upper canine tooth. The anterior margin of the film should not project beyond the mesial surface of the lateral incisor, which is included in this view.

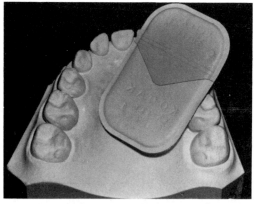

Figure 4–19 Placement of film for exposure of maxillary cuspid area.

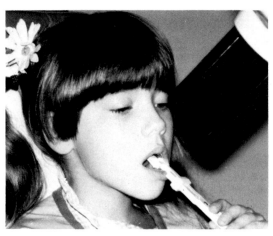

Figure 4–18 Angulation of cone in relation to patient and film for exposure of maxillary cuspid area.

Figure 4–20 Resulting radiograph of maxillary cuspid area.

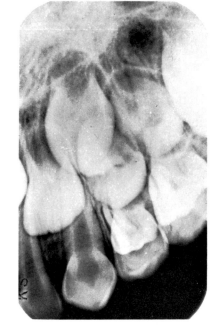

I.   INTRAORAL RADIOGRAPHY *Continued*

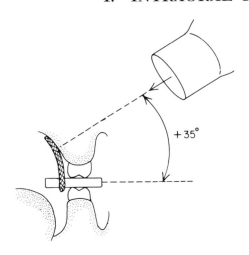

Figure 4-21 *Maxillary Molar Apical View* *(+35°)*. The film holder is used and is held with a gentle biting pressure by the molar teeth. The film should not project beyond the mesial surface of the canine tooth.

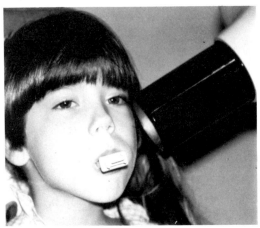

Figure 4-22 Angulation of cone in relation to patient and film for exposure of maxillary posterior area.

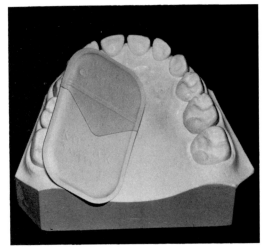

Figure 4-23 Placement of film for exposure of maxillary posterior area.

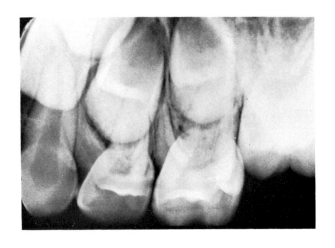

Figure 4-24 Resulting radiograph of maxillary posterior area.

I. INTRAORAL RADIOGRAPHY *Continued*

Figure 4-25 *Mandibular Occlusal View* (−55°). The x-ray tube is positioned at an angle of −55° to the plane of the film. (This is the only view in which the occlusal plane is not parallel to the floor.) The film should be held with only a *gentle* biting pressure.

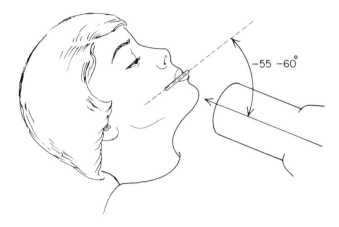

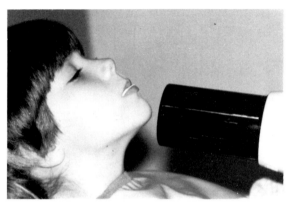

Figure 4-26 Angulation of cone in relation to patient and film for mandibular occlusal exposure. The vertical cone angulation for this exposure is dependent upon how far back the patient's head is tipped.

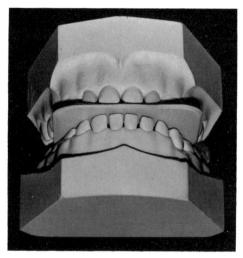

Figure 4-27 Placement of film for mandibular occlusal exposure.

Figure 4-28 Resulting radiograph of mandibular occlusal exposure.

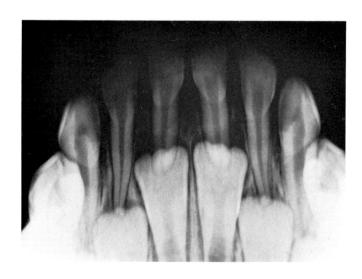

I. INTRAORAL RADIOGRAPHY *Continued*

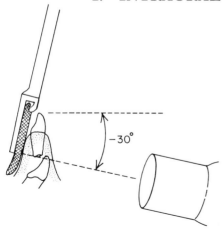

Figure 4–29 *Mandibular Incisor — Periapical View (−30°).*   The film holder may be used for this view. The patient should bite lightly on the ribbed bite plane of the holder while holding the end and exerting slight pressure toward the face.

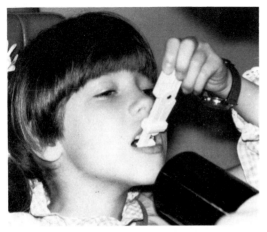

Figure 4–30 Angulation of cone in relation to patient and film for exposure of mandibular central and lateral incisors.

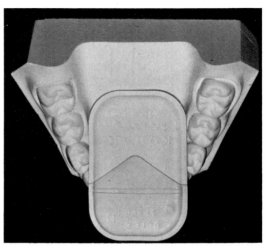

Figure 4–31 Placement of film for exposure of mandibular central and lateral incisors.

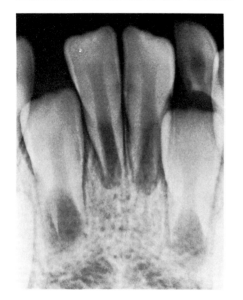

Figure 4–32 Resulting radiograph of mandibular central and lateral incisors.

I. INTRAORAL RADIOGRAPHY *Continued*

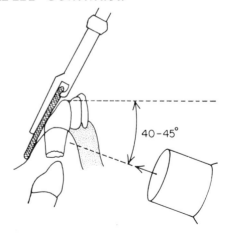

Figure 4–33 *Mandibular Canine (40 to 45°).* The film holder may be used for this view. The long axis of the film should be placed parallel to the long axis of the lower canine tooth. The lateral incisor is included in this view.

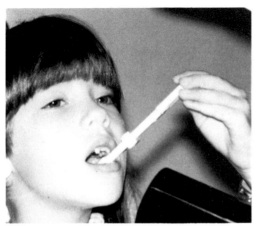

Figure 4–34 Angulation of cone in relation to patient and film for exposure of mandibular cuspid area.

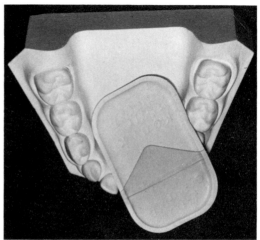

Figure 4–35 Placement of film for exposure of mandibular cuspid area.

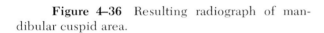

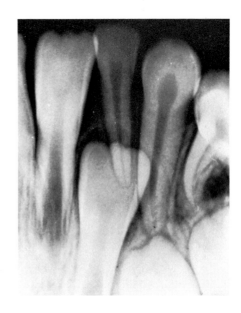

Figure 4–36 Resulting radiograph of mandibular cuspid area.

I. INTRAORAL RADIOGRAPHY *Continued*

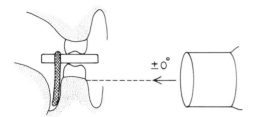

Figure 4–37 *Mandibular Molar Apical View (O°).* The film holder is used and is held by a firm biting pressure from the molar teeth. The film should not project beyond the mesial surface of the canine tooth.

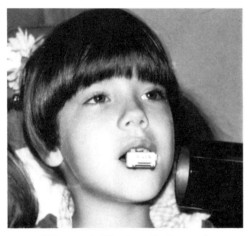

Figure 4–38 Angulation of cone in relation to patient and film for exposure of mandibular posterior area.

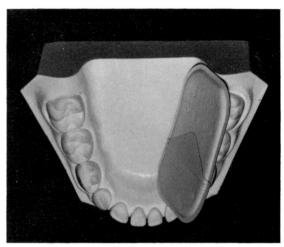

Figure 4–39 Placement of film for exposure of mandibular posterior area.

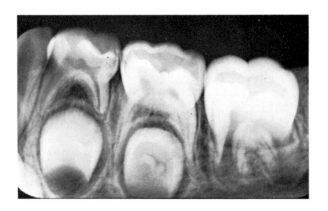

Figure 4–40 Resulting radiograph of mandibular posterior area.

I. INTRAORAL RADIOGRAPHY *Continued*

Figure 4–41 *Molar   Bitewing   View (+10°).* The film is held as close as possible to the lingual surfaces of the teeth and is held with a firm biting pressure on the bitewing loop tab. The cone should be directed through the contact of the first and second primary molars. The distal surface of the canine tooth is included in this view.

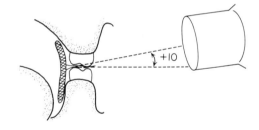

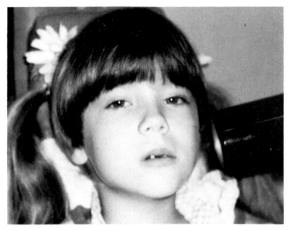

Figure 4–42 Angulation of cone in relation to patient and film for posterior bitewing exposure.

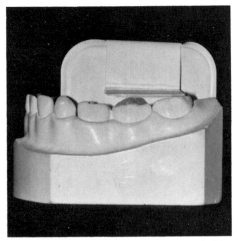

Figure 4–43 Placement of film for posterior bitewing exposure.

Figure 4–44 Resulting   radiograph of posterior bitewing exposure.

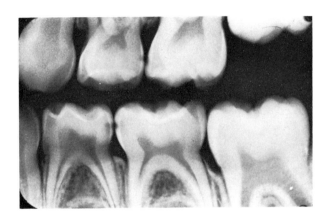

I. INTRAORAL RADIOGRAPHY *Continued*

Common Errors

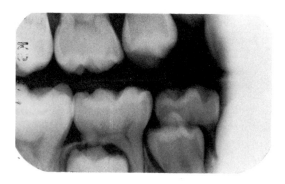

Figure 4–45 *Part of Film Not Exposed (Clear Area).* This is caused by cone cutting — this portion of the film was not in the x-ray beam. Care should be taken to center the cone in the middle of the film pack.

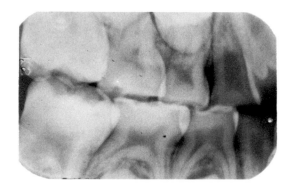

Figure 4–46 *Overlapping of Tooth Contact Areas.* This is caused by an improper horizontal angle of tube. The central ray should be directed through the appropriate contact area.

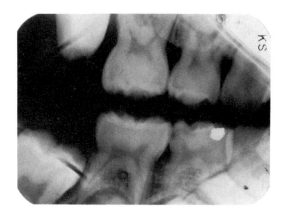

Figure 4–47 *Black Lines on Exposed Film.* Creasing the film causes damage to the emulsion coating. Corners should be rolled, not sharply creased.

I. INTRAORAL RADIOGRAPHY *Continued*

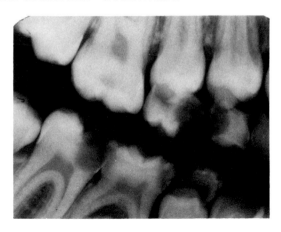

Figure 4–48 *Tipped Bitewing Film.* This is caused by the teeth not being closed firmly on the bitewing tab or by the film not being drawn tightly to the lingual surface of the teeth.

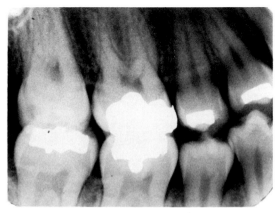

Figure 4–49 *Occlusal Plane Not Centered on Film.* This is caused by the bitewing tab not being centered on the film.

II. EXTRAORAL RADIOGRAPHY

LATERAL JAW RADIOGRAPH

This radiograph is very useful in evaluating osseous structures as well as erupted and unerupted teeth in the posterior dental arch.

Figure 4–50 Diagrammatic sketch of patient illustrating placement of film and horizontal cone angulation for a lateral jaw radiograph. (From O'Brien, R.C.: *Dental Radiography:* An Introduction for Dental Hygienists and Assistants, 3rd ed., W. B. Saunders Co., Philadelphia, 1977, p. 141.

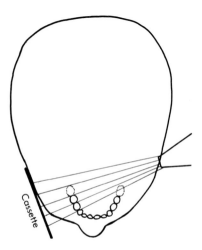

II. **EXTRAORAL RADIOGRAPHY** *Continued*

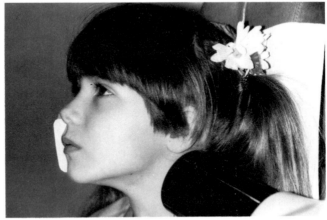

Figure 4–51   Position of the patient, film, and cone for a lateral jaw radiograph. The central ray should pass 1 cm below and 1 cm posterior to the angle of the mandible. Note that in the young patient, this exposure may be made on an occlusal film packet attached to the face with tape.

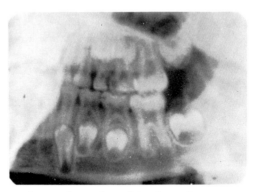

Figure 4–52   Radiograph produced by lateral jaw exposure. (From O'Brien, R. C., *Dental Radiography*, 2nd ed., W. B. Saunders Co., Philadelphia, 1966, p. 104.)

III.   PANORAMIC RADIOGRAPHY

Panoramic radiography is widely used in pedodontic practices today. The technique offers the ability to evaluate radiographically those orofacial structures outside the range of intraoral periapical films. Panoramic radiographs are especially valuable in detecting anomalies of tooth development, eruption, and fractures of osseous structures, and in assessment of postsurgical or post-traumatic healing. They do not replace intraoral radiographs for caries detection or arch length analysis. As a new patient screening procedure, this type of radiography requires less exposure to radiation for the patient than does a conventional full mouth series (see Table 4–1).

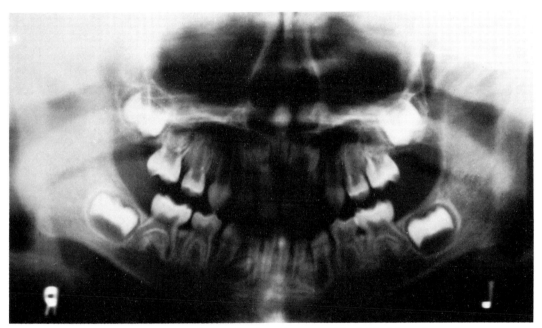

Figure 4–53   Panoramic radiograph of a 2½-year-old child. Note the value of this type of x-ray in assessing the multiple missing teeth. (Courtesy Dr. Douglas J. Fogle.)

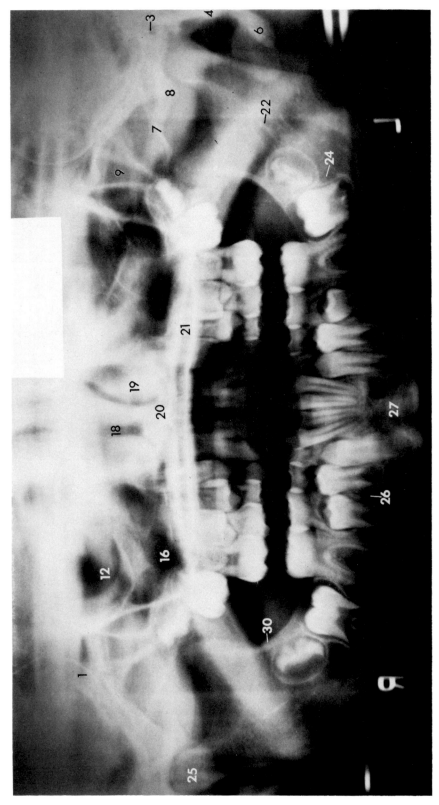

Figure 4–54 Panoramic radiograph. (See Figure 4–55 for designation of each numbered landmark.)

III. PANORAMIC RADIOGRAPHY *Continued*

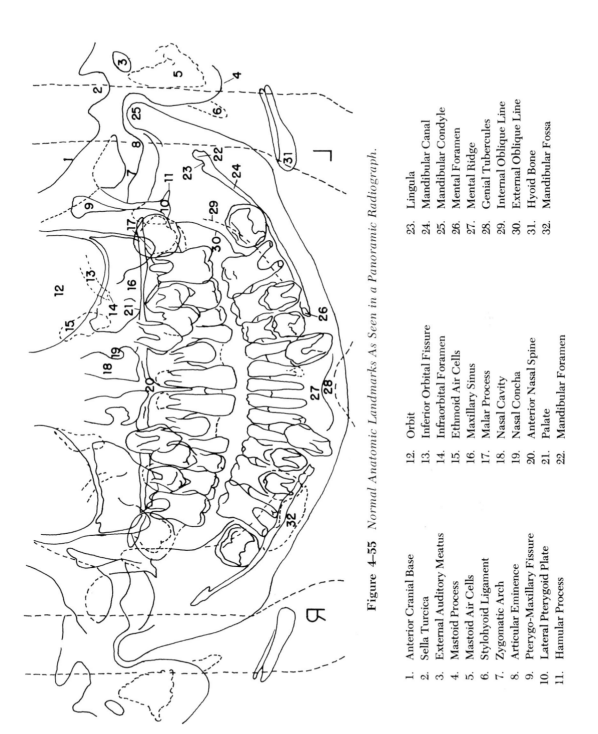

Figure 4-55 *Normal Anatomic Landmarks As Seen in a Panoramic Radiograph.*

1. Anterior Cranial Base
2. Sella Turcica
3. External Auditory Meatus
4. Mastoid Process
5. Mastoid Air Cells
6. Stylohyoid Ligament
7. Zygomatic Arch
8. Articular Eminence
9. Pterygo-Maxillary Fissure
10. Lateral Pterygoid Plate
11. Hamular Process
12. Orbit
13. Inferior Orbital Fissure
14. Infraorbital Foramen
15. Ethmoid Air Cells
16. Maxillary Sinus
17. Malar Process
18. Nasal Cavity
19. Nasal Concha
20. Anterior Nasal Spine
21. Palate
22. Mandibular Foramen
23. Lingula
24. Mandibular Canal
25. Mandibular Condyle
26. Mental Foramen
27. Mental Ridge
28. Genial Tubercules
29. Internal Oblique Line
30. External Oblique Line
31. Hyoid Bone
32. Mandibular Fossa

III. PANORAMIC RADIOGRAPHY *Continued*

There are currently three major types of panoramic radiography machines available. Variation among these three types is related to the number of centers of rotation of the radiation source.

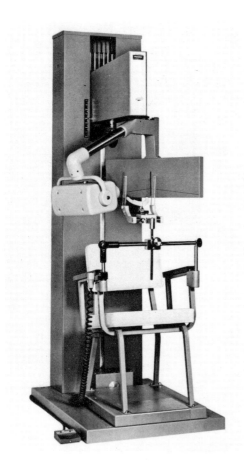

Figure 4-56 The S. S. White Panorex is a system that uses two pivotal points for the radiation source.

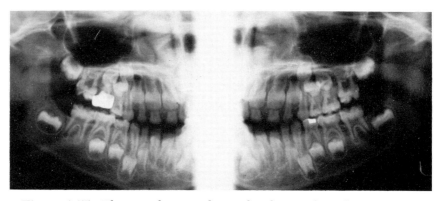

Figure 4-57 The resulting radiograph shows the characteristic "white band" in the spinal column area. (X-ray courtesy S. S. White.)

III.   PANORAMIC RADIOGRAPHY *Continued*

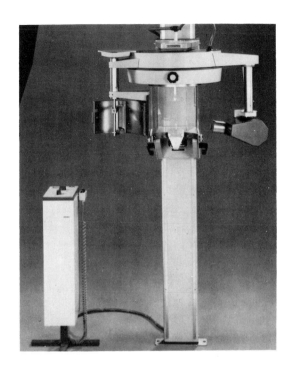

Figure 4–58 The Siemens Orthopantomograph uses three pivotal points for the radiation source.

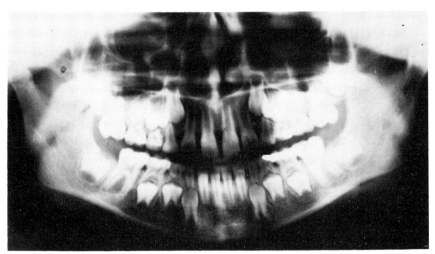

Figure 4–59 A typical patient's dentition as shown by the Orthopantomograph. (X-ray courtesy Siemans.)

III. PANORAMIC RADIOGRAPHY *Continued*

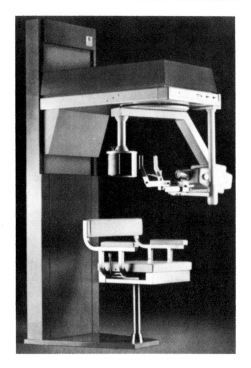

Figure 4–60 The General Electric Panelipse uses an adjustable elliptical arc of rotation for the radiation source.

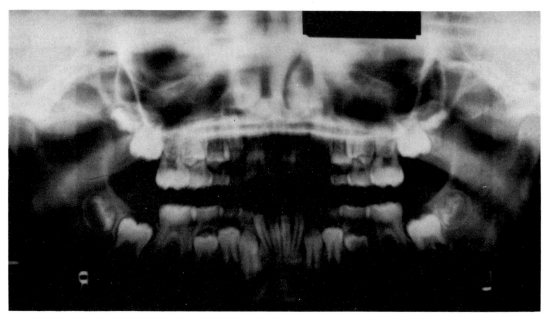

Figure 4–61 A mixed dentition as shown by the Panelipse.

III. PANORAMIC RADIOGRAPHY *Continued*

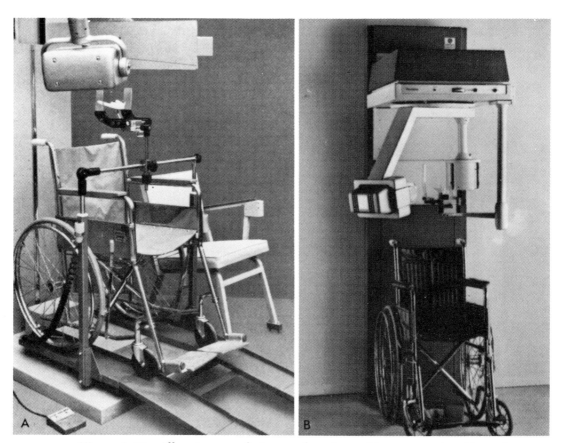

Figure 4–62 All major manufacturers of equipment for panoramic radiography offer provisions to accommodate patients confined to wheelchairs.

III. PANORAMIC RADIOGRAPHY *Continued*

SOME ANOMALIES DEMONSTRATED BY PANORAMIC RADIOGRAPHY

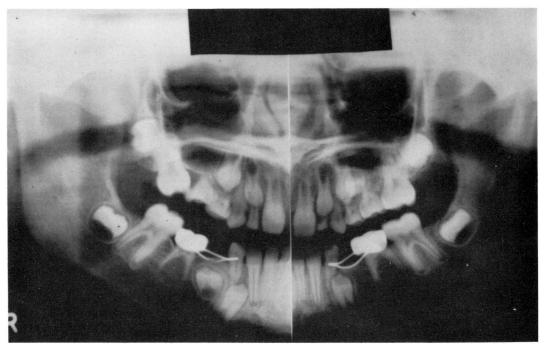

Figure 4–63   Ectopic eruption of maxillary right first permanent molar.

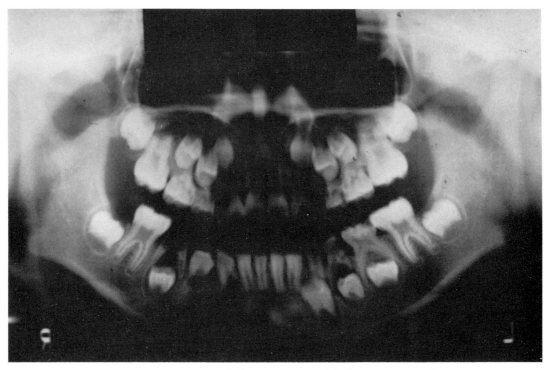

Figure 4–64   Periapical abscess on mandibular primary molar.

III. PANORAMIC RADIOGRAPHY *Continued*

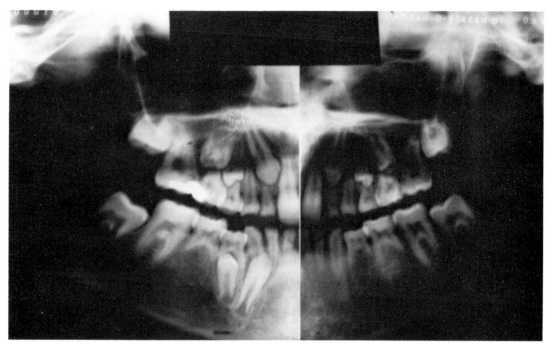

Figure 4–65 Oligodontia (partial anodontia). Patient underwent extensive orthodontic and restorative treatment in later years.

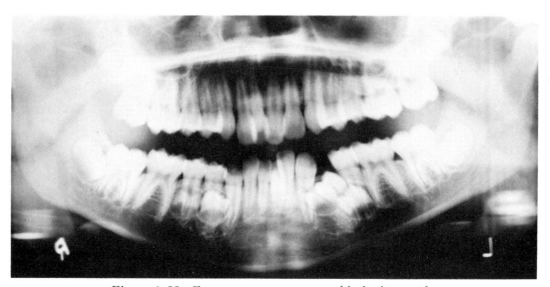

Figure 4–66 Four supernumerary mandibular bicuspids.

III. PANORAMIC RADIOGRAPHY *Continued*

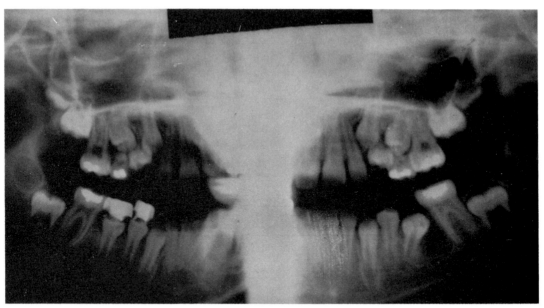

Figure 4–67   Dentigenous cyst in mandibular left quadrant was not revealed by routine bitewing film.

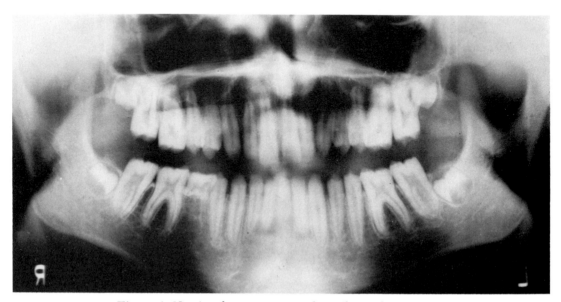

Figure 4–68   Amelogenesis imperfecta (hypoplastic type).

III. PANORAMIC RADIOGRAPHY *Continued*

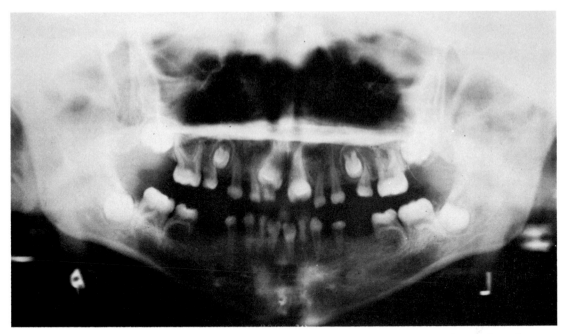

Figure 4–69 Patient with ectodermal dysplasia showing malformed and missing teeth.

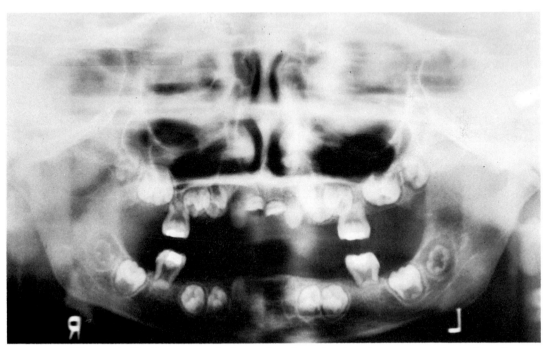

Figure 4–70 Patient with hypophosphatasia showing noneruption of teeth and dental malformations.

IV. CEPHALOMETRIC RADIOGRAPHY

Cephalometrics is the process of exposure and interpretation of oriented lateral and posteroanterior skull radiographs. Interpretation of cephalometric radiographs provides information on the relative contribution of underlying skeletal structures to malocclusion. This information is vital in orthodontics, longitudinal growth studies, and craniofacial surgery.

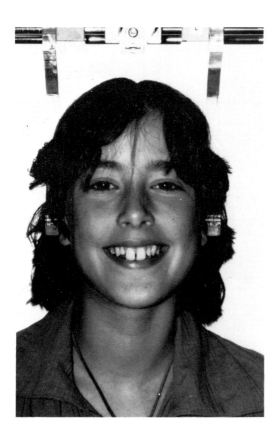

Figure 4–71   Anterior view of patient in position for lateral cephalometric radiograph.

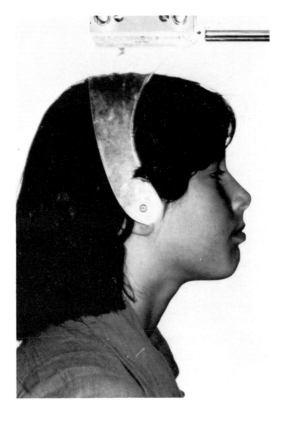

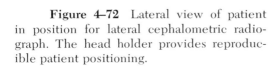

Figure 4–72 Lateral view of patient in position for lateral cephalometric radiograph. The head holder provides reproducible patient positioning.

IV.   CEPHALOMETRIC RADIOGRAPHY *Continued*

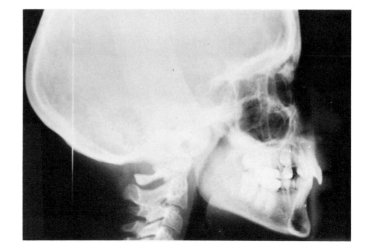

Figure 4–73 Resulting lateral cephalometric radiograph.

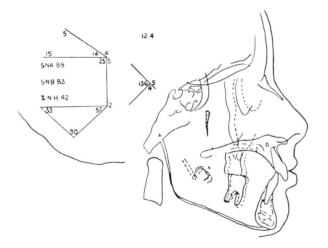

Figure 4–74 Tracing of lateral cephalometric radiograph. Angles marked on the left denote the skeletal and/or dental contribution to a malocclusion.

Figure 4–75 Serial cephalometric tracings may be superimposed on relatively stable planes to provide valuable information on the direction, amount, and timing of craniofacial growth. The technique illustrated shows an overall superimposition plus individual superimpositions of the maxilla and mandible.

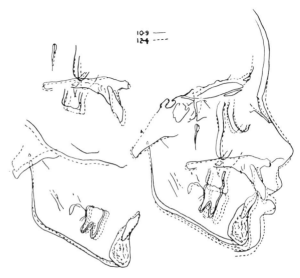

Radiation Hygiene

It is imperative that all personnel operating radiographic equipment be both well informed on the hazards of radiation and adequately protected from exposure. Proper equipment and techniques, in conjunction with correct shielding, will protect patients. All radiographic exposures should be made only when the patient is wearing a lead apron. The responsibility lies with the dental practitioner to minimize the number of radiographic views taken; only those necessary to yield the required diagnostic information should be considered.

The tubehead of the intraoral machine must be equipped with an aluminum disc filtration, which absorbs the biologically destructive long wavelength rays. A lead collimator should restrict the beam to the minimum area needed for diagnostic exposure.

Current research is being conducted on beam collimation of panoramic radiography machines. Restriction of radiation to the maxilla and mandible will result in less exposure to structures that are not of primary diagnostic interest. With the increased concern about radiation exposure to nondental structures, some sources recommend that patients wear a thyroid shielding collar in addition to the lead apron when undergoing any dental radiographic examination.

Radiation monitoring badges should be worn by all dental office personnel. All control units should be protected with lead shielding and should be located a minimum of 6 feet from the radiation source. Recommendations on adequate filtration of units and protective structures in the office vary from state to state. Both the local radiographic equipment dealer and the state radiation protection agency should be consulted prior to the installation or relocation of radiographic equipment.

TABLE 4-1 REFERENCE CHART SHOWING RADIATION EXPOSURES

The values given in this table indicate relative radiation exposure for each type of survey; some variation from these values may be expected in specific machines' output.

Site Exposures Reported in Mrad° per Radiograph
(from Manson-Hing[2])

	PANOREX	PANELIPSE	ORTHOPANTOMOGRAPH
Eye	2.8–27	9	8.1–50
Thyroid	5–37	6.4	9.9
Gonads	.01–.48	–	.03–.21
Parotid gland	12.7–485	17	118
Sella turcica	6.7–100	10	23

Mean Bone Marrow Dose (Mrem°) by Site in Mandible (from White and Rose[4])

SITE	PAN-OREX	PAN-ELIPSE	ORTHOPAN-TOMOGRAPH	INTRA-ORAL†	COLLIMATED INTRAORAL†	LATERAL CEPHALO-METRIC
Right third molar	22.00	56.3	29.9	510	183	33.80
Right first molar	12.10	17.5	26.7	821	261	25.60
Right first premolar	9.02	16.7	20.2	1143	326	29.00
Symphysis	8.71	16.0	19.3	988	422	17.70
Left first premolar	9.13	20.1	18.2	1080	299	9.84
Left first molar	13.20	25.2	22.0	826	284	7.74
Left third molar	24.80	71.0	30.9	580	192	7.57
Mean	14.10	31.8	23.9	850	282	18.80

Exposure Range in Milliroentgens° per Bitewing Radiograph
(Adapted from Alcox and Jameson[5])

	50 kVp	70 kVp	90 kVp
Target film distance	8″	16″	16″
Child‡	80–84	51.1–52.2	34.7–47.2

° For dental x-rays, the terms millirad, millirem, and milliroentgen are essentially synonymous.

† Intraoral series of 21 films (17 periapicals and 4 bitewings) 80 kVp, 15 mA, with 24 impulses (2/5 sec) for the anteriors and 30 impulses (½ sec) for the posterior exposures.

‡ Calculated as two-thirds of the adult exposure.

REFERENCES

1. X-rays in Dentistry: Eastman Kodak Company, Radiography Markets Division, Rochester, New York, 1977.
2. Manson-Hing, L. R.: Panoramic Dental Radiography, Charles C Thomas, Springfield, Illinois, 1976.
3. O'Brien, R. C.: Dental Radiography, 3rd ed., W. B. Saunders Co., Philadelphia, 1977.
4. White, S. C., and Rose, T. C.: Absorbed bone marrow dose in certain dental radiographic techniques. J.A.D.A., 98: 553–558, April, 1979.
5. Alcox, R. W., and Jameson, W. R.: Patient exposure from intraoral radiographic examination. J.A.D.A. 98: 568–579, May, 1979.
6. Simpson, W. J., MacRae, P., and Simons, A.: A University of Alberta Pedodontic Technique Manual, 1978.

CARIES PREVENTION

Chapter 5 _____

Caries control is an essential part of the practice of preventive dentistry for children. It is especially important that dentists keep abreast of scientific advances in this area if they are to offer the best service to their patients. Research has reinforced certain observations about the role of sugars, particularly sucrose, in the production of carious lesions. The utmost effort should therefore be made to educate parents and children on the need for the children to curtail their consumption of food with high sugar content, particularly cookies, candy, jams, jellies, and other adhesive carbohydrates. Frequency of eating can be a decisive factor in rampant caries, as can the habit of eating before bedtime.

The importance of the dental plaque in the caries process has likewise received renewed attention. Oral hygiene procedures correctly taught and practiced after mealtime can help to reduce plaque accumulation on accessible surfaces.

The use of fluoride probably represents the most promising approach to caries control when incorporated in a program that also includes sugar restriction and emphasis on oral hygiene. Community water fluoridation is the most effective means of providing for fluoride ingestion during the formative years. If it is not available, the dentist should prescribe a daily dietary supplement of fluoride. Systemic ingestion of fluoride results in incorporation of the ion in enamel and dentin. This leads to the formation of a more stable crystal that is more resistant to demineralization. It is recommended that all children, whether or not they are ingesting fluoride, should have twice yearly topical treatments. (Fluoride at a concentration of one part per million in drinking water does not saturate the outer enamel layer; the topical treatments provide a desirable supplementation.) Stannous or acidulated fluoride may be used depending upon the preference of the dentist.

Oral rinses of fluoride affect the plaque primarily and must be continued to be of significant benefit. The action of fluorides on plaque metabolism is not clear, although there is some evidence that they may inhibit polysaccharide formation. Epidemiological studies conclusively demonstrate that all fluorides are more effective in reducing smooth surface caries than in inhibiting pits and fissure lesions.

Water Fluoridation

The presence of fluoride in the water supply during and after the development of the dentition favors the formation of teeth more resistant to dental caries. Lifelong residents of communities whose water supply contains 1 ppm of fluoride ion have incorporated fluoride into the apatite structure of the teeth during the calcification period, the pre-eruptive period, and the post-eruptive period. Overall reduction of caries by 50 to 60 per cent has been demonstrated in a number of long-term investigations in the United States, Canada, and other countries. Anterior teeth are protected to a greater degree than posterior teeth. Benefits accrue both to the deciduous dentition and to the permanent teeth.

Dietary Supplements of Fluoride

In communities not served with fluoridated water, caries prevention is in part a matter of how dedicated parents and children are to the use of daily supplements of fluoride ion prescribed by the dentist. With sufficient individual cooperation, benefits comparable to those cited above can be expected (to some extent, it is the fact that no such cooperation is needed in community fluoridation programs that accounts for their success). Fluoride is available in liquid form, tablets, and chewable lozenges, and is an added ingredient in some vitamin preparations. Dosage must be adjusted to the age and approximate body weight of the infant or child to prevent excessive intake and enamel mottling.

It should be pointed out that in some communities fluoride may be present in the water in amounts below 1 ppm. This can be verified by the local water department or, in the case of well water sources, by water analysis. When community water is found low in fluoride (<1 ppm), the prescription for fluoride should be adjusted accordingly (see Table 5–1).

If there is *no* fluoride in the water, the following dosages are suggested:

birth to 2 years of age: Prescribe 0.25 mg fluoride daily. This can be added in the form of drops to fluids that the infant consumes or may be placed directly on the tongue.

2 to 3 years of age: Prescribe 0.5 mg fluoride daily.

3 years of age and older: Prescribe 1.0 mg fluoride daily.
(on through time of
eruption of permanent
teeth)

For children over 3 years of age, fluoride lozenges are highly recommended as an alternative to drops. Chewing these tablets raises the saliva's fluoride concentration. With fluoride present and perhaps able to permeate the plaque, a benefit in addition to the desired systemic effect is possible.

TABLE 5–1   ADMINISTRATION OF FLUORIDE SUPPLEMENTS °

Proper daily allowance of fluoride ion for a child 3 years or over. Reduce these amounts by one-half for children 2 to 3 years old. For children under 2 years of age, use prepared bottled water, 1 ppm fluoride concentration, in formula and food preparation.

| FLUORIDE IN H_2O | ADJUSTED ALLOWANCE | |
| | Sodium Fluoride | Provides Fluoride Ion |
ppm	mg per day	mg per day
0.0	2.2	1.0
0.2	1.8	0.8
0.4	1.3	0.6
0.6	0.9	0.4

°From *Accepted Dental Remedies*, 37th ed., American Dental Association, Chicago, January, 1977, p. 294.

Topical Application of Fluorides

A number of studies have demonstrated that the topical application of fluoride solutions to freshly cleaned teeth results in caries reduction in children. Semi-annual topical applications of fluoride solutions, studied in communities not served by fluoridated water, provide children with reported caries reductions of 30 to 40 per cent. The topical application of acid phosphate fluoride solutions once a year for three years, studied in a city *with* fluoridated water, provides children with a reported 20 per cent reduction in caries. In addition, findings in one study point to a significant increase in fluoride concentration in comparable enamel layers of both deciduous and permanent teeth in children who have consumed fluoridated water and have also had a topical acid phosphate gel treatment. Although the mechanism of action of topical fluorides is considered similar to that of ingested fluoride, it is also thought that topically applied fluorides permeate the plaque to some extent and possibly exert some inhibiting effect.

Three topical fluoride solutions have been extensively investigated: 2 per cent aqueous sodium fluoride, 8 per cent stannous fluoride, and acidulated phosphate fluoride. The latter two preparations have been demonstrated to be superior to aqueous sodium fluoride, probably because of their low pH, which favors a greater fluoride reaction on the apatite crystal. Topical fluorides should be applied semi-annually on a professional basis.

Fluoride Rinses

Studies have shown an increased resistance to caries in persons using neutral sodium fluoride mouth rinses, whether the program they have followed is one of rinsing with 0.2 per cent neutral sodium fluoride once every two weeks or one of rinsing daily with 0.05 per cent neutral sodium fluoride. Fluoride is accumulated in the plaque as a result of fluoride rinses, and probably is bound to precipitated calcium phosphate. Clinical studies demonstrating caries reductions of 25 to 37 per cent when sodium fluoride rinses have been used over several years indicate that continuing usage is necessary for rinses to have an optimal effect on caries activity. Since rinsing depends upon patient cooperation, it has been found most effective where carried out under supervision, such as in a school or institution.

Fluoride Dentifrices

Dentifrices containing sodium fluoride, stannous fluoride, and sodium monofluorophosphate have been tested for their caries-reducing properties and have been found effective when used daily under supervised or unsupervised conditions. The amount of caries reduction recorded varies from 10 to 40 per cent. Since most people use a dentifrice of some kind in daily oral hygiene practices, it would seem obvious to encourage the use of a fluoride-type formulation.

Fluoride Varnishes

There is growing evidence to support the conclusion that effective caries inhibition can be obtained through professional application of fluoride-containing varnishes to the accessible surfaces of the teeth. The slow release of fluoride ion by the varnishes offers a means of greatly increasing the fluoride concentration of the external enamel surface.

Text continued on page 156

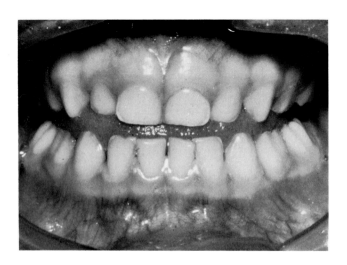

Figure 5–1 A caries-free mouth in the primary dentition. This is the goal of an adequate program of prevention started in the first year of life.

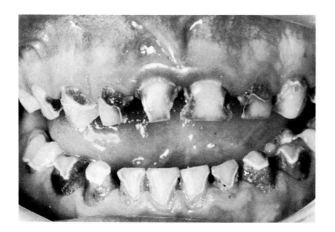

Figure 5–2 Rampant caries in the primary dentition. This condition has resulted from a combination of factors, including a high sugar diet, lack of oral hygiene, and lack of professional care and supervision

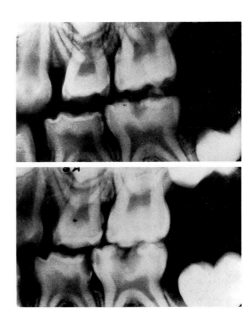

Figure 5–3 Radiographs showing 1 year's progress of carious lesions in a preschool child. Periodic recalls are essential if the child is to be kept free of serious dental problems.

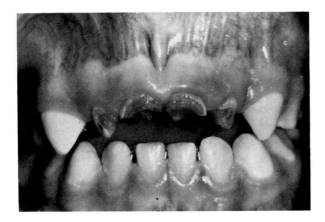

Figure 5–4 Anterior primary incisors involved with extensive carious lesions, sometimes called "baby bottle syndrome." In this case the maxillary cuspids are not affected because the bottle was discontinued just prior to their eruption. Parents should be counseled on the need to avoid adding sweet jucies or other sugar-containing substances to the baby's nursing bottle.

Figure 5–5 Gingival caries in the primary molars. Adequate brushing after meals will materially aid in preventing caries in such accesible areas.

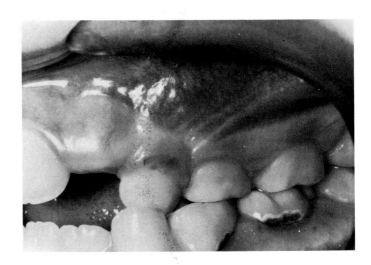

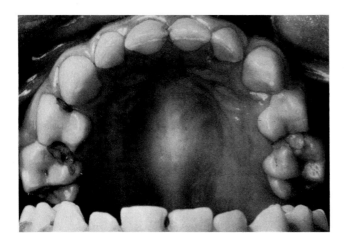

Figure 5–6 Interproximal carious lesions in the maxillary primary molars. These lesions should have been detected in the early stages of the disease and restorations placed to prevent further tooth destruction.

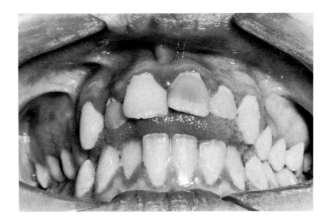

Figure 5–7 Anterior view of a teenager with poor oral hygiene practices. Note debris around gingiva of maxillary incisors permitting the formation of a bacterial plaque.

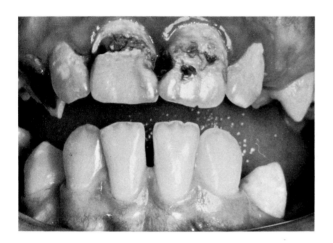

Figure 5–8 Anterior view of a teenager who neglected oral hygiene and consumed large quantities of highly cariogenic foods. Carious lesions are evident in areas easily accessible to the toothbrush.

Figure 5–9 Interproximal caries in lower permanent incisors in a 9-year-old boy. These teeth are the least susceptible to caries. In such a case the child should be placed on a stringent program of oral hygiene, sugar restriction, and fluoride therapy.

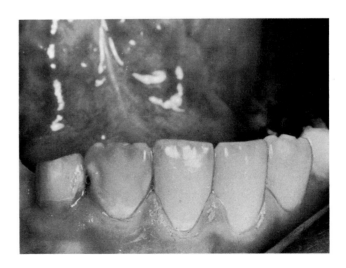

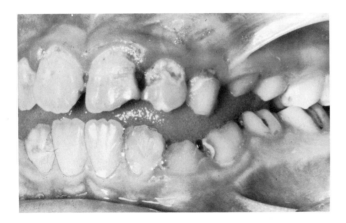

Figure 5–10 An open bite prevented this child from getting the benefit of masticatory scouring action on the left side. Increased susceptibility to caries resulted. Careful brushing of these areas is necessary.

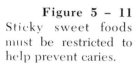

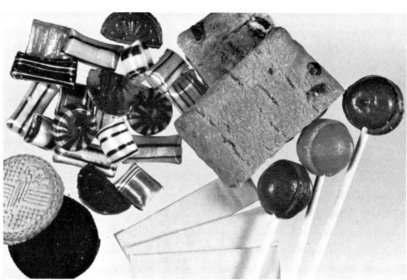

Figure 5 – 11 Sticky sweet foods must be restricted to help prevent caries.

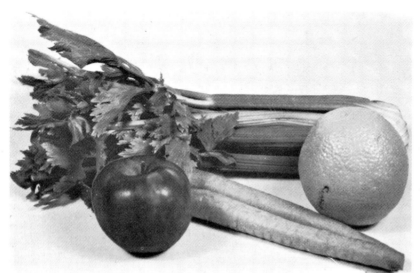

Figure 5 – 12 Raw vegetables and fresh fruits are acceptable substitutes for sweets and have considerable cleansing action as well.

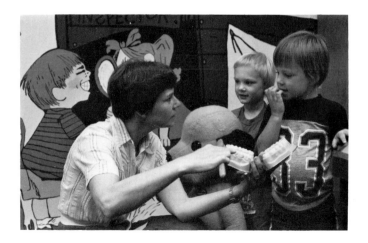

Figure 5–13 Demonstration of tooth-brushing using large models. Note initial apprehension of children.

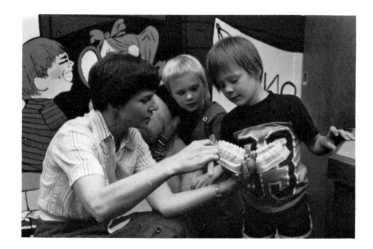

Figure 5–14 Demonstration continued. Note that children are now more interested in procedures.

Figure 5–15 After demonstration, child is now participating in procedure.

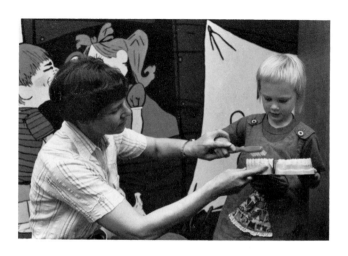

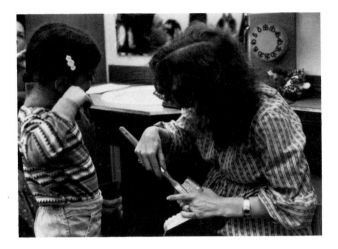

Figure 5–16 Child brushing while dental auxiliary is demonstrating proper technique.

Figure 5–17 Dental auxiliary observes and coaches child on proper tooth-brushing as mother observes.

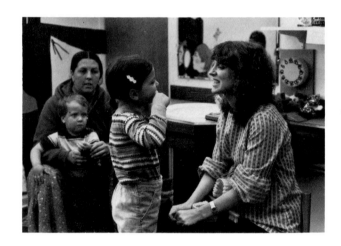

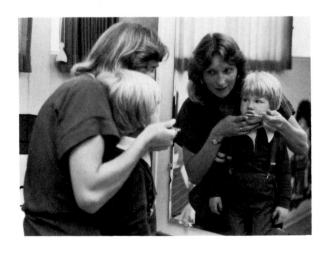

Figure 5–18 Mother brushing child's teeth in front of mirror.

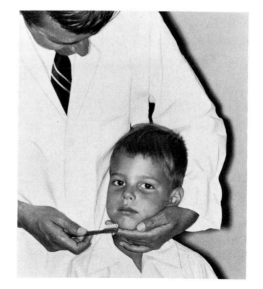

Figure 5–19 Correct position of parent and child in preparation for brushing the child's teeth. The head is cradled between the body and arm, and the fingers of the left hand retract the lips.

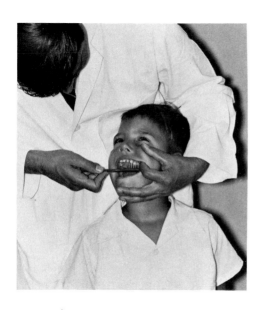

Figure 5–20 Correct position of parent and child in preparation for brushing the child's upper teeth.

Figure 5–21 Correct position of parent and child in preparation for brushing the child's lower teeth.

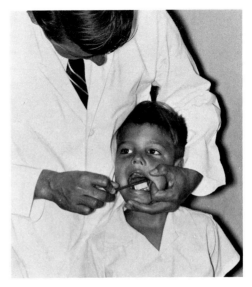

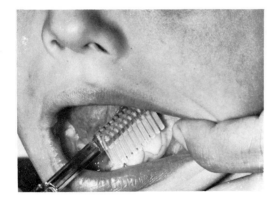

Figure 5–22 Brushing the occlusal surfaces of the lower molars.

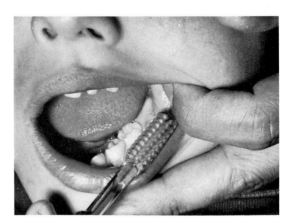

Figure 5–23 Brushing the buccal surfaces of the lower molars. Note lip retraction.

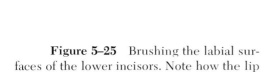

Figure 5–24 Brushing the lingual surfaces of the lower molars.

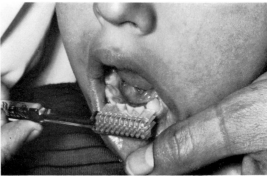

Figure 5–25 Brushing the labial surfaces of the lower incisors. Note how the lip is retracted.

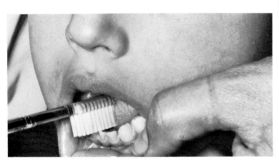

Figure 5–26 Brushing the lingual surfaces of the lower incisors.

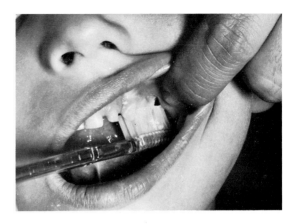

Figure 5–27 Brushing the occlusal surfaces of the upper molars.

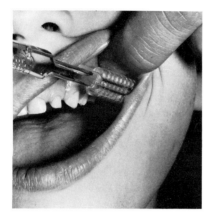

Figure 5–28 Brushing the buccal surfaces of the upper molars. Note lip retraction.

Figure 5–29 Brushing the lingual surfaces of the upper molars.

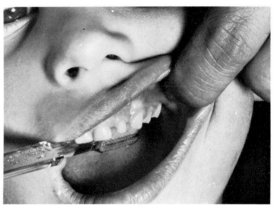

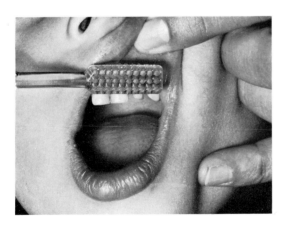

Figure 5–30 Brushing the labial surfaces of the upper incisors. Note how the lip is retracted.

Figure 5–31 Brushing the lingual surfaces of the upper incisors.

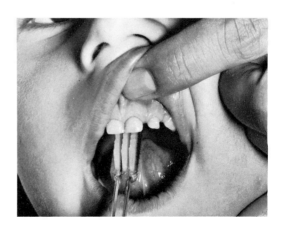

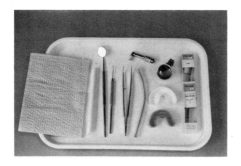

Figure 5–32 Tray set-up for examination and prevention. Note bib, mouth mirror, explorer, cotton pliers, saliva ejector, prophylaxis angle with rubber cup, container for prophylaxis paste, fluoride trays, and a toothbrush.

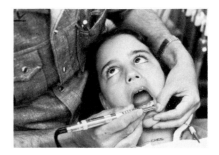

Figure 5–33 Polishing of teeth with a prophylaxis cup and fluoride paste. This is done prior to topical application of fluoride.

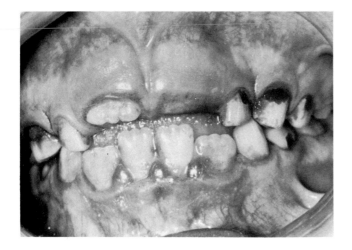

Figure 5–34 Disclosing solution applied to the teeth before prophylaxis. This is a convenient aid for indicating areas of plaque formation which must be removed during prophylaxis.

Figure 5–35 Patient seen in Figure 5–34 following prophylaxis and reapplication of disclosing solution. The solution should be applied after the prophylaxis in order to expose any uncleaned areas. It is also recommended that children use disclosing tablets periodically at home. This is a good aid in determining whether all areas have been cleaned thoroughly.

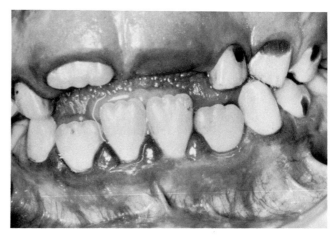

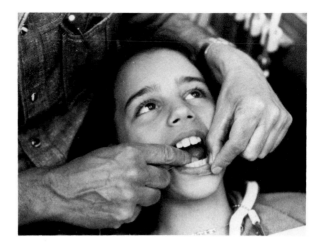

Figure 5–36 Flossing immediately after prophylaxis.

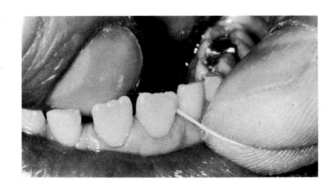

Figure 5–37 Dental floss (preferably unwaxed) with paste is used to polish the interproximal contact areas.

Figure 5–38 Child flossing in front of a mirror.

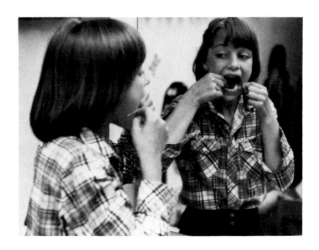

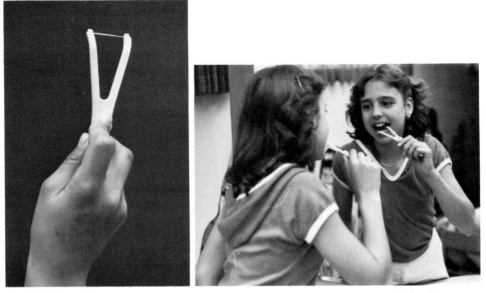

Figure 5–39 The flossing fork, rather than wrapping floss around the fingers, is preferred by some children.

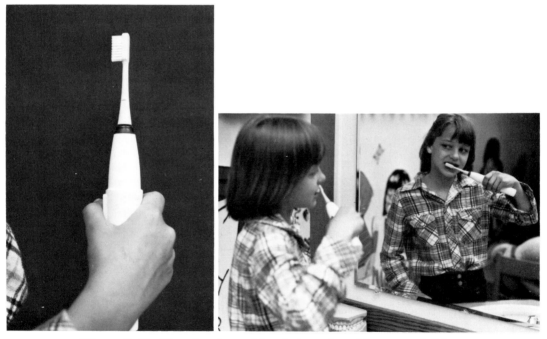

Figure 5–40 The electric toothbrush is preferred by some children.

Figure 5–41 Condit Jr. cotton roll holder used to keep teeth dry while topical fluoride is applied. A cotton roll may be used to obstruct the flow of saliva from Stenson's duct (parotid gland) and a saliva ejector to remove excess saliva. Topical fluoride treatment is given every 6 to 12 months. Acidulated sodium fluoride and sodium fluoride solutions must be stored in polyethylene containers. Stannous fluoride solutions must be prepared fresh immediately prior to treatment.

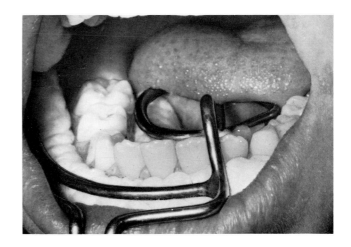

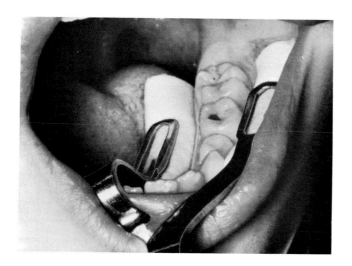

Figure 5–42 Garmer cotton roll holder used to keep teeth dry while topical fluoride is applied.

Figure 5–43 Application of fluoride solution; cotton ball is held by cotton pliers.

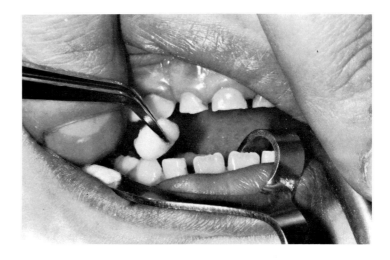

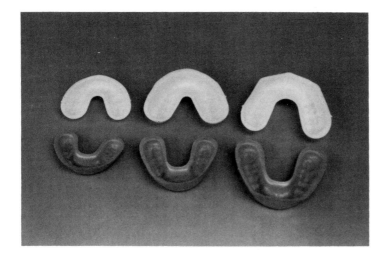

Figure 5–44 Adaptable trays may be used for the application of topical fluoride. The size that most closely fits the patient's dental arch should be used.

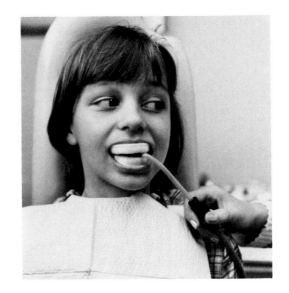

Figure 5–45 Fluoride trays in the mouth with a saliva ejector used to remove excess fluids. Child should be warned against swallowing while fluoride is in contact with teeth during the 4-minute application. Following treatment child should be instructed not to eat or drink for 30 minutes.

Pit and Fissure Sealants

The use of polymerized resin sealants has been demonstrated to be effective in the prevention of pit and fissure caries in both primary and permanent dentitions. They may be utilized as a routine part of the preventive program. Sealants require periodic evaluation — and, if necessary, replacement — by the dentist.

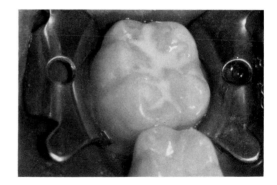

Figure 5–46 A pigmented pit and fissure sealant used to protect the occlusal surface of the permanent molar. Either a translucent or pigmented sealant may be used depending upon the preference of the dentist.

Conclusion

No preventive program will be effective unless the child is seen by the dentist on a regular basis. Recall visits permit early radiographic detection of caries, application of topical fluorides, placement of sealants, and reinforcement of home care procedures. If the dentist sees the child on a semi-annual basis after the child's first visit at two to three years of age, significant benefits will be realized.

REFERENCES

1. Aasenden, R., et al.: Effects of daily rinsing and ingestion of fluoride solutions upon dental caries and enamel fluoride. Arch. Oral Biol. *17*:1705–1714, Dec., 1972.
2. Brandt, R. S., et al.: The use of sodium fluoride mouthwash in reducing dental caries increments in eleven-year-old English school children. Proc. Brit. Paedont. Soc. 2:23, 1972.
3. Englander, H. R., et al.: Residual anticaries effect of repeated topical sodium fluoride applications by mouthpieces. J.A.D.A. 78:783–787, Apr., 1969.
4. Hilleboe, H. E., et al.: Newburgh Kingston caries-fluoride study. First report. I.A.D.R. 52:290–325, March, 1956.
5. Horowitz, H. S., and Doyle, J.: The effect on dental caries of topically applied acidulated phosphate-fluoride: results after three years. J.A.D.A. 82:359–365, Feb., 1971.
6. Isaac, S., et al.: The relation of fluoride in the drinking water to the distribution of fluoride in enamel. Intl. Dent. Res. 37:318–326, 1958.
7. Koch, G.: Caries increment in school children during and two years after end of supervised rinsing of the mouth with sodium fluoride solution. Odont. Rev. *20*:323–330, 1969.
8. Monthaler, T. M.: Confidence limits of clinical tests with fluoride administration. Caries Res. 4:343–372, 1971.
9. Mellberg, J. R., et al.: Acquisition of fluoride in vivo by enamel from repeated topical sodium fluoride applications in a fluoridated area: final report. J. Dent. Res. 49(Suppl.): 1473–1477, Nov.–Dec., 1970.
10. Silverstone, Leon M.: *Preventive Dentistry*. Update Books, London, 1978, pp. 97–133.
11. Simonsen, R. J.: Fissure sealants in primary molars: retention of colored sealants with variable etch times, at 12 months. J. Dent. Child. 46:382–384, Sept.–Oct., 1979.
12. Weiss, S., et al.: Influence of various factors on polysaccharide synthesis in S. *mitis*. Ann. N.Y. Acad. Sci. *131*:839–850, Sept., 1965

ANESTHESIA

Chapter 6 _____

Local Anesthesia

Skillful administration of a local anesthetic affords the practitioner an excellent opportunity to give the child the optimum advantage of modern dentistry. When a child has a painful injection experience or if no anesthetic at all is used during operative procedures, patient management problems are more likely to occur. After a pleasant injection experience, however, a child will become more confident in the dental environment and accept local anesthesia as part of routine dental treatment. A smooth injection technique is the cornerstone to painless dentistry and successful patient management.

Among the requirements basic to a good local anesthetic technique are:

1. An appropriate case history to ensure that the child can physically withstand a local anesthetic procedure.

2. A knowledge of the type of anesthetic most appropriate to the specific operation that is to be performed.

3. An awareness of the type of injection needed to fulfill the goal of anesthesia.

4. Sterile and sharp needles.

5. A technique which will minimize the child's fear and condition him or her favorably for future treatment.

The anesthetic of choice is the one which is the least toxic, most profound, and of shortest duration for the particular procedure at hand. Undesirable side effects, such as lip biting, may occur if the anesthetic is of long duration.

For most injections in children, short needles are desirable. A 1¼ inch stainless steel disposable needle of a fine gauge (27 or 30) can be successfully used to obtain suitable anesthesia for most treatment involving the primary and mixed dentitions.

Drying of the injection site (with air or a 2 × 2 sponge) and the application of a topical anesthetic will result in a more comfortable injection. Other techniques for minimizing the discomfort of an injection may include use of nitrous oxide analgesia (see Chapter 19) or a pressure injection device such as the Syrijet (see Figures 6–17 and 6–18).

The child's acceptance of local anesthetics can best be obtained if the operator makes all motions gracefully and with a sense of confidence. The dentist should forewarn the child — preferably immediately prior to the injection — so there is not much time for the child to speculate about the procedure. The child should not be allowed to actually see the instruments used. It has been found most helpful to have the patient's eyes open though, so that the operator may, by the use of facial expression as well as words, offer reassurance and instill confidence in spite of the fact that some discomfort may be experienced.

There is always a possibility that a dental emergency might arise from the use of a local anesthetic. Consequently, it is important to have oxygen resuscitation equipment close at hand. All personnel in the dental office should be taught the use of the equipment and know where it is kept.

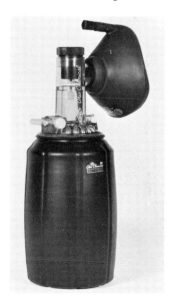

Figure 6–1   Resuscitation equipment should always be close at hand whenever a local anesthetic is used. Oxygen should be available for connection to this type of apparatus.

General Anesthesia

The use of general anesthesia in the treatment of certain children has gained wide acceptance. Patients for whom this method is used should be rigidly selected and the method and place of administration carefully determined. It is possible that complications may arise from the use of a general anesthetic. Therefore it should be employed on those children who are either severely physically handicapped or mentally unable to cooperate under a local anesthetic. Occasionally the extent of necessary treatment, combined with the distance between the child's residence and the professional office, makes general anesthesia the method of choice. In some cases involving very young children, it is the only method by which treatment can be accomplished satisfactorily. General anesthesia for children should be carried out only in a location where complete emergency and recovery facilities and trained professional personnel are available. In most instances, the ideal facilities are found in a hospital. The desirable team of professional personnel includes a pediatrician, anesthesiologist, registered nurse, and dentist. When these individuals work in close harmony in a well-equipped hospital, the ideal environment is established for rendering full-mouth restorative care of children under general anesthesia.

TABLE 6–1   NERVES AND AREAS INNERVATED*

Inferior alveolar n.	Mandibular teeth to midline. Frequently the central incisor and its labial investing soft tissues are innervated by fibers of the opposite inferior alveolar nerve.
Lingual n.	Lingual investing soft tissues to midline and anterior two-thirds of tongue.
Long buccal n.	Mucosa of the lower cheek and the buccal investing soft tissues of the mandibular posterior teeth.
Posterior superior alveolar (zygomatic) n.	Maxillary permanent molars and their buccal investing soft tissues with the exception of the mesiobuccal root of the first permanent molar.
Middle superior alveolar n.	Mesiobuccal root of the first permanent molar, primary molars, premolars, the buccal investing soft tissues of these teeth as well as a part of the labial investing soft tissues of the canine.
Anterior superior alveolar n.	Incisors and canine and their labial investing soft tissues.
Anterior palatine n.	Palatal investing soft tissues of the primary and permanent molars and premolars and a portion of the palatal investing soft tissues of the canine.
Nasopalatine n.	Palatal investing soft tissues of the incisors and a portion of the palatal investing soft tissues of the canine. Contributes to the innervation of the central and lateral incisors.

*Modified from Mink, J. R., and Spedding, R. H.: An injection procedure for the child dental patient. Dental Clin. North Amer., July, 1966, p. 315.

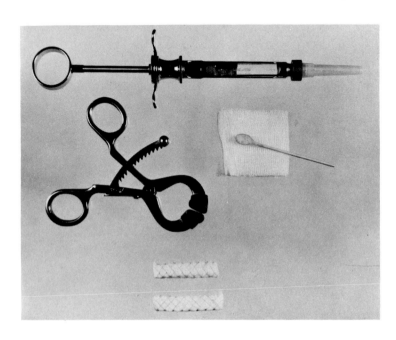

Figure 6–2 Suggested equipment for local anesthesia. Note aspirating syringe, disposable 27 gauge needle, topical anesthetic, 2 × 2 gauze sponge, mouth prop, and cotton rolls. The aspirating syringe enables the operator to reposition the needle if blood is aspirated in the anesthetic Carpule, avoiding intravascular injection of anesthetic fluid.

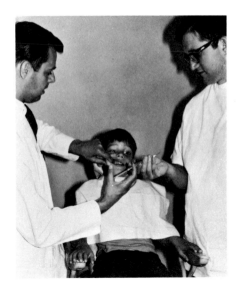

Figure 6–3 Passing the syringe in front of the child before injecting anesthetic should be avoided since it frequently causes management problems.

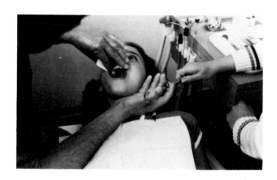

Figure 6–4 Passing syringe out of child's direct vision for maxillary injection.

Figure 6–5 Passing syringe out of child's direct vision for mandibular injection.

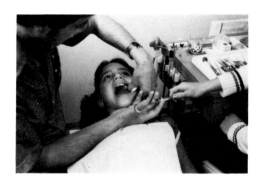

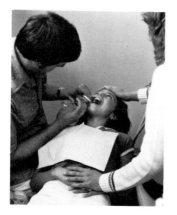

Figure 6–6   Stabilization of patient's hands and forehead by dental assistant during injection. This is necessary only if it is anticipated that the child will move around during the injection. Note child's eyes looking up at ceiling. If there are interesting posters or objects above the chair, the patient can be encouraged to look up at them during the injection.

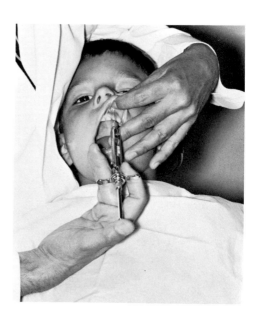

Figure 6–7   Position of operator's arms for injecting the maxillary anterior area. Fingers are used for stabilization.

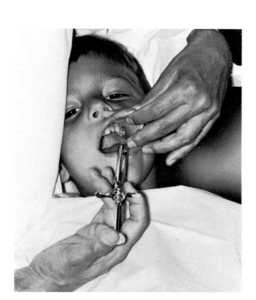

Figure 6–8   Position of operator's arms for injecting maxillary posterior area. Arms are used to stabilize operator and patient. Note finger and forearm position of the dentist.

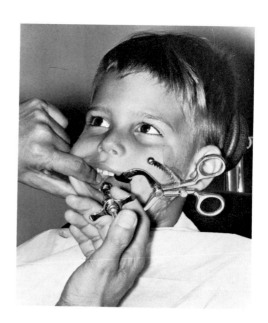

Figure 6–9   For the handicapped child who has difficulty in keeping his mouth open, the Molt mouth prop may be used during the inferior alveolar block injection.

Figure 6–10 Procedure for the inferior alveolar injection. The index finger or thumb is moved up and down along the anterior border of the ramus until the greatest concavity is palpated (the coronoid notch). The finger is then moved lingually onto the internal oblique ridge. The needle is inserted from the opposite side of the mouth and should bisect the fingernail as the tissue is penetrated. A very small amount of anesthetic is injected upon entering the tissue and continued until the needle gently touches bone (the lingual nerve is usually anesthetized at this time). When bone is touched the needle should be withdrawn slightly, the syringe aspirated, and anesthetic injected slowly provided no blood is aspirated. All injections should be made slowly, taking at least 1 minute. When this is done the injection is almost painless and produces a more profound state of anesthesia. Arrow designates area of mandibular foramen.

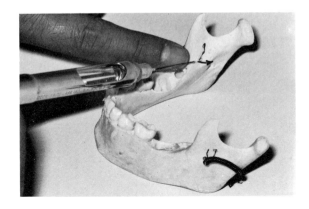

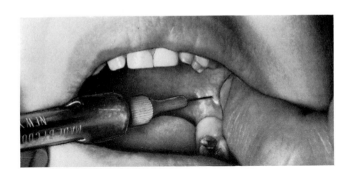

Figure 6–11 Inferior alveolar injection in 4-year-old child.

Figure 6–12 Long buccal injection. Note path of insertion of needle.

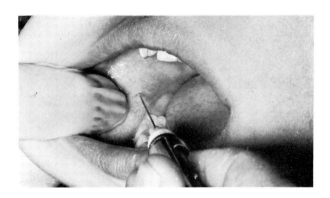

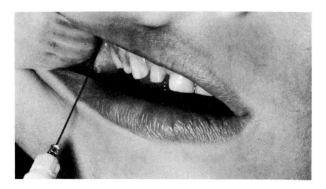

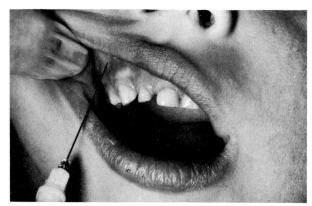

Figure 6–13 Posterior superior alveolar injection. A long needle is used in this figure and in Figure 6–14 for demonstration purposes only. A short needle is usually adequate for injections on children.

Figure 6–14 Middle superior alveolar injection.

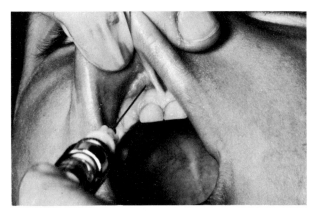

Figure 6–15 Anterior superior alveolar injection.

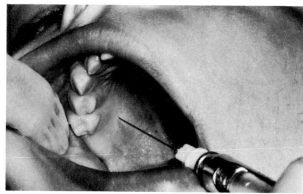

Figure 6–16 Palatal injection. This may be a painful injection. Both topical and pressure anesthesia from the cotton applicator held in place during the injection will reduce the sensation of pain considerably.

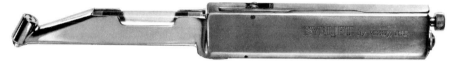

Figure 6–17 Pressure injection device (Mizzy Syrijet) for forcing anesthetic solution into superficial tissues. Useful in obtaining painless topical anesthesia prior to needle injection.

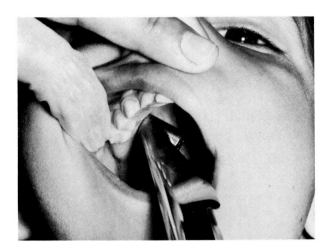

Figure 6–18 Same instrument as seen in Figure 6–17 being used on the lingual aspect of the maxillary right first primary molar.

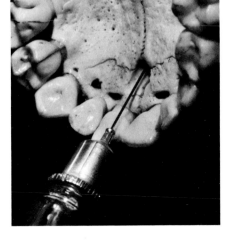

Figure 6–19 Anatomy of nasopalatine injection. Note how the needle parallels the long axis of the anterior teeth in order to enter the foramen.

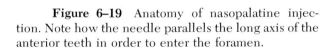

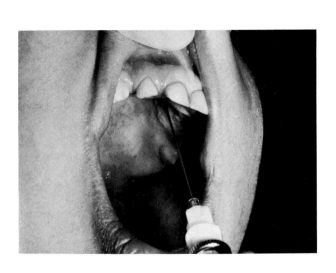

Figure 6–20 Nasopalatine injection. This can also be a painful injection and the same technique as presented in Figure 6–16 or 6–18 may be used.

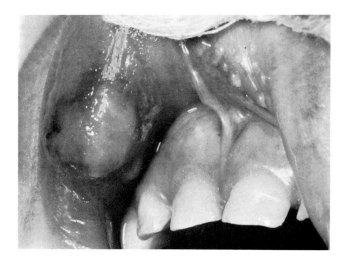

Figure 6–21 Trauma resulting from biting the upper lip after infiltration with local anesthetic was made over the maxillary right primary cuspid. If the area is still anesthetized when the child is dismissed, the parent and patient should be told of the trauma which will ensue if the child bites on the lip as the anesthetic wears off.

Figure 6–22 Trauma resulting from biting the lower lip. An inferior alveolar block injection was given prior to treatment, and after dismissal the child chewed on the lips as the anesthetic was wearing off. It usually takes from 5 to 7 days for these traumatized areas to heal.

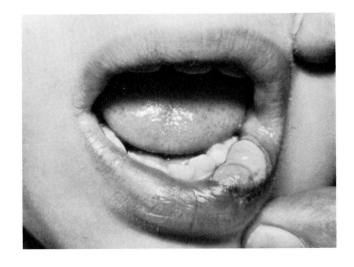

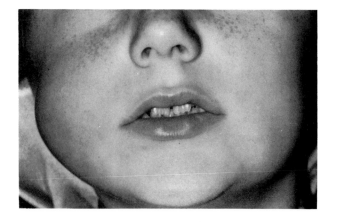

Figure 6–23 Hematoma of the right cheeck resulting from a posterior superior alveolar injection performed without aspiration. Aspiration is necessary when injecting in the area of the posterior superior alveolar nerve.

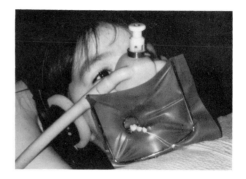

Figure 6–24 Use of nitrous oxide and oxygen analgesia with an apprehensive child. (See Chapter 19 concerning details of use of this procedure.)

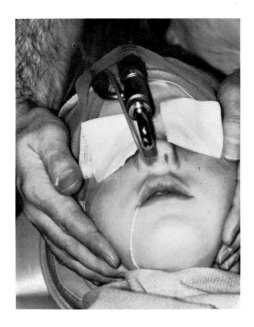

Figure 6–25 Nasotracheal intubation. This is the intubation method of choice for full-mouth dental treatment under general anesthesia.

Figure 6–26 Orotracheal intubation. On rare occasion the anesthesiologist will not be able to pass a nasal tube and instead will have to intubate through the oral cavity. Note how the operating area in the oral cavity is restricted for the dentist when this method of intubation is used.

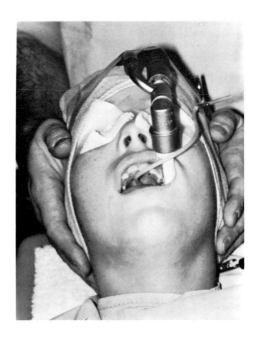

RUBBER DAM

Chapter 7 _____

The use of the rubber dam provides many advantages in treating children, most important of which is the high degree of patient control during operative procedures. Involuntary movements of the mandible and associated muscles combine to make other techniques less satisfactory than the rubber dam. With some children, if it is not used the area of operation becomes contaminated with saliva despite all efforts of the dentist to keep it dry. In addition to moisture control, use of the rubber dam results in the following:

1. A greater degree of protection for the patient against swallowing or aspirating foreign bodies that may come in contact with the posterior areas of the mouth. This is especially important during general anesthesia.

2. Better restriction of the tongue, cheeks, and lingual muscles from involuntary movements as in cases of cerebral palsy.

3. Decreased operating time because of better patient control and operator visibility.

4. Improvement in parent education, since the dentist can more clearly illustrate to the parent his or her specific treatment.

The use of the rubber dam has been found to be well received by children. They are able to swallow and to make themselves understood with the dam in place. The speed and accuracy in completion of the operation with the use of the rubber dam easily offset any inconvenience to the patient at the beginning of treatment. The psychological effect upon the dentist is to make procedures seem easier to accomplish.

The following technique has been found to be the most expedient and practical for the dam's placement and maintenance:

1. Use 5 × 5 inch rubber dam.

2. Largest hole is used for rubber dam clamp.

3. Holes are punched close together — 2 mm. between outsides of holes.

4. Only those teeth that must be involved in the treatment are included. The second primary molar is usually the best tooth to clamp because of its configuration.

5. Desirable clamps for most pedodontic cases include Ivory (carbon steel) number 00, 4, 8A, 14, and 14A.

6. Clamp is placed on dam and dam on frame before inserting into the mouth. The dam is secured on the frame by exerting tension in the vertical direction to permit maximum flexibility in the horizontal direction.

7. Dental floss is used to depress the dam around the gingivae of the teeth and to ligate where needed.

8. Wooden wedges are used if needed to depress interproximal areas. The wedges may be left in position throughout the cavity preparation phase of the operation.

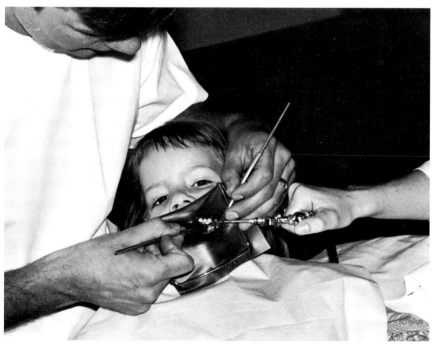

Figure 7–1 Rubber dam in place and patient ready for restorative procedures in the maxillary left quadrant. Note how the rubber dam isolates the teeth and provides a clean dry field of operation.

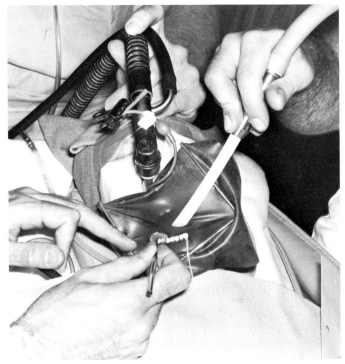

Figure 7–2 Rubber dam in place for routine operative procedures under general anesthesia. Throat pack should be placed prior to seating rubber dam.

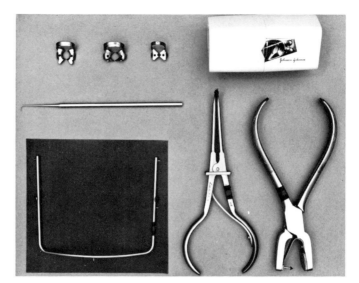

Figure 7–3 Tray setup for placement of rubber dam.

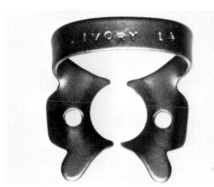

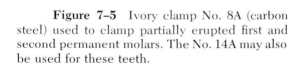

Figure 7–4 Ivory clamp No. 14 (carbon steel) used to clamp second primary molar and first permanent molar (erupted). The No. 4 may also be used for these teeth.

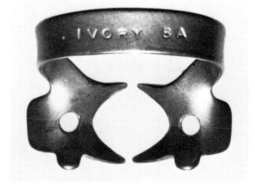

Figure 7–5 Ivory clamp No. 8A (carbon steel) used to clamp partially erupted first and second permanent molars. The No. 14A may also be used for these teeth.

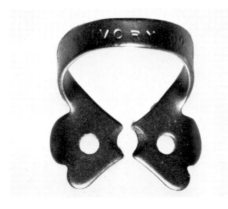

Figure 7–6 Ivory clamp No. 00 (carbon steel) used to clamp primary cuspids and first primary molars.

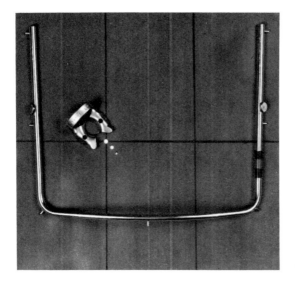

Figure 7–7 Holes punched in a 5 × 5 inch rubber dam for routine operative work in the mandibular arch (right side). This same punched rubber dam may be used on the left side of the mandibular arch by turning it over. Note the following:

1. The largest hole of the punch is used for the tooth to be clamped.

2. Holes are punched 2 mm. apart (outside measurements).

3. Holes are punched at a 45-degree angle.

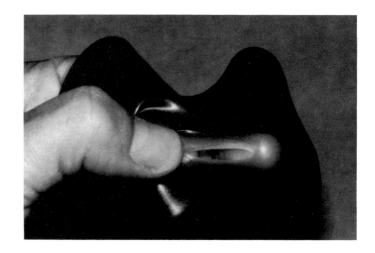

Figure 7–8 Dam stretched for insertion of clamp. The thumb and index finger are used to hold the dam while the middle finger stretches it.

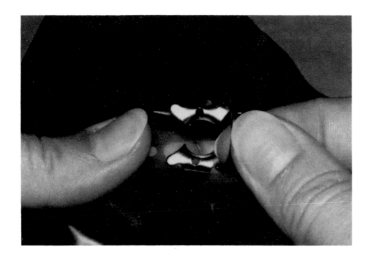

Figure 7–9 Wings of clamp inserted in rubber dam.

Figure 7–10 Rubber dam and clamp ready to be carried to the mouth attached to the Young's frame. Note that the frame is held to the dam by a slight tension in the vertical direction so as to permit maximum flexibility in the horizontal direction for easier placement in the mouth.

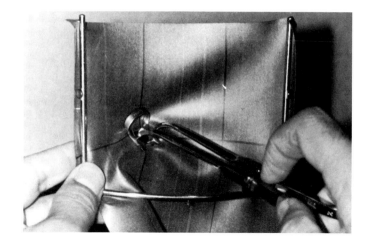

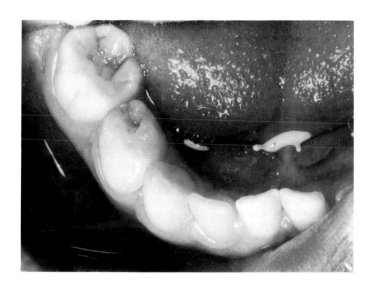

Figure 7–11 Right mandibular quadrant in a preschool child. Rubber dam will be placed on the second primary molar, first primary molar, and primary cuspid to facilitate operative procedures.

Figure 7–12 Rubber dam, clamp, and Young's frame carried to the mouth. The clamp is always on the outside, with the wings engaged only in the dam. This prevents accidental aspiration of the clamp in the event that it slips off the tooth during placement.

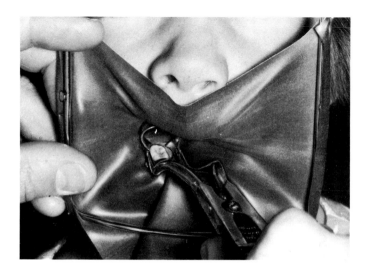

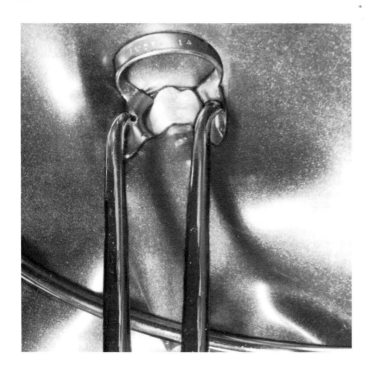

Figure 7–13 Clamp is seated on tooth with firm pressure. Minimal tissue damage is assured by carefully sliding clamp down the tooth.

Figure 7–14 Upon releasing clamp, the operator must use thumbs or forefingers to further seat clamp firmly on the tooth. Such action will prevent the clamp from snapping off.

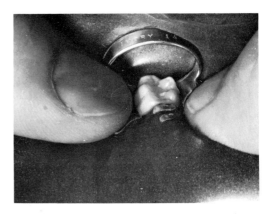

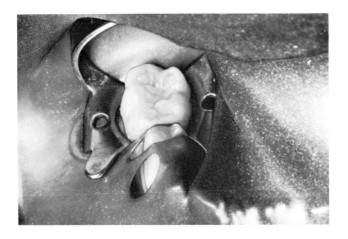

Figure 7–15 Clamp and dam in position prior to adjustment of rubber around teeth. Note that the rubber has not been snapped under the clamp yet.

Figure 7–16 Rubber dam is snapped under the clamp and stretched around the remaining teeth by use of the fingers and dental floss. The edges of the dam around the teeth are then tucked into the gingival crevice with an explorer. Warm air blown around the teeth as the dam is tucked facilitates this procedure.

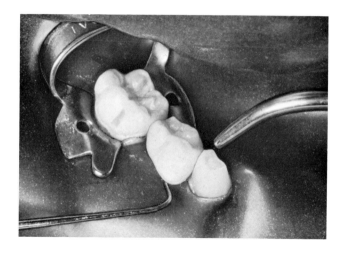

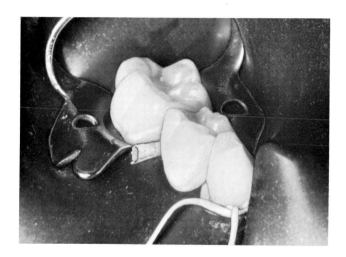

Figure 7–17 An interproximal wedge and simple ligature (dental floss) may be used to retract the dam and prevent it from slipping off the teeth. The gingival constriction of primary teeth makes ligature application very effective. When preparing Class II cavities, preparation may be carried into the wedge itself.

Figure 7–18 Rubber dam in position assuring a clean, dry field. The mouth is held open and accessory actions of tongue and lips are controlled. The Young's frame does not restrain the child unduly, and he is able to move his head without disturbing the placement of the dam. If it is desirable to cover the nose with the rubber dam, the series of holes is punched in the same direction, but ½ to 1 inch lower on the dam.

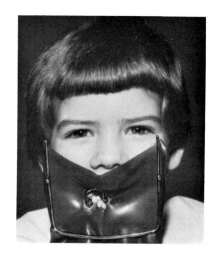

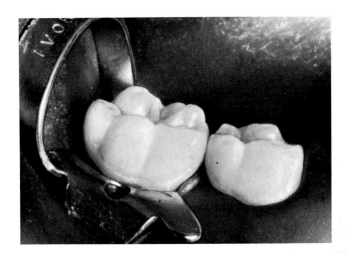

Figure 7–19 Buccal view of rubber dam when only two teeth are included. In many cases it is desirable to include in the dam only those teeth that are to be treated plus the tooth to be clamped.

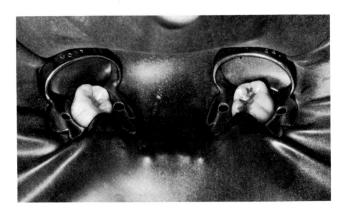

Figure 7–20 Bilateral clamping of mandibular first permanent molars to accomplish occlusal restorations in a single appointment. This procedure is particularly effective when a patient is treated under general anesthesia.

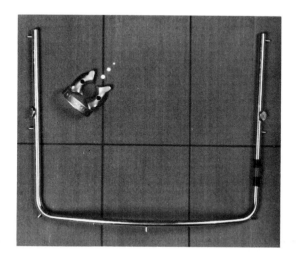

Figure 7–21 Holes punched in a 5 × 5 inch rubber dam for routine operative work in the maxillary arch (right side). This same punched rubber dam may be used on the left side of the maxillary arch by turning it over (see Figure 7–1). Note close proximity of holes to one another and 45-degree inclination toward center of dam.

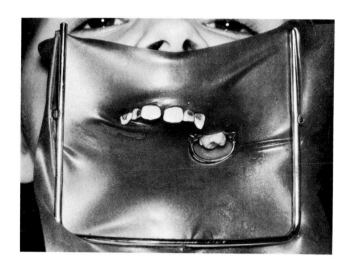

Figure 7–22 Position of rubber dam for treatment of anterior teeth. Stability of dam is best achieved by clamping a molar tooth. Wedges and ligatures are frequently used.

OPERATIVE
DENTISTRY

Chapter 8 _____

   Historically, restorative procedures for the child patient have constituted a major consideration for the practicing dentist. The rapidity of onset of caries in the primary dentition has always presented a challenge to the serious operator concerned with providing functional, durable, and esthetic restorations. Over the years, better understanding of child behavior, plus the use of local anesthetics, has enabled the motivated practitioner to accomplish operative procedures in the child that are equal to those in the adult. In addition, there has been the impact of the advent of new materials. It can be predicted, however, that with the wider use of fluoride and other caries-control agents now being tested, operative procedures in the child patient will gradually become less necessary, and a shift will be seen in the direction of greater emphasis on other problems of the early years, such as occlusal disharmonies.

   It is the purpose of this chapter to display and discuss many of the common restorative needs seen in children. Amalgam, composite, and stainless steel crown restorations will be discussed extensively. However, it is not the intent to go into detail concerning the various dental materials. For more information on this subject, the reader is referred to the current textbooks on dental materials.

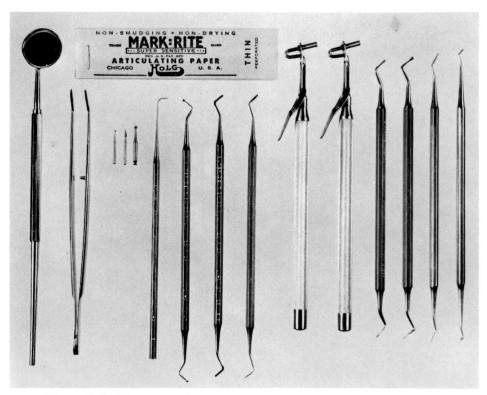

Figure 8–1 Tray setup for routine operative procedures includes mirror, cotton forceps, inverted cone bur, fissure bur, round bur, explorer, double-ended spoon excavator, enamel hatchets, amalgam carriers, amalgam condensers, and amalgam carvers.

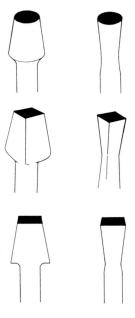

Figure 8–2 Suggested modification of amalgam condensers to achieve better adaptation to cavity walls. (Courtesy Dr. Joseph M. Sim, from Finn, S. B.: *Clinical Pedodontics*. 3rd ed., W. B. Saunders Co., Philadelphia, 1967, p. 187.)

Conventional   Altered

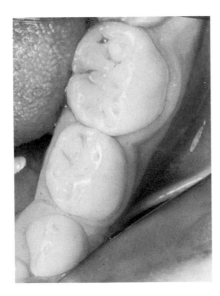

Figure 8–3 Anatomy of the primary mandibular molars. Note typical flat contacts. Numerous supplementary fissures are characteristic of the occlusal surface of the mandibular second primary molar.

Figure 8–4 Illustration of the occlusal view of the mandibular right first and second primary molars. Note suggested outline of cavity preparation.

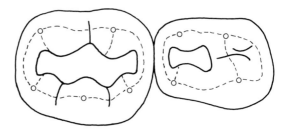

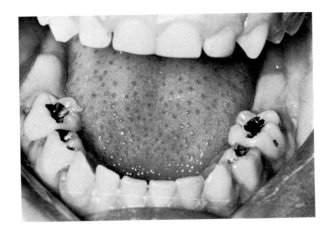

Figure 8–5 Occlusal amalgam restorations on mandibular second primary molars.

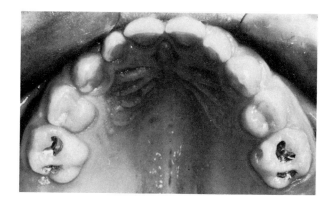

Figure 8–6 Occlusal amalgam restorations on maxillary second primary molars. Outline form is minimal because of absence of supplementary grooves.

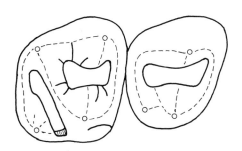

Figure 8–7 Illustration of occlusal view of maxillary right first and second primary molars. Note suggested outline of cavity preparations.

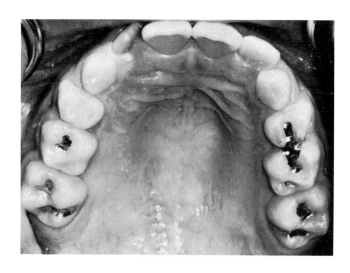

Figure 8–8 Polished amalgam restorations in the maxillary arch.

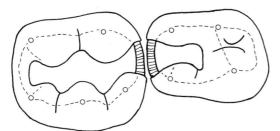

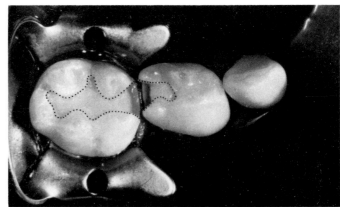

Figure 8–9 Illustration of occlusal view of mandibular right first and second primary molars. Note suggested outline of cavity preparations.

Figure 8–10 Clinical view of mandibular right first and second primary molars. Note occlusal outline, isthmus width, interproximal extension, interproximal box form, and width of gingival floor. The choice of burs is left to the preference of the clinician; however, some of the most popular burs for these preparations are the friction grip 33, 56, 169, 245 and 330.

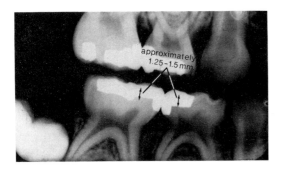

Figure 8–11 Radiograph of same patient as in Figure 8–10. Note suggested depth for these preparations.

Figure 8–12 Distal view of mandibular right first primary molar. Note outline of cavity preparation in this area.

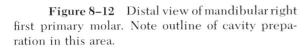

Figure 8–13 Tofflemire matrix holder prior to insertion of amalgam.

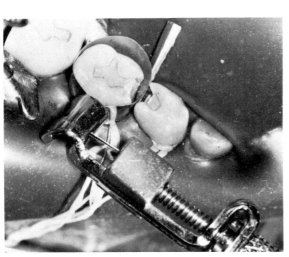

182

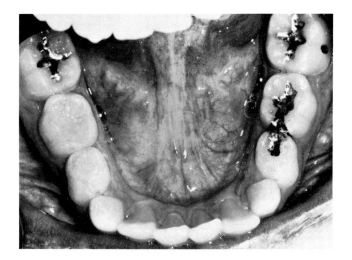

Figure 8–14 Mandibular arch with finished amalgam restorations.

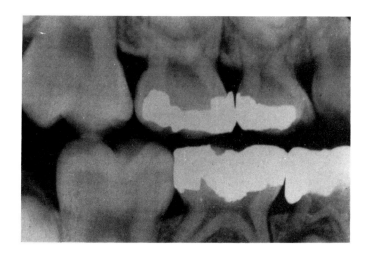

Figure 8–15 Radiograph showing the effect of faulty wedging during matrix adaption, resulting in amalgam overhang.

Figure 8–16 Radiograph illustrating result of faulty matrix. Wedging is necessary to prevent overhangs at gingival margin.

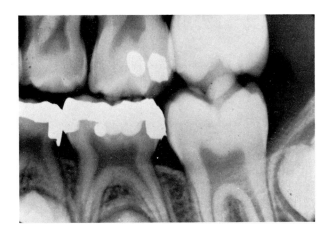

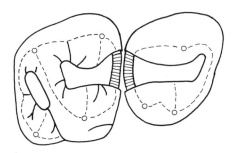

Figure 8–17 Illustration of occlusal view of maxillary right first and second primary molars. Note suggested outline of cavity preparations.

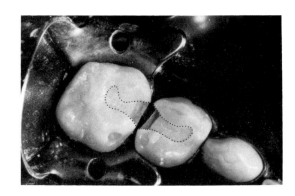

Figure 8–18 Clinical view of maxillary right first and second primary molars. Note occlusal outline, isthmus width, interproximal extension, interproximal box form, and width of gingival floor.

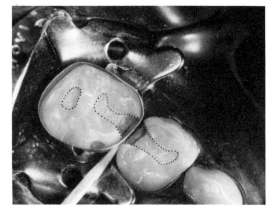

Figure 8–19 T-Band matrix adapted, and wedge placed, for same patient as in Figure 8–18. The T-Band, Tofflemire, and spot-welded matrices are used when restoring primary molars. The type of matrix selected is left to the preference of the clinician.

Figure 8–20 Polished restorations in the primary dentition. Note that anatomy is not deep.

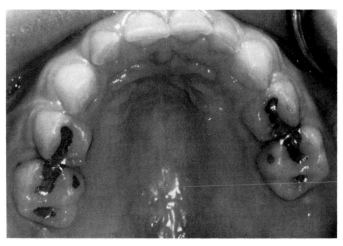

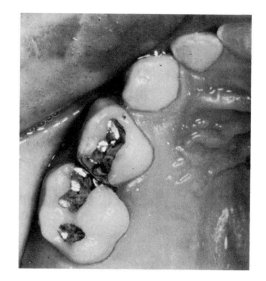

Figure 8–21 Properly finished approximating amalgam restorations.

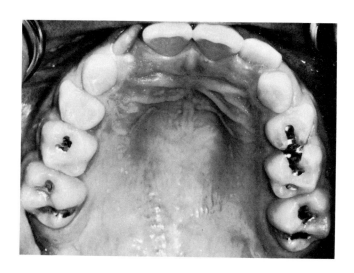

Figure 8–22 Another example of the conservative isthmus in the proximo-occlusal amalgam restoration.

Figure 8–23 Occlusal amalgam restoration on mandibular first permanent molar. Note anatomical carving of the amalgam. This is important in the young permanent teeth to maintain proper cuspal interdigitation.

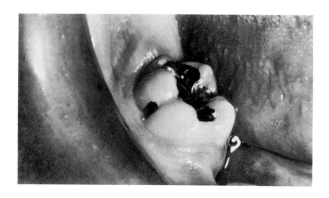

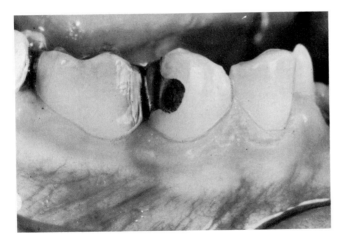

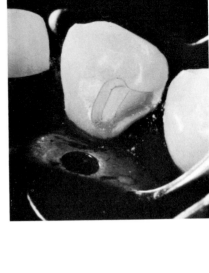

Figure 8–24 Labial dove-tail amalgam restoration, for the distal surface of the mandibular cuspid.

Figure 8–25 Lingual dovetail cavity preparation on a primary cuspid. The incisal edge should not be undercut if later fracture is to be avoided.

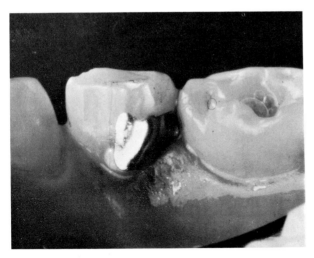

Figure 8–26 Restoration placed. Same tooth as shown in Figure 8–25.

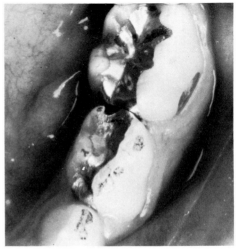

Figure 8–27 Fracture of the marginal ridge of a disto-occlusal amalgam restoration in a mandibular first primary molar. This usually occurs from traumatic interdigitation of the lingual cusp of the maxillary first primary molar.

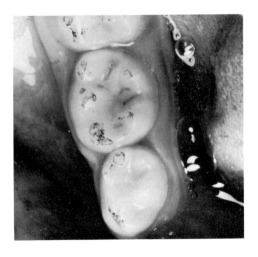

Figure 8–28 Carbon markings on the mandibular arch prior to beginning operative procedures. Markings on marginal ridge denote need for reduction of opposing cusp.

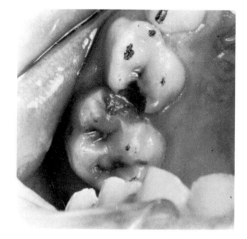

Figure 8–29 Opposing teeth in case illustrated in Figure 8–28. Sharp lingual cusp of first primary molar should be reduced.

Figure 8–30 Marginal deterioration or ditching in proximo-occlusal amalgam restorations. Overcarving or undercarving can cause this, as can rough enamel walls or, in some cases, poor manipulation of alloy and mercury.

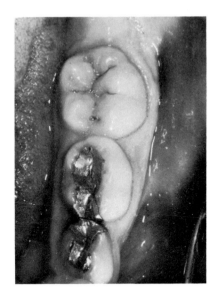

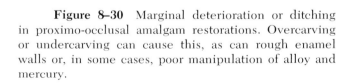

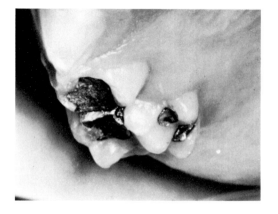

Figure 8–31 Marginal ditching that may be the result of a wide flaring cavity preparation.

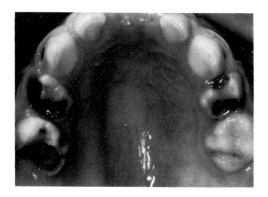

Figure 8–32 Extensive caries in the maxillary arch. Stainless steel crowns are indicated for most of these primary molars.

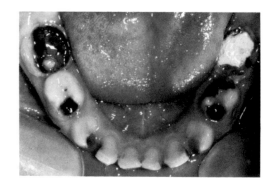

Figure 8–33 Owing to extensive caries, these primary mandibular molars are indicated for stainless steel crowns.

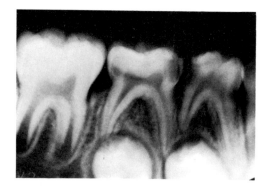

Figure 8–34 Preoperative radiograph of patient with caries probably involving the pulp. Stainless steel crowns are usually indicated after pulp therapy in primary teeth (see Figures 10–20 through 10–22).

Figure 8–35 Rubber dam in place prior to preparation of the first and second primary molars for stainless steel crowns.

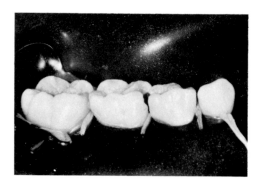

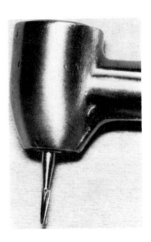

Figure 8–36 The No. 170 friction grip carbide bur is used for the occlusal reduction and buccal and lingual bevels. Numerous other burs may be used for this procedure depending on the preference of the clinician.

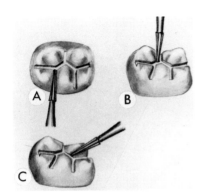

Figure 8–37 The occlusal reduction: (a) Depth cuts are established by placing the bur on its side. The occlusal reduction should be approximately 1.5 mm. This is easily established by cutting into the tooth slightly deeper than the diameter of the bur. (b) Depth cuts are established in occlusal grooves. (c) Completion of occlusal reduction is made by reducing tooth structure between depth cuts.

Figure 8–38 The occlusal depth cuts made on the second primary molar. These act as a guide in determining the proper amount of reduction of tooth structure on the occlusal surface.

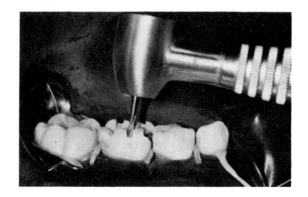

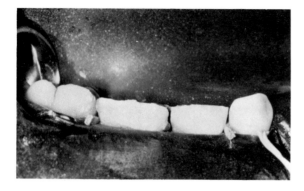

Figure 8–39 Occlusal reduction of both primary molars as viewed bucally.

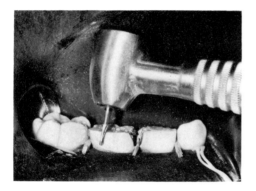

Figure 8–40 The buccal bevel extends to tissue level but not below it. The only exception to this is the subgingival reduction of the buccal bulge on the mandibular and maxillary first primary molars (see Figures 8–42 and 8–43).

Figure 8–41 Subgingival reduction of the buccal bulge on the mandibular first primary molar using a large, flat instrument to depress tissue in this area (see Figure 8–42).

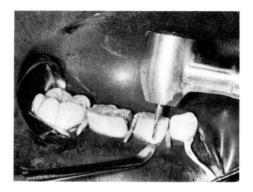

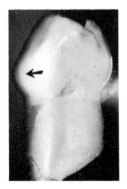

Figure 8–42 Mesial view of mandibular right first primary molar showing buccal and lingual outline. (Note large buccal bulge. This must be partially reduced during preparation for a stainless steel crown; otherwise, the crown will not slide over the tooth in this area (see Figure 8–41).

Figure 8–43 Mesial view of maxillary right first primary molar showing buccal and lingual outline. (Note large buccal bulge.) The bulge on this tooth must be partially reduced also, for the same reason described in Figure 8–42.

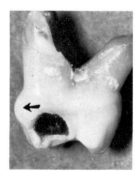

Figure 8–44 Mesial view of tooth before and after occlusal reduction and buccal and lingual bevels. Note the prepared tooth on the right. Tooth structure was not reduced below the buccogingival or linguogingival tissue. As previously stated, the only place tooth structure is reduced below the gingiva is on the maxillary and mandibular first primary molars in the area of the buccal bulge. Note that there is no finish line on the tooth prepared for a stainless steel crown.

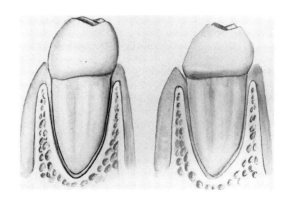

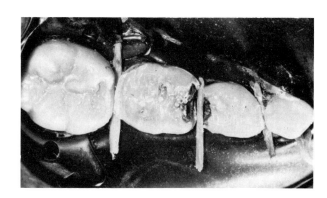

Figure 8–45 Placement of interproximal wedges to depress the papilla. The proximal slice is made into the wooden wedge rather than the papilla, thereby avoiding unnecessary hemorrhage.

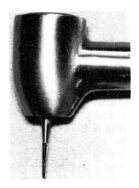

Figure 8–46 The No. 169L friction grip carbide bur is used for the proximal slice.

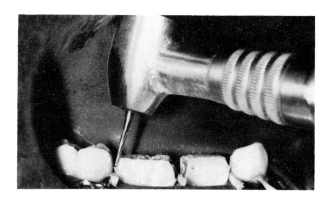

Figure 8–47 Preparation of the proximal slice with the No. 169L friction grip carbide bur. By angling the bur and starting with a ledge, the proximal surface of the adjacent tooth is not cut accidentally.

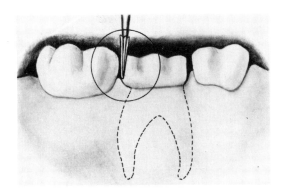

Figure 8–48 The No. 169L friction grip bur reducing tooth structure to height of papilla. The proximal slice must be extended below tissue in this area in order to avoid leaving a ledge. If a ledge is left, it will not be possible for the crown to slide over the tooth far enough to have the margins of the crown under tissue (see Figure 8–54).

Figure 8–49 This type of ledge must *not* be left in the proximal area. See Figure 8–50 for correct reduction of the proximal surface.

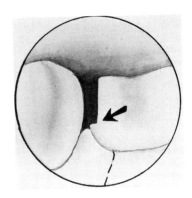

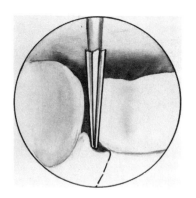

Figure 8–50 The No. 169L friction grip carbide bur must extend below tissue and end with a proximal slice in this area.

Figure 8–51 After the slices are made, the wedges are removed and the proximal is checked to make sure no ledges exist. An explorer or the No. 169L friction grip bur may be used for this purpose; however, the bur must not be rotating. It must pass up and down through the proximal area without any interference. If a ledge is detected, it must be removed before proceeding to the next step.

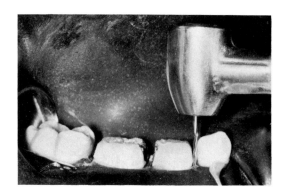

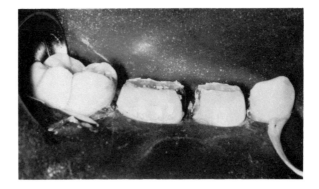

Figure 8–52 Appearance of teeth after they have been prepared for placement of stainless steel crowns. The teeth are now ready for caries removal and formocresol pulpotomies; however, pulpotomies are usually done *before* the crown preparation is completed.

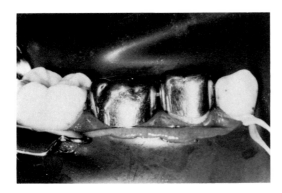

Figure 8–53 Failure of the stainless steel crown to seat on the first primary molar. Whenever this occurs, it is usually an indication of a ledge in the interproximal area.

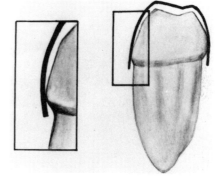

Figure 8–54 Initial placement of a stainless steel crown. If it extends too far gingivally it must be trimmed (see Figure 8–55).

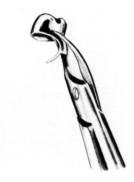

Figure 8–55 Trimming excess material from crown. The gingival margin of the crown should be finished to a fine edge, as shown on the enlarged gingival view in Figure 8–58. The edge should be polished with a rubber wheel.

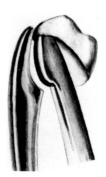

Figure 8–56 Crimping the gingival one third of the crown with a No. 114 plier.

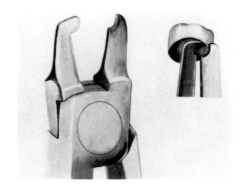

Figure 8–57 Crimping of the crown may also be accomplished with a No. 109 plier.

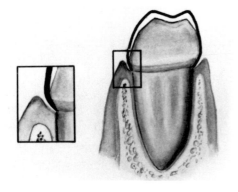

Figure 8–58 A cross-sectional view of finished stainless steel crown in place. Isolation prior to cementation may be accomplished with the rubber dam or cotton rolls. After all excess cement has been removed, the gingival one third of the crown may be polished with pumice to remove any remaining small particles of cement.

Figure 8–59 Use of knotted dental floss to remove excess cement in the interproximal area. This must be passed interproximally before the cement has completely hardened.

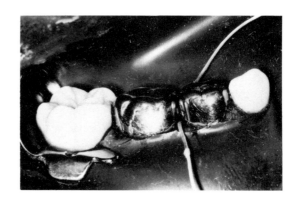

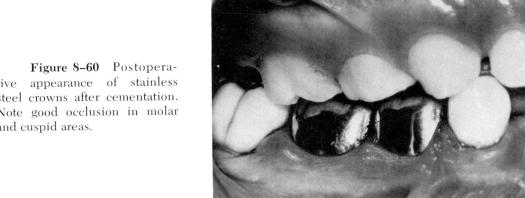

Figure 8–60 Postoperative appearance of stainless steel crowns after cementation. Note good occlusion in molar and cuspid areas.

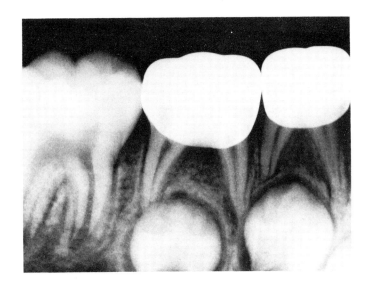

Figure 8–61 Postoperative radiograph of same patient as in Figure 8–60.

Figure 8–62 A stainless steel crown imbedded in a large glob of hard, sticky candy. Although a well-adapted crown should not come off under these circumstances, patients and parents should be warned of the possibility.

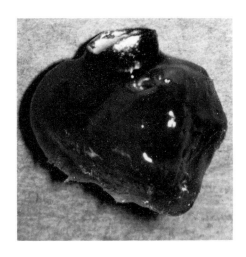

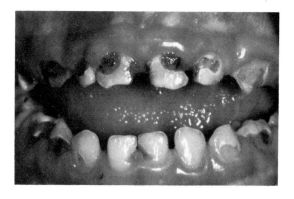

Figure 8–63 Rampant caries in the primary dentition (see Figures 8–64 through 8–70).

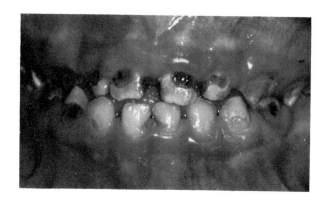

Figure 8–64 Same patient as in Figure 8–63. Note occlusion prior to treatment. See Figure 8–68 for occlusion after treatment.

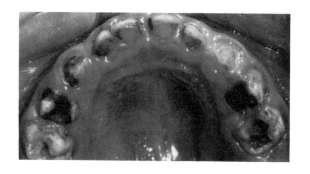

Figure 8–65 Maxillary view of same patient as in Figures 8–63 and 8–64.

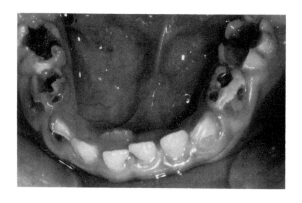

Figure 8–66 Mandibular view of same patient as in Figures 8–63 through 8–65. Note position of permanent incisor prior to extraction of the primary central incisors (see Figures 8–67 through 8–70).

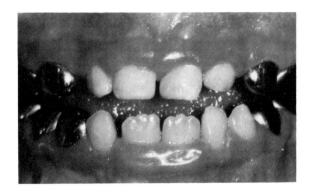

Figure 8–67 Anterior view of same patient as in Figures 8–63 through 8–66 after restorations were placed.

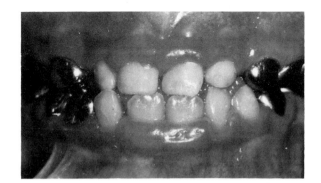

Figure 8–68 Same patient as in Figures 8–63 through 8–67. Note occlusion.

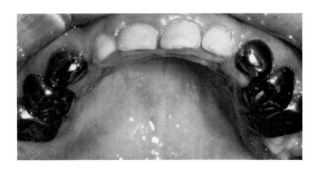

Figure 8–69 Maxillary view of same patient as in Figures 8–63 through 8–68. Note that stainless steel crowns were placed on all primary cuspids and molars, and the incisors were restored with composite restorations after acid etching.

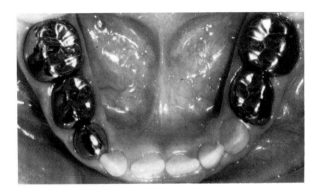

Figure 8–70 Mandibular view of same patient as in Figures 8–63 through 8–69. Note that stainless steel crowns were placed on all primary molars and the right cuspid. The left cuspid and the lateral incisors were restored with composite restorations. (Courtesy Dr. Gary Bell.)

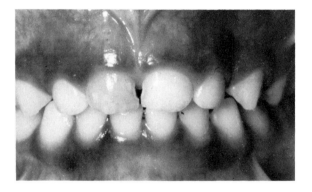

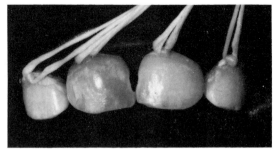

Figure 8–71 Labial view of interproximal caries of maxillary right and left primary central incisors (see Figures 8–72 through 8–74).

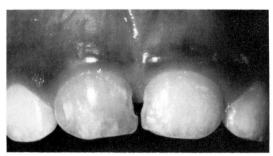

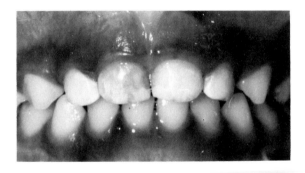

Figure 8–72 Close-up view of patient in Figure 8–71.

Figure 8–73 Rubber dam in place prior to treatment of carious lesions. Note use of dental floss for ligation.

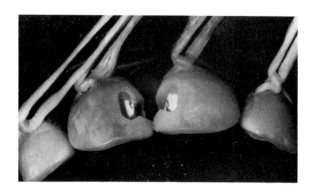

Figure 8–74 Class III cavity preparations. Since the labial walls were weakened, dovetails were placed for retention of composite material.

Figure 8–75 Labial view of patient in Figures 8–71 through 8–74 after placement of composite restorations.

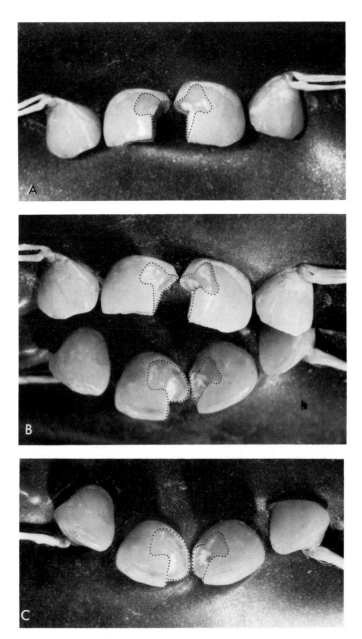

Figure 8–76 Class IV cavity preparation. Whenever an incisal angle of a primary incisor is weakened, a preparation as demonstrated here is suggested. This may be necessary because of caries that extend into the area or because of an overextension of a Class III preparation that has weakened the incisal angle. *A*. Labial view. *B*. Labiolingual view. Note outline and placement of dovetail. It is in the gingival half of the tooth. This reduces the risk of weakening support of incisal enamel. *C*. Lingual view. Note amount of incisal angle reduction and placement of dovetail.

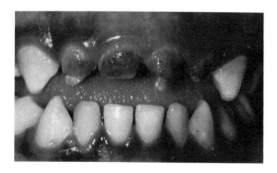

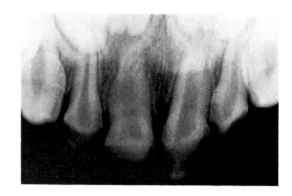

Figure 8–77 Extensive decay of the maxillary primary incisors as a result of "baby bottle syndrome" (see Figures 8–78 through 8–80).

Figure 8–78 Radiograph of same patient as in Figure 8–77. Fortunately, caries did not extend into any of the pulp chambers.

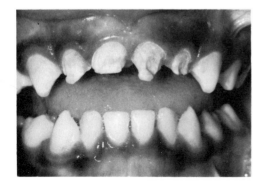

Figure 8–79 Same patient as in Figures 8–77 and 8–78 after caries removal. A sedative base was placed over dentin, the teeth were etched with phosphoric acid, then rinsed and dried, after which a resin was placed and then restored with composite restorations. The composite was placed on the teeth with a celluloid crown form.

Figure 8–80 Same patient as in Figures 8–77 through 8–79 after acid etching and placement of composite crowns. The mandibular right cuspid is next in the sequence of treatment.

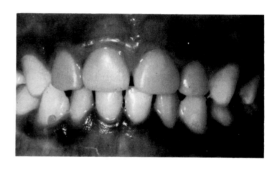

Figure 8–81 Because of extensive caries, stainless steel crowns were placed on these primary incisors. When subgingival retention is the only means of retaining an anterior restoration, stainless steel crowns are preferred by many clinicians. To improve esthetics, the labial surface of the crown is removed and filled in with composite (see Figures 8–84 through 8–86).

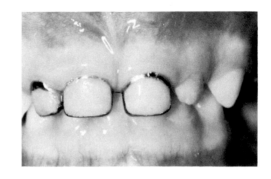

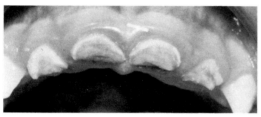

Figure 8–82 Extensive decay of the maxillary primary incisors as a result of "baby bottle syndrome." Because of minimal remaining coronal tooth structure, these teeth were restored with stainless steel crowns and a labial window of composite (see Figures 8–83 through 8–86). Courtesy Dr. Daniel N. O'Brien.)

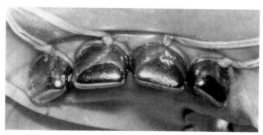

Figure 8–83 Stainless steel crowns were cemented on the involved teeth.

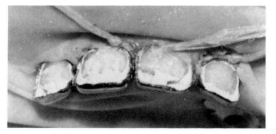

Figure 8–84 The labial surfaces of the crown were removed with a friction grip fissure bur.

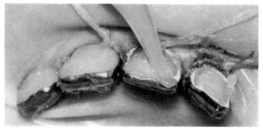

Figure 8–85 Convenient placement of material is with a composite syringe.

Figure 8–86 Discs were used for final finish of composite restorations.

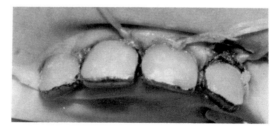
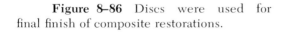

PULP THERAPY

Chapter 9 _____

Conservation of the vitality and health of the dental pulp is one of the most important preventive aspects in the practice of dentistry for children. No space-maintaining appliance can equal the natural tooth during the developmental years, nor can the psychological value of the retention of natural teeth be overestimated. Some differences exist in the approach to clinical management of the exposed or nearly exposed dental pulp in the primary and immature permanent dentition as contrasted to the fully formed adult dentition.

The primary teeth exhibit special morphologic characteristics that make conventional endodontic procedures somewhat difficult. The root canals tend to be flatter and ribbon-like, particularly as the tooth becomes more mature. Root resorption presents problems in obtaining a good apical seal. In spite of these complicating factors there is increased interest in utilizing endodontic procedures in the nonvital primary tooth during the preschool years. By far the most common pulpal problem in children is carious exposure of the vital primary tooth. This is best treated by pulpal amputation and sealing off at the canal orifices with a suitable agent that will promote healing and maintain viable tissue in the root canal. Thus far, formocresol has proved to be far more successful in this regard than calcium hydroxide in treating the primary teeth. Other agents will undoubtedly be developed that may prove even more effective, but in the long run, prevention of the carious lesion is still the most rewarding approach to the problem.

There is little justification for so-called capping in carious exposures in primary teeth. Pulpotomy has been demonstrated to be much more successful, and the extra time required is not significant. Indirect pulp capping has demonstrated considerable usefulness in recent years. In this procedure, a drug such as calcium hydroxide or zinc oxide and eugenol is placed over partially excavated carious dentin to inhibit bacterial activity and stimulate

203

dentin calcification. Although it is of greater value in treating doubtful cases in the immature permanent dentition, the operator may elect to utilize this procedure on primary teeth in selected instances.

Special considerations surround the problem of pulp exposure in the young immature permanent tooth. In most cases, the apical foramen is still open, complicating endodontic procedures. Often, the dentition is still in a state of adjustment and transition, and tooth loss is especially undesirable. Here again, the clinician must elect to perform the procedure that is most likely to conserve and protect the involved tooth. Traumatic injury is one of the most frequent causes of exposure in the immature permanent tooth, and these cases have responded quite successfully to pulpotomy with calcium hydroxide. When apical completion has occurred, endodontics must be weighed against the pulpotomy procedure. The decision remains with the operator to determine which will be most successful over a period of years.

Indirect pulp capping is the sealing in of a suitable drug over partially excavated carious dentin. The purpose is to arrest the existing caries process and stimulate sclerosis and hardening in the remaining vital dentin. Calcium hydroxide has been used successfully, as have zinc oxide and eugenol and also camphorated monochlorophenol. Indications include deep carious lesions approaching the pulp, especially in young permanent teeth with incompletely formed root ends. Contraindications include a history of dental pain, frank dental exposure, or periapical pathology.

Pulp capping is the direct placement of a drug or medication over small, "pin point," pulpal exposures. It is primarily recommended for accidental operative exposures, although it is used by some clinicians for small carious exposures of 1 mm. or less. Numerous different drugs have been suggested for this procedure, calcium hydroxide being the most widely utilized at present. Capping has never been a consistently successful approach to pulp management and should be employed sparingly.

Pulpotomy implies the complete amputation of the vital coronal pulp and the placement of a suitable drug over the remaining exposed tissue. The objective is to maintain the vitality of the pulp remaining in the root canals so that the restored tooth can function as a healthy biological unit. A variety of drugs have been used in the pulpotomy procedure, including zinc oxide and eugenol, calcium hydroxide, formocresol, and other combinations. Current research indicates formocresol to be the preparation of choice in treating carious exposures in primary teeth, whereas calcium hydroxide is preferred for the immature permanent tooth, such as the traumatically injured incisor.

Pulpectomy, or complete extirpation of the pulp tissue from the crown and root canals of teeth, may be employed in the treatment of necrotic primary teeth. The root canal sealant must be capable of being resorbed. Best results will be achieved in pulpectomy on primary teeth when performed on single rooted teeth or on molars during the preschool years before secondary calcification has taken place. Success can also be attained in pulpectomy on immature permanent teeth. Recent developments indicate an advantage in using calcium hydroxide and camphorated monochlorophenol filling material in these cases to promote root end closure.

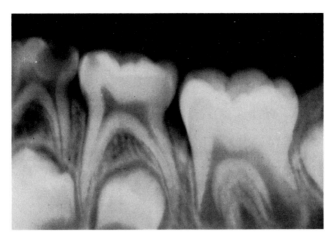

Figure 9–1 Deep carious lesion (almost pulpal exposure) in occlusal surface of the mandibular first primary molar. In a mouth with multiple lesions similar to this the *indirect pulp capping* technique may be used to great advantage. In one visit, all severely affected areas may be temporarily treated and caries arrested, and at a later visit, permanent restorations may be placed. The procedure is as follows:

1. Remove all soft, leathery carious dentin (harder carious dentin is not removed in order to avoid exposing the pulp).
2. Cover the harder carious dentin with a paste of calcium hydroxide and place a temporary amalgam restoration over it.
3. Remove the amalgam and calcium hydroxide and extirpate any remaining carious dentin in 3 to 6 months. By this time most of the underlying carious dentin has become hard.

This technique enables the dentist to temporarily treat multiple areas in one sitting and usually prevent pulpal exposures when the permanent restorations are placed.

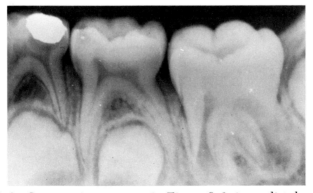

Figure 9–2 Same patient as seen in Figure 9–1, immediately after treatment. Note radiolucency under the amalgam. This is calcium hydroxide, which normally has a radiolucent appearance in a radiograph.

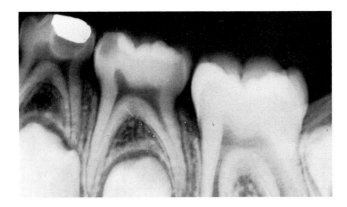

Figure 9–3 Same patient as shown in Figures 9–1 and 9–2, 6 months after indirect pulp capping. Note increased radiopacity under the calcium hydroxide. This is a reflection of the increased density of the vital dentin. The tooth is now ready for a permanent restoration.

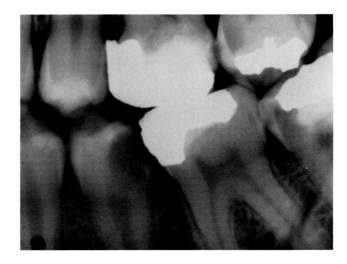

Figure 9–4 Deep carious lesion in a mandibular second bicuspid. Tooth was treated with an indirect pulp capping, as described in Figure 9–1.

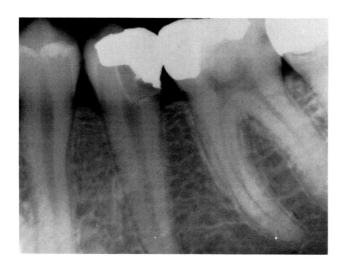

Figure 9–5 Same patient as seen in Figure 9–4, 6 months after indirect pulp capping. Note increased radiopacity of tooth structure adjacent to calcium hydroxide. Pulpal exposure was avoided and the tooth successfully treated.

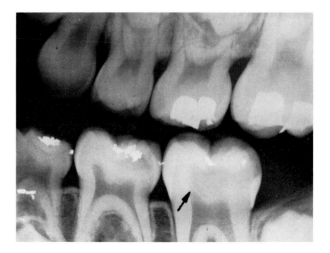

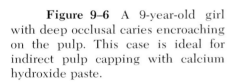

Figure 9-6 A 9-year-old girl with deep occlusal caries encroaching on the pulp. This case is ideal for indirect pulp capping with calcium hydroxide paste.

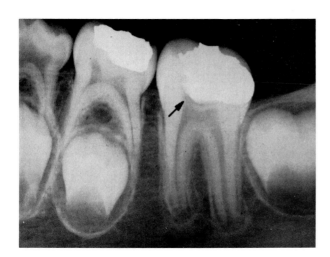

Figure 9-7 Postoperative radiograph of tooth seen in Figure 9-6, showing partial removal of caries and placement of calcium hydroxide under a temporary amalgam restoration. Note incomplete root apices.

Figure 9-8 Radiograph of tooth shown in Figure 9-6, 7 months postoperatively. Note radiopaque line under calcium hydroxide base. This represents a layer of sound dentin of increased density.

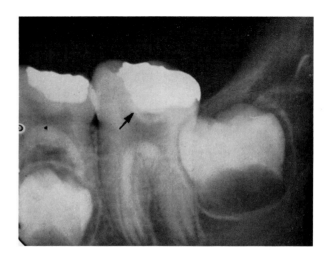

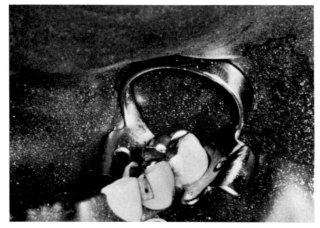

Figure 9–9 A minute surgical exposure on the mesial surface of a mandibular primary molar. Small *surgical* exposures may be capped with a paste of calcium hydroxide.

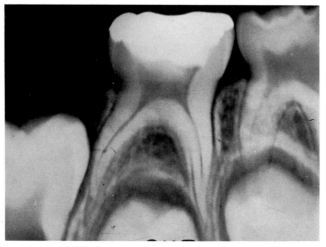

Figure 9–10 Radiograph of successful calcium hydroxide capping on mesial horn of mandibular second primary molar.

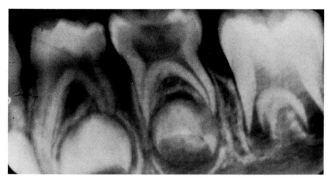

Figure 9–11 A large carious exposure in a primary second molar. *A formo-cresol pulpotomy* is the treatment of choice for this tooth. Contraindications for the formocresol pulpotomy are the following:

On clinical evaluation:
1. History of spontaneous pain.
2. Pain from percussion.
3. Suppuration.

On radiographic evaluation:
1. Calcified globules in the pulp.
2. Internal resorption.
3. Pathologic bifurcation radiolucency.
4. Pathologic periapical radiolucency.

None of the contraindications listed were observed in this case, so the formo-cresol pulpotomy was performed with success. Formocresol pulpotomy is done on primary teeth only.

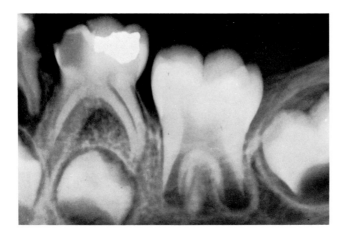

Figure 9–12 Primary second molar with a carious exposure on the mesial surface. Clinical and radiographic findings were normal. Formocresol pulpotomy was the treatment of choice.

Figure 9–13 Pulp exposures in adjacent primary molars. Hyperplasia of the pulp is not a contraindication for pulp treatment as long as the clinical and radiographic findings are normal. (See contraindications listed in Figure 9–11.)

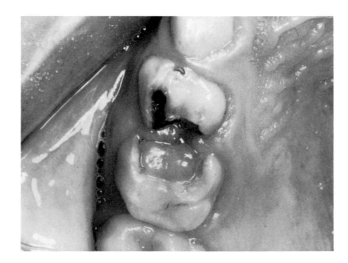

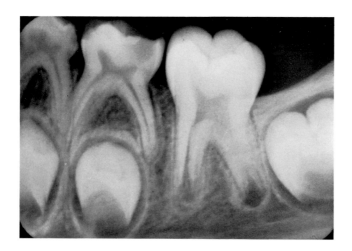

Figure 9–14 Radiograph of a carious exposure in a primary second molar. Formocresol pulpotomy is the treatment of choice.

Figure 9–15 Two primary molars with pulp exposures resulting from deep interproximal caries. There is questionable radiolucency in the bifurcation area and possible beginning internal resorption in the distal root of the second molar. In such cases, additional films should be taken varying the exposure time. It is also helpful to examine comparable radiographs from the opposite side to determine what is normal for the patient.

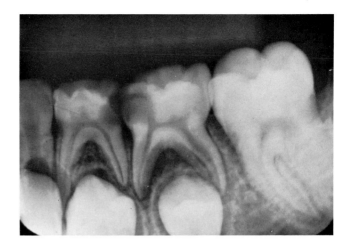

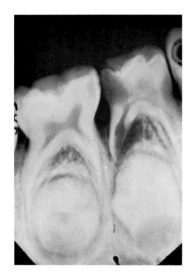

Figure 9–16 Radiograph of a primary first molar with a large carious exposure. Note the internal resorption in the distal canal and the radiopaque calcific body lying just above the orifice of the distal canal. These are indications of advanced degenerative changes of the pulp. Successful pulpotomy therapy is dependent upon proper selection of cases; with these degenerative changes it is definitely contraindicated.

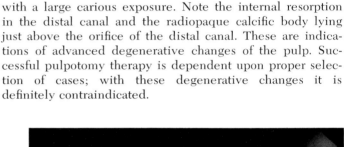

Figure 9–17 A 5-year-old child with advanced caries in both first and second primary molars. Note the pathological calcification above the distal canal of the first primary molar (a contraindication for pulp therapy).

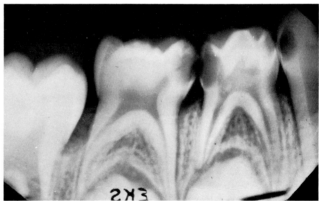

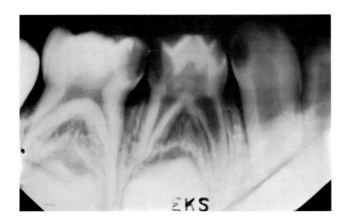

Figure 9–18 Same patient as seen in Figure 9–17, 6 weeks later. There is marked internal resorption of the first primary molar, indicating advanced degenerative changes. These changes were forecast in the earlier radiographs.

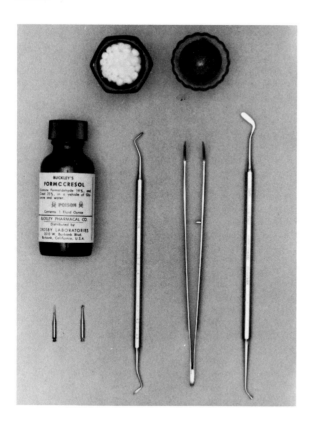

Figure 9–19 Tray setup for a formocresol pulpotomy; small cotton pellets, dish for formocresol liquid (Dappen dish), formocresol liquid (19 per cent formaldehyde, 35 per cent tricresol in a vehicle of 15 per cent glycerin plus water), fissure bur (high or low speed), round bur (low speed No. 4 or No. 6), excavator, cotton pliers, applicating instrument. The procedure for treatment of primary teeth with the 5-minute formocresol pulpotomy is described in Figures 9–20 through 9–24.

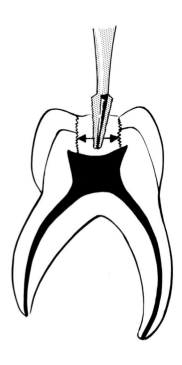

Figure 9–20 After the tooth is anesthetized, rubber dam is placed and the roof of the pulp chamber is removed with a fissure bur.

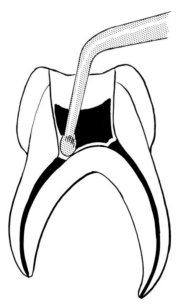

Figure 9–21 Excavator used to remove coronal portion of dental pulp. A round bur may also be used to remove the coronal pulp; however, extreme care must be taken to avoid perforating floor of pulp chamber with the round bur. Walls of pulp chamber must be exposed and no dentin must hang over to constrict the chamber. Pulp chamber is then flushed with sterile water.

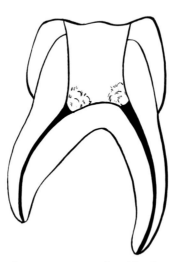

Figure 9–22 Hemorrhage is stopped with dry cotton pellets or a cotton pellet moistened with epinephrine. Hemorrhage must be stopped before placing cotton pellets impregnated with formocresol over pulp stumps.

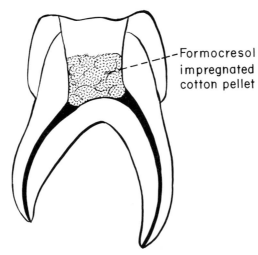

Figure 9–23 Cotton pellets moistened with formocresol are placed over pulp stumps and left in place for 5 minutes. Cotton pellet must not be so thoroughly saturated with formocresol that excess liquid might leak out under the dam onto the tissue. Formocresol is a caustic liquid and will cause tissue necrosis (see Figure 9–26). Excess liquid in the pellet should be absorbed by another pellet before it is placed in the pulp chamber. If hemorrhage has stopped after the formocresol-impregnated cotton pellet has been in place for 6 minutes, proceed to the steps given in Figure 9–24 for the final step in the one-stage formocresol pulpotomy treatment. If, however, hemorrhage has not stopped after 5 minutes or time is lacking to complete the restoration of the tooth, a two-stage formocresol pulpotomy may be performed. The formocresol-impregnated cotton pellets are sealed in over the pulp stumps with a zinc oxide and eugenol temporary filling. The patient is then scheduled for completion of treatment within 5 to 7 days. On the second visit, the cotton pellets are removed and treatment is completed as described in Figure 9–24.

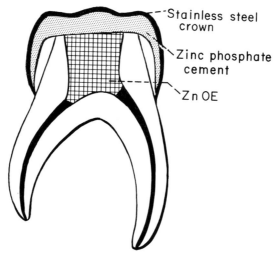

Figure 9–24 The formocresol pellet is removed and the area is left slightly moist with the drug. The pulp chamber is slightly overfilled with a paste consisting of zinc oxide powder and a liquid prepared by mixing equal parts of formocresol and eugenol. The preparation for a stainless steel crown is then finished.

Figure 9–25 Graph depicting yearly success rate in two clinical studies of 434 formocresol pulpotomies performed on primary teeth. Teeth treated with formocresol pulpotomy should be evaluated clinically and radiographically on the recall visit for success or failure. (From Law, D. B., and Lewis, T. M.: Formocresol pulpotomy in deciduous teeth. J.A.D.A. 69:601–607, 1964.)

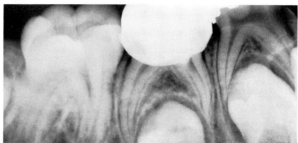

Figure 9–26 Formocresol burn from liquid that leaked out onto the tissue during pulpotomy procedure.

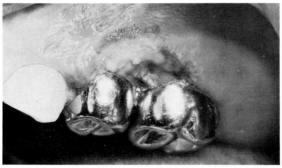

Figure 9–27 Radiograph of a mandibular second primary molar 2½ years after formocresol pulpotomy. This tooth was restored with a stainless steel crown. These teeth will often fracture because of the brittleness of the dentin from dehydration. Therefore, a stainless steel crown is the restoration of choice.

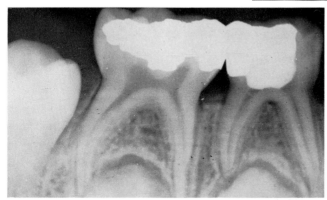

Figure 9–28 A first primary molar that exhibits a dentin bridge in the distal canal. This tooth underwent formocresol pulp therapy. Usually this drug does not stimulate calcification at the site of pulpal amputation.

Figure 9–29 An obvious formocresol pulpotomy failure of the mandibular first primary molar caused by degenerative changes around the distal root. Tooth had to be extracted.

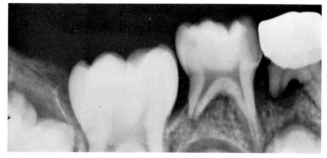

215

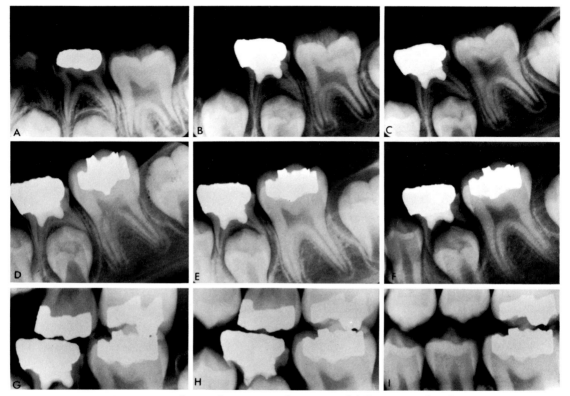

Figure 9–30 Radiographic series of a successful formocresol pulpotomy on a second primary molar over a 5-year period. Pulpotomy was performed when the child was 7 years of age. (Courtesy Dr. Donald R. Dietz.)

A, Preoperative radiograph of a 7-year-old child prior to formocresol pulpotomy of the second primary molar. B, Six months after pulpotomy. C, One year after pulpotomy. D, Two years after pulpotomy. E, Three years after pulpotomy. F, Three and one-quarter years after pulpotomy. G, Three and one-half years after pulpotomy. H, Four years after pulpotomy. I, Five years after pulpotomy.

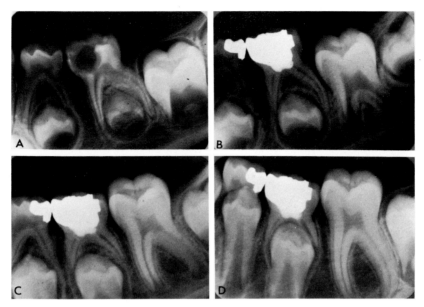

Figure 9–31 Radiographic series of a successful formocresol pulpotomy on a second primary molar. (Courtesy Dr. Donald R. Dietz.)

A, Preoperative radiograph of a 4½-year-old child prior to formocresol pulpotomy of the second primary molar. B, One year after pulpotomy. C, Three years after pulpotomy. D, Five years after pulpotomy.

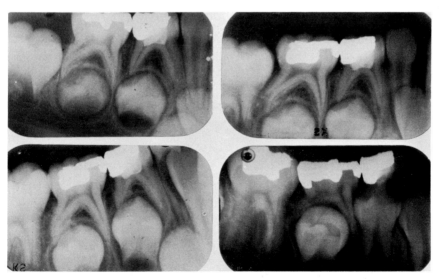

Figure 9–32 The first primary molar illustrated here received a formocresol pulpotomy when the child was 4 years of age. The tooth remained healthy and exfoliated at the usual time.

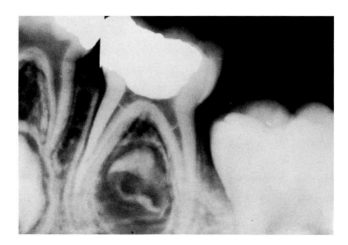

Figure 9–33 Successful pulpotomy using calcium hydroxide in a second primary molar. Dentin bridging can be seen in roots. Such bridging may not always be present in a calcium hydroxide pulpotomy.

Figure 9–34 Internal resorption in the mesial canal of a second primary molar following calcium hydroxide pulpotomy. This is frequently the cause of failure in calcium hydroxide pulpotomies.

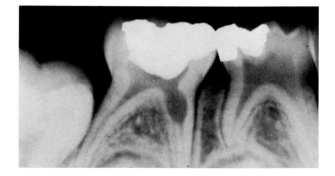

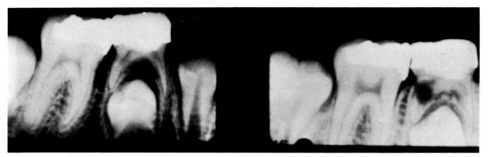

Figure 9–35 Rapid internal resorption in the distal canal of a second primary molar following calcium hydroxide pulpotomy. This occurred in less than 9 months. The tooth had to be extracted.

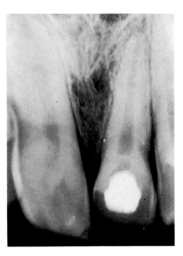

Figure 9–36 Radiograph of a fractured maxillary incisor showing a dentin bridge formed 3 months after a calcium hydroxide pulpotomy. See Chapter 17 for calcium hydroxide pulpotomy procedure on permanent incisors with pulpal exposures.

Treatment Procedure for Inducing Root End Closure of Nonvital Permanent Teeth

Acute symptoms of the involved tooth must be controlled before beginning root end induction procedures. For example, if an acute abscess is present, the tooth must be opened for drainage, antibiotics must be prescribed if necessary, and root end induction procedures must be postponed until the tooth is clinically asymptomatic.

FIRST APPOINTMENT

1. After access to the root canal is established, the coronal half of the canal is debrided with large reamers or files.
2. The canal is thoroughly irrigated and dried.
3. A cotton pellet moistened with CMCP is placed in the pulp chamber and sealed with a temporary restoration.

SECOND APPOINTMENT (7 DAYS LATER)

1. The temporary restoration is removed and the canal irrigated.
2. An approximation is made of tooth length in order to avoid any instrumentation of the thin apical dentinal walls. All instrumentation should be 3 mm. short of the radiographic apex. The dentinal walls are cleaned by peripheral filing. The apical portion of the canal should be avoided to preserve tooth structure and prevent disturbance of any apical cellular organization that may be present.
3. The canal is then irrigated, dried, and filled with a paste of calcium hydroxide U.S.P. and CMCP. The calcium hydroxide and CMCP are mixed together on a sterile glass slab to a consistency resembling that of silicate cement that is ready for placement. A small plunger-type analgam carrier may

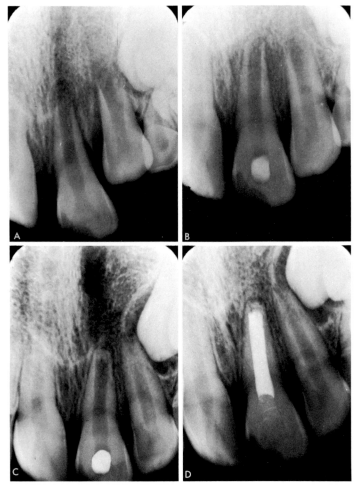

Figure 9–37   Treatment of a *nonvital* maxillary left central incisor with an incompletely formed apex in an 8-year-old boy. (From Steiner, J. C., Dow, P. R., and Cathey, G. M.: Inducing root end closure of non-vital permanent teeth. J. Dent. Child. 35:47–54, 1968.)

A, Fractured maxillary left central incisor with periapical lesion. *B*, Fractured incisor filled temporarily with calcium hydroxide and camphorated monochlorophenol (CMCP). *C*, Note root end closure of fractured incisor with calcium hydroxide and CMCP temporary filling. *D*, Permanent root canal filling with gutta percha 13 months later.

be used to insert the paste into the canal. The paste is then forced down into the canal with the blunt end of a large gutta percha cone or plugger. Overfilling does not seem to be a cause for concern, since the excess is apparently absorbed. The primary objective is to·completely fill and obturate the canal with paste.

4. A radiograph is taken to determine how well the canal has been obturated. Any adjustments to the root canal filling should be made at this time.

5. The excess paste is then removed from the pulp chamber. A small cotton pellet is placed over the canal orifice, and the remainder of the pulp chamber is filled with composite.

RECALL APPOINTMENT

The patient should be seen in 6 months and a radiograph taken at that time to check for any evidence of root end closure. If closure is occurring but is incomplete and the coronal seal is adequate, the paste should not be disturbed. If no evidence of closure is seen, the old paste should be removed and new material inserted into the canal. The patient should be continually supervised in this manner until the root end has closed sufficiently to permit placement of a conventional endodontic filling. This may take 12 to 16 months.

FINAL APPOINTMENT

When the apex appears to be closed on the radiograph, the paste is removed from the root canal. The walls are freshened with peripheral filing, and the root canal is prepared 1 mm. short of the radiographic bridge. It is then irrigated, dried, and filled with gutta percha using the lateral condensation technique. The patient should be followed every 6 months to make sure of continued success. It has been observed that failure with this technique has resulted when the paste of calcium hydroxide U.S.P. and CMCP was not left in the tooth long enough.

ENDODONTIC THERAPY IN THE PRIMARY DENTITION

Chapter 10 _____

Endodontic treatment of nonvital primary teeth has been successfully practiced by numerous dentists for many years. It is a rapid and uncomplicated procedure for treating those teeth for which a formocresol pulpotomy is contraindicated and that would otherwise be extracted. Endodontic treatment is an effective way to retain primary teeth and to avoid the necessity for a space maintainer. There are, however, contraindications that must be considered in order to prevent damage to the underlying permanent tooth or to the general health of the patient. Consequently, successful treatment will be achieved when based on proper case selection.

Indications

Teeth for which a formocresol pulpotomy is contraindicated because of pulpal necrosis may be considered for primary endodontics.

CONTRAINDICATIONS

The following are poor risks for treatment when long-term success is desired:
1. Perforation of the pulpal floor opening into the bifurcation.
2. Radiographic evidence of extensive internal resorption.

222

3. Coronal or root breakdown that could ultimately affect the long-term success of treatment.

4. Pathological resorption of bone over the permanent tooth.

5. A patient with a history of any chronic systemic disease.

6. A patient with a history of rheumatic fever.

Armamentarium

In addition to the usual dental armamentarium available for routine restorative procedures, suggested instruments and materials include:

1. Hedstrom files (stainless steel, 21 mm. long) sizes 15, 20, 30, 40, 50, 60, 70, and 80.

2. Silicone stops.

3. A plastic bottle of zinc oxide U.S.P.

4. A glass bottle of eugenol.

5. Irrigating solution (70 per cent isopropyl alcohol, sodium hypochloride, or hydrogen peroxide).

Procedure

1. Adequate *anesthesia* must be obtained so that the child will not experience any discomfort.

2. The *rubber dam* is placed.

3. Occlusal *access* is made with a high-speed fissure bur.

4. The *length of root* is obtained from the preoperative x-ray. Hedstrom files are marked with rubber stoppers to the estimated length for instrumentation (approximately 1 to 1½ mm. short of the apex).

5. *Irrigation* is performed after initial instrumentation (70 per cent isopropyl alcohol, hydrogen peroxide, or sodium hypochloride may be used, depending upon the preference of the clinician). Debris is evacuated with high-velocity suction.

6. *Filing* is performed with Hedstrom files in a pull-back direction to enlarge canals. The operator should be able to clearly visualize the orifice of each canal at the end of this procedure.

7. *Irrigation* is once again performed. NOTE: This may be the stopping point for a two-appointment procedure. A cotton pellet of formocresol is placed over the orifice to each canal and a temporary filling is placed. Two appointments are usually necessary when a draining fistula from the infected tooth is present.

8. The *root canal* filling is a soft, putty-like consistency of zinc oxide U.S.P. and eugenol mixed on a glass slab. A large amalgam carrier is suitable to transport the mixture to the tooth. A cotton pellet, held with cotton pliers, is placed over the zinc oxide–eugenol, and pressure is exerted on the material

to push it down the canals. A root canal plugger may also be used for condensation (this is an optional step). Other methods of filling primary root canals are equally effective, such as the pressure syringe or lentulo spirals.

9. *Recall evaluation* for children with endodontically treated primary teeth should be performed every 6 to 12 months.

Antibiotics

The use of antibiotics is seldom necessary.

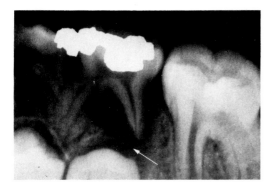

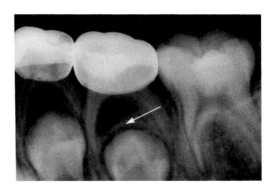

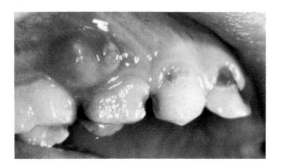

Figure 10-1 Note soft tissue lesion buccal to maxillary primary molars. This tooth has undergone pulpal degeneration and extraction could be considered. Removal is not always necessary, however.

Figure 10-2 Pathological bony resorption in bifurcation of second primary molar. If there is a solid layer of bone over the underlying permanent tooth, endodontics may be considered. However, when the continuity of the bone is invaded (see Figure 10-3), endodontics should not be attempted.

Figure 10-3 Endodontic procedures for this primary molar are contraindicated because it has caused pathological bone resorption over the permanent tooth. It would be a very poor risk for long-term success and should be extracted (see Figures 10-27 through 10-36).

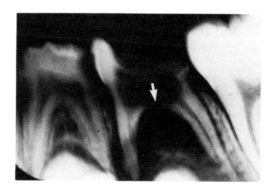

Figure 10–4 A perforation from the pulp chamber into the bifurcation or trifurcation is a contraindication for primary endodontics.

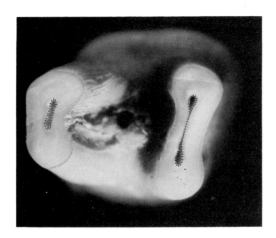

Figure 10–5 A mandibular second primary molar sectioned through the middle third of the roots — note ribbon-shaped canals. Although these canals cannot be completely filed, they can be effectively filled.

Figure 10–6 A maxillary second primary molar sectioned through the middle third of the roots — note shape of canals.

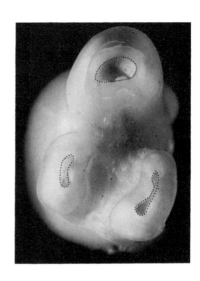

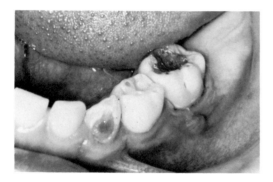

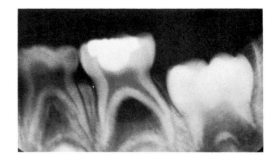

Figure 10–7 Same patient as seen in Figure 10–8 prior to endodontic procedures. Note soft tissue lesion buccal to the second primary molar.

Figure 10–8 Radiograph of same patient seen in Figure 10–7. Note pathologic condition in bifurcation and continuity of bone over permanent tooth. Endodontic therapy is indicated for this tooth.

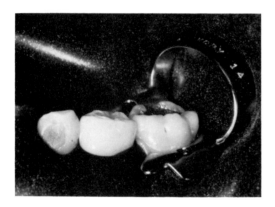

Figure 10–9 After adequate anesthesia has been obtained, the rubber dam is placed. Some children are more comfortable with their teeth resting against a mouth prop during the procedure.

Figure 10–10 Note access made in occlusal surface prior to instrumentation. Adequate access is necessary for visualization and manipulation during the procedure.

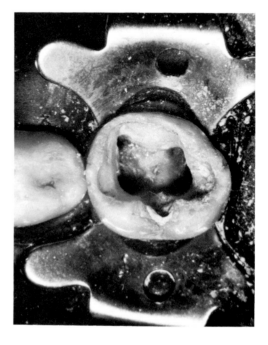

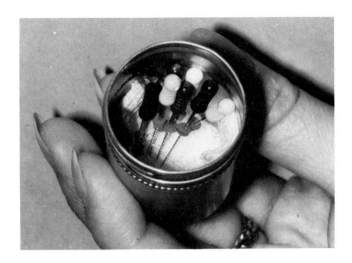

Figure 10–11 A small container is convenient for storing the Hedstrom files rather than mixing them with the large sizes used for permanent endodontics.

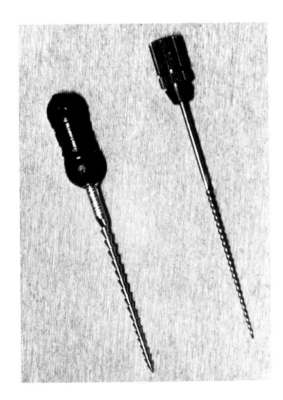

Figure 10–12 Note Hedstrom file on left used for primary endodontics (21 mm. long). The shorter length is preferred, since children have a difficult time opening their mouths wide enough to accommodate the standard 25-mm. file seen on the right.

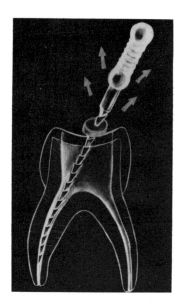

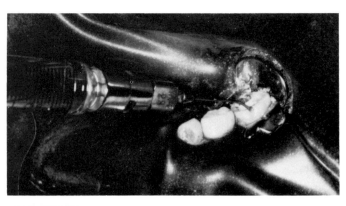

Figure 10–13 Diagram demonstrating action used with Hedstrom files. Cutting is accomplished by pulling the instrument out of the canal against the walls. Instrumentation is started with a size 15 Hedstrom file used to a depth of approximately 1 to 1½ mm. short of the apex. Cutting to a point at which a size 40 or 50 file can be used is usually adequate for most canals. However, the maxillary incisors and lingual canals of the maxillary molar usually require larger files, since they have wider canals.

Figure 10–14 The canals are irrigated after instrumentation with whichever irrigating solution happens to be the preference of the clinician — 70 per cent isopropyl alcohol, hydrogen peroxide, or sodium hypochloride.

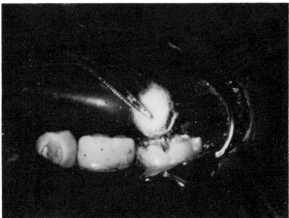

Figure 10–15 Zinc oxide–eugenol root canal filler is mixed to a soft putty consistency. When mixed this way it dissolves at approximately the same rate as the normal resorption of the root prior to exfoliation. It is carried to the pulp chamber and then condensed gently down the canals with a cotton pellet. Other methods of filling the canals, such as the pressure syringe or lentulo spirals, are equally effective.

Figure 10–16 Condensation of zinc oxide–eugenol with a cotton pellet.

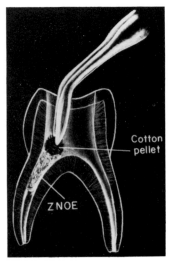

Figure 10–17 Postoperative appearance of second primary molar of patient seen in Figures 10–7 through 10–10, 10–14, and 10–15. Note the following:

1. *The distance that zinc oxide–eugenol condenses down canals.* This is considered adequate for primary endodontic procedures.

2. *The extrusion of zinc oxide–eugenol into bifurcation.* Whenever uncontrolled hemorrhage is encountered during instrumentation, there may be a perforation somewhere down the canal. This should be remembered, as excess zinc oxide-eugenol will likely be extruded out the perforation if excessive pressure is used during condensation.

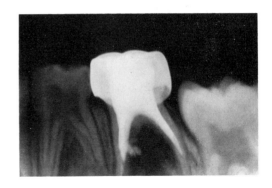

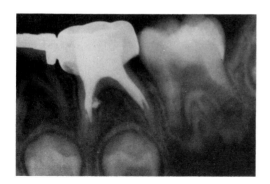

Figure 10–18 Postoperative appearance at 1 year of second primary molar of patient in Figure 10–17. Note the following:

1. Position of erupting 6-year molar.
2. Bony healing in bifurcation area.
3. Resorbing zinc oxide-eugenol.

Figure 10–19 Postoperative appearance at 2 years of second primary molar of patient in Figures 10–17 and 10–18. Note the following:

1. Position of 6-year molar.
2. Bony healing in bifurcation area.
3. Resorbing zinc oxide-eugenol.

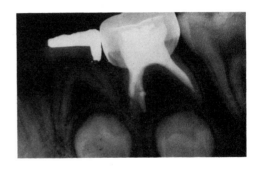

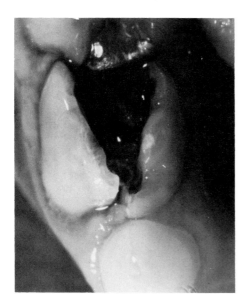

Figure 10–20 Unfortunately, endodontically treated posterior teeth become brittle and run the risk of fracturing. Consequently, for long-term success a stainless steel crown is preferred over a large amalgam restoration.

Note mesiodistal fracture of the mandibular right first primary molar. This tooth was treated endodontically. The fracture could have been prevented if a stainless steel crown had been placed (see Figures 10–21 and 10–22).

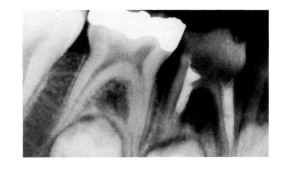

Figure 10–21 Radiograph of same patient seen in Figure 10–20. Note that endodontic treatment was adequate.

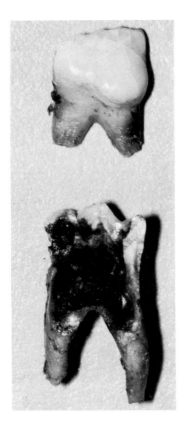

Figure 10–22 Extracted tooth of same patient seen in Figures 10–20 and 10–21. The fracture extended too far down the roots to save the tooth.

Figure 10–23 Endodontically treated maxillary left central incisor. Zinc oxide–eugenol was the root canal filling material. It was mixed to a hard putty consistency. A thick mixture of zinc oxide–eugenol should *not* be used, as it resorbs much slower than normal root resorption prior to exfoliation (see Figures 10–24 and 10–25). Note that the adjacent central incisor was treated with a formocresol pulpotomy.

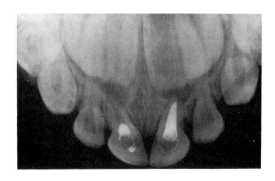

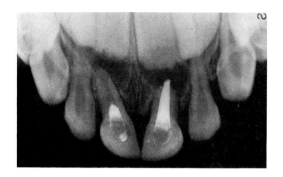

Figure 10–24 Same patient as seen in Figure 10–23. Note that zinc oxide–eugenol is not resorbing as fast as the root.

Figure 10–25 Same patient as seen in Figures 10–23 and 10–24. Note the delayed resorption of zinc oxide–eugenol. When the primary incisor exfoliated, it was necessary to curette the remaining zinc oxide–eugenol that had not resorbed.

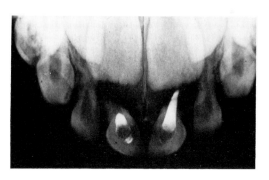

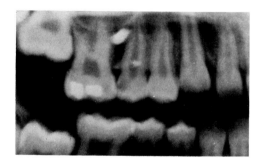

Figure 10–26 Unresorbed zinc oxide–eugenol between the maxillary first molar and second bicuspid. This remaining material is from an endodontically treated maxillary second primary molar that has long since resorbed and exfoliated. The zinc oxide–eugenol was obviously mixed too thick in this case. Note unrestored caries.

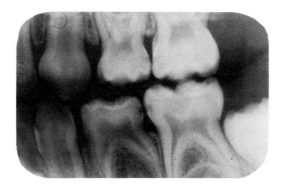

Figure 10–27   A routine bitewing was taken of this 4-year-old child to evaluate interproximal caries (see Figures 10–28 through 10–36 for ensuing problems related to the treatment of this patient).

Figure 10–28   Radiographic appearance of primary molars in same patient seen in Figure 10–27 at 6 years of age (several years after restorations were placed).

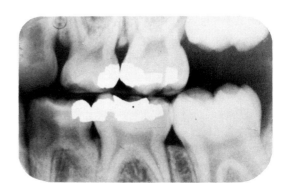

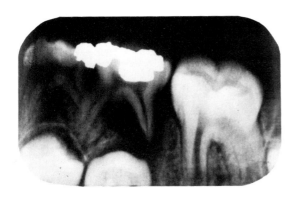

Figure 10–29   Same patient as seen in Figures 10–27 and 10–28 at 8 years of age. Note pathological bony resorption over second bicuspid. The second primary molar should have been extracted and a space maintainer placed. However, the second primary molar was treated endodontically, with resulting ill-effects (see Figures 10–30 through 10–36).

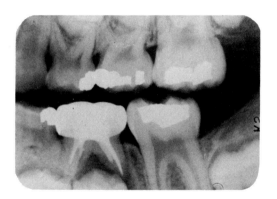

Figure 10–30 Radiograph of same patient seen in Figures 10–27 through 10–29 after endodontic treatment of the mandibular left second primary molar (age 8 years).

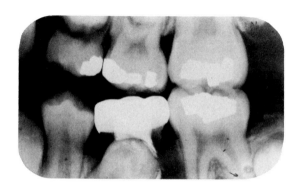

Figure 10–31 Same patient seen in Figures 10–27 through 10–30 at 10 years of age. The success of this root canal procedure is questionable, and a periapical radiograph should be taken (see Figure 10–32).

Figure 10–32 Periapical radiograph of same patient seen in Figure 10–31 taken on same day as bitewing in that figure. Note large cystic area around underlying permanent tooth. Primary endodontics should not be considered on a long-term basis whenever bone is resorbed over the permanent tooth as demonstrated in Figure 10–29. If left undetected, there is a chance that the pathologic condition may continue until it engulfs the underlying permanent tooth, with its subsequent loss. The involved primary tooth was extracted and the tissue was biopsied. The pathology report of the involved area indicated an apical inflammatory cyst.

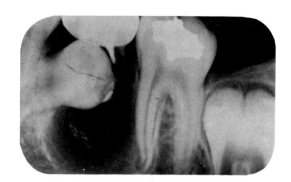

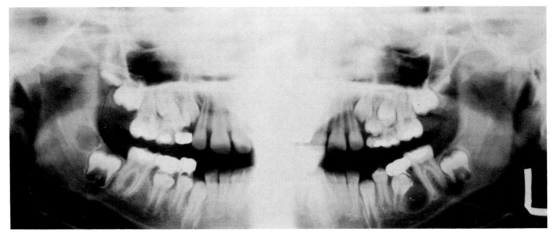

Figure 10–33 Panoramic radiograph of patient seen in Figure 10–32 at 10 years of age.

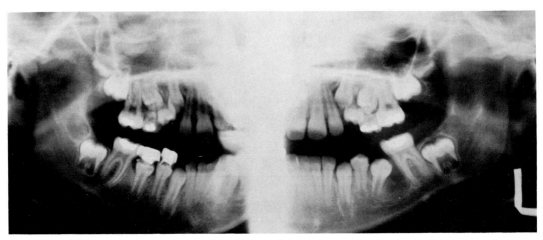

Figure 10–34 Panoramic radiograph of patient seen in Figure 10–32 after mandibular left second primary molar was extracted (age 10 years).

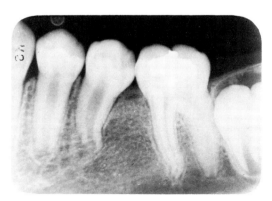

Figure 10–35   Periapical radiograph of same patient seen in Figure 10–32 (age 11 years) one year after the primary molar was extracted. Note position of permanent tooth and bony repair of former cystic area. There was no evidence of hypocalcification or hypoplasia of the second bicuspid.

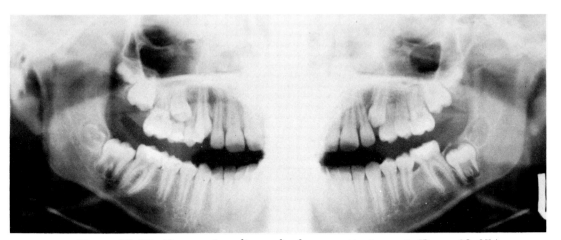

Figure 10–36   Panoramic radiograph of same patient seen in Figure 10–35 (age 11 years). Note maxillary crowding, which was subsequently treated.

REFERENCES

1. Cartwright, H. V., and Bevans, J. L.: Management of two abscessed primary molars in a four-year-old child: Report of interesting case. J. Dent. Child. 37:230–232, 1970.
2. Gerlach, E: Root canal treatment for deciduous teeth. J.A.D.A. 25:711–717, 1938.
3. Gould, J. M.: Root canal therapy for infected primary molar teeth — preliminary report. J. Dent. Child. 39:269–273, 1972.
4. Starkey, P. E.: Pulpectomy and root canal filling in a primary molar: Report of a case. J. Dent. Child. 40:49–53, 1973.

EXODONTIA IN THE PRIMARY DENTITION

Chapter 11 _____

The extraction of primary teeth is an integral part of any dental practice that includes children. Fear, the main deterrent to seeking dental care, reaches its maximum in a child anticipating any form of oral surgery. For this reason alone it is very desirable that the dentist who has successfully carried the youngster through many previous experiences (the first visit to the dental office, dental x-ray examinations, prophylaxis, and operative procedures) be the person to perform the extraction. Whenever possible, the child should be informed several days in advance that he or she has an appointment for a tooth extraction. If this is not done, he or she will be apprehensive of every visit to the dental office. Baldwin has indicated that a period of 4 to 7 days' prior notice of impending surgery is adequate for children, and that such a period of advance warning is a deterrent to adverse psychological reactions.

Recognition of an abnormality and diagnosis of the condition is a prerequisite to the correct resolution of any oral surgical problem. Good dental radiographs, therefore, are of prime importance before any surgery is undertaken. They are also essential for protection against medicolegal action.

The most frequent oral surgical problem in children is the extraction of one or more carious teeth. Good radiographs will determine if the roots of the primary molars are still fully formed and encircle the developing tooth bud. If so, extra care must be taken to separate the roots and prevent dislodgment of the succedaneous tooth. If a carious tooth whose roots are partially resorbed is to be extracted, the radiographs will denote the areas of resorption and potential areas of root fracture.

Dentists frequently see children when they are in pain from a toothache. If this is the case, the offending tooth is generally easy to identify

237

because of its mobility and sensitivity to percussion. Lymphadenopathy often exists along with soft tissue swelling and reddening around the affected area. Radiographs are essential as part of the diagnosis and should be retained as a permanent record.

The use of antibiotics in children needing dental extractions is an important consideration. A good rule to follow is if the dental abscess is well resolved and a fistulous tract established, and if the patient is asymptomatic and in good general health, an antibiotic is not mandatory. If, however, there is pain or fever or periapical swelling and adenopathy, and the infection apparently has not reached its maximum limit, or if the child has a chronic debilitating condition such as congenital heart disease, proper antibiotic therapy should be instituted.

One of the tenets of good surgery is profound anesthesia. Inasmuch as good operative dentistry is based on the same premise, the dentist should be able to provide this quite readily. Chapter 6 illustrates the procedures for local anesthesia. In some cases, especially with the very young child, extraction of teeth is best performed under general anesthesia. It should be pointed out that the decision to perform more complex operations, such as frenectomies, removal of impacted teeth, and the like, will depend entirely on the dentist's training and feeling of competency. He or she should, however, be able to diagnose these conditions, understand their implications, relate them to the parent, and render acceptable judgments as to when surgery should take place.

In all procedures with children, slow, smooth, and graceful movements as opposed to fast, jerky, and awkward movements are the most desirable. This is particularly true during extractions. Not only will such actions be conducive to good patient management, but they also will minimize breaking the roots of primary teeth, which are frequently thin and fragile. If a root should be fractured, it is advisable to be cautious in removing the root tips, so that the permanent tooth bud will not be jeopardized. Frequently, the better part of valor is to leave the embedded root tip and let it be exfoliated or resorbed. In such a case, the parent should be advised that the root tip remains. This should be recorded in the patient's chart, and the area should be rechecked at periodic intervals.

Young children seldom have any problems with healing of extraction sites postoperatively. So-called dry sockets are rarely encountered. Some discomfort, however, may be experienced when the local anesthetic wears off. It is a good procedure to have children bite on a gauze pack for at least ½ hour following surgery. In addition, the child should keep his or her head elevated and avoid eating or drinking for several hours. Soft diets are recommended for the first day, avoiding such foods as peanuts and popcorn so that food debris will not be trapped in the sockets. The prevention of lip biting can be a problem, but with the use of short-acting anesthetic agents and an appropriate warning to the child and the parent, trauma to the cheeks and lips should be infrequent.

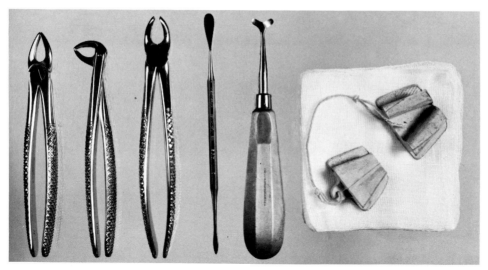

Figure 11–1 Suggested tray for routine extractions of primary teeth: Ash 37, universal maxillary pedodontic forceps; Ash 123, universal mandibular pedodontic forceps; Ash 157 forceps; periosteal elevator; Forsyth elevator (optional); 4 × 4 gauze sponges; two rubber mouthprops.

A mouthprop should be used during extraction of mandibular primary molars when excessive stress is applied to the opposite mandibular condyle.

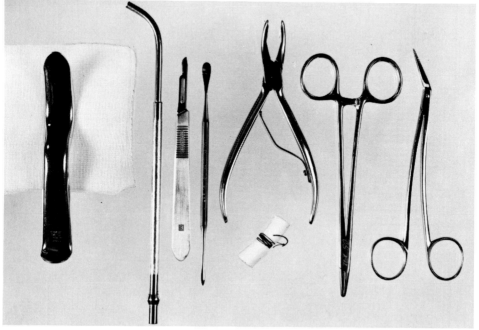

Figure 11–2 Suggested tray for tissue flap procedures: lip retractor, suction tip, scalpel and blade, periosteal elevator, rongeur, suture material with needle, hemostat, scissors, and 4 × 4 gauze sponges.

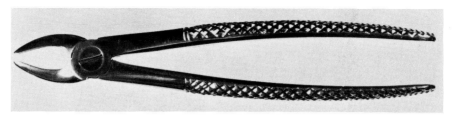

Figure 11–3 Ash 37 forceps used in extraction of maxillary primary centrals, laterals, and cuspids.

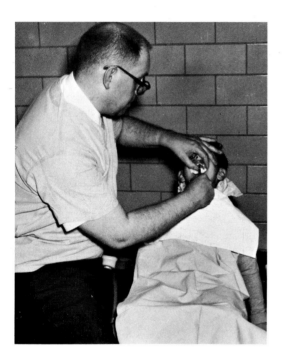

Figure 11–4 Position of dentist and patient for extraction of maxillary primary anterior teeth.

Figure 11–5 Placement of forceps for extraction of maxillary primary anterior teeth. Note position of dentist's fingers.

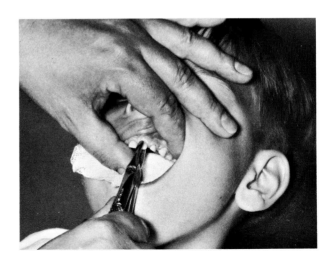

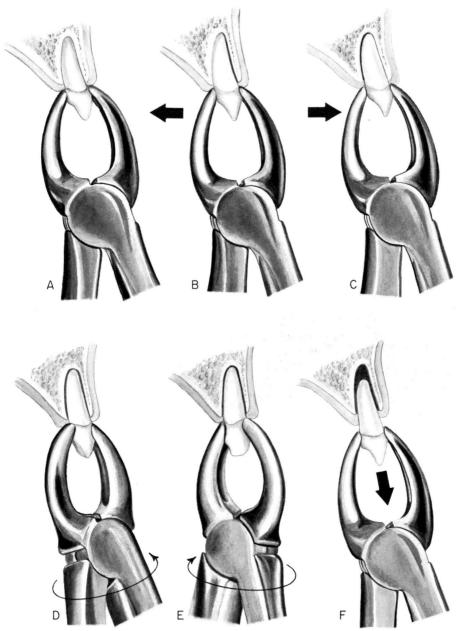

Figure 11–6 Movements used in extracting maxillary primary centrals, laterals, and cuspids. *A*, Placement of forceps. *B*, Movement to lingual and hold. *C*, Movement to labial and hold. *D*, Rotary movement. *E*, Rotary movement reversed. *F*, Extraction of tooth in path of least resistance.

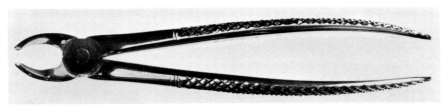

Figure 11–7 Ash 157 forceps used in extraction of maxillary primary molars.

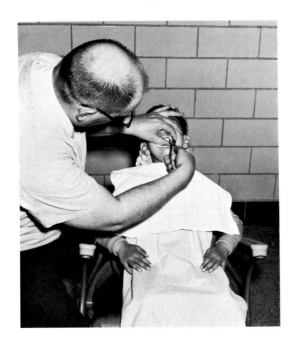

Figure 11–8 Position of dentist and patient for extraction of maxillary primary molars.

Figure 11–9 Placement of forceps for extraction of maxillary primary molar. Note position of dentist's fingers.

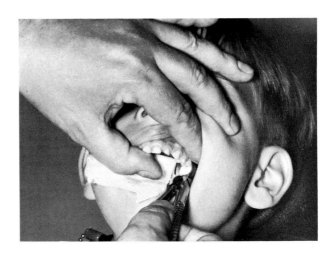

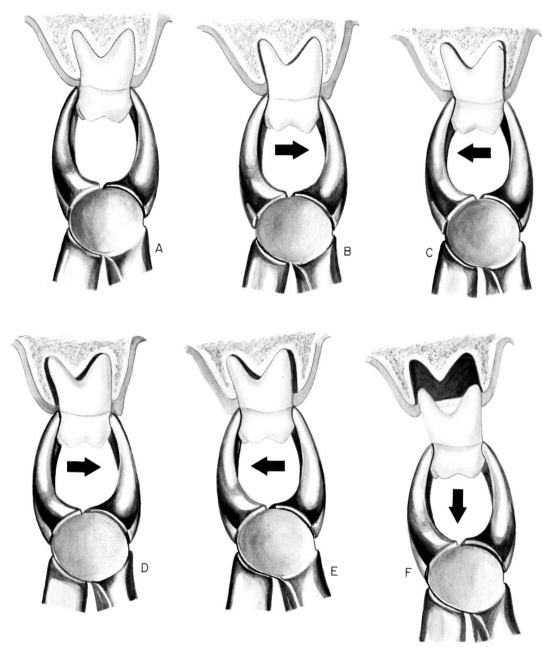

Figure 11–10 Movements used in extracting maxillary primary molars. *A*, Placement of forceps. *B*, Movement to buccal and hold. *C*, Movement to lingual and hold. *D*, Stronger movement again to buccal. *E*, Stronger movement again to lingual. *F*, Extraction of tooth in path of least resistance.

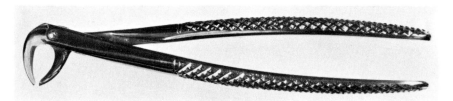

Figure 11–11 Ash 123 forceps used in extraction of mandibular primary centrals, laterals, and cuspids.

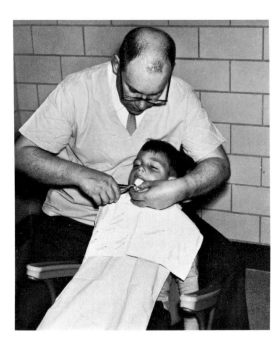

Figure 11–12 Position of dentist and patient for extraction of mandibular primary anterior teeth.

Figure 11–13 Placement of forceps for extraction of mandibular primary anterior teeth. Note position of dentist's fingers.

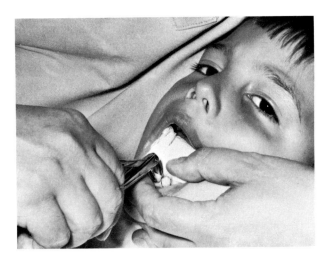

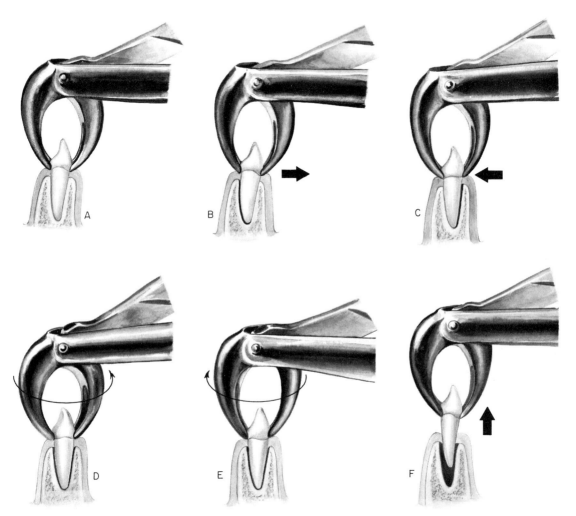

Figure 11–14 Movements used in extracting mandibular primary centrals, laterals, and cuspids. A, Placement of forceps. B, Movement to labial and hold. C, Movement to lingual and hold. D, Rotary movement. E, Rotary movement reversed. F, Extraction of tooth in path of least resistance.

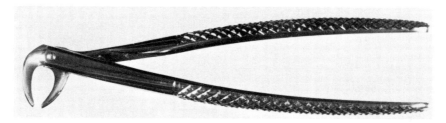

Figure 11–15 Ash 123 forceps used in extraction of mandibular primary molars.

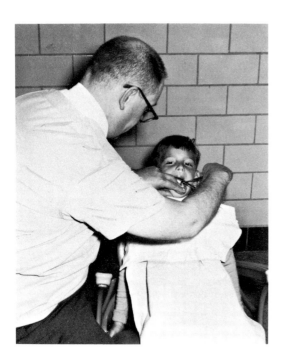

Figure 11–16 Position of dentist and patient for extraction of mandibular primary molars.

Figure 11–17 Placement of forceps for extraction of mandibular primary molars. Note position of dentist's fingers.

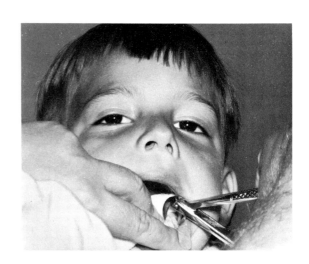

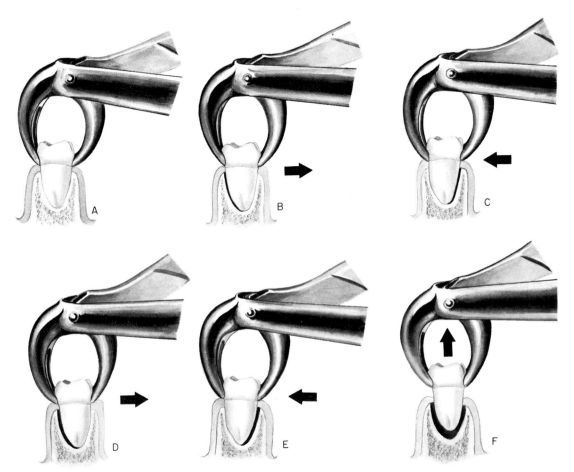

Figure 11–18   Movements used in extracting mandibular primary molars. *A*, Placement of forceps. *B*, Movement to buccal and hold. *C*, Movement to lingual and hold. *D*, Stronger movement again to buccal. *E*, Stronger movement again to lingual. *F*, Extraction of tooth in path of least resistance. Slight rotary movement may be used; however, when solid resistance is felt this movement should be diminished.

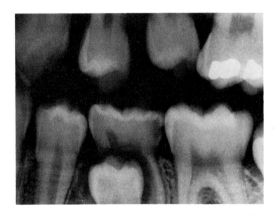

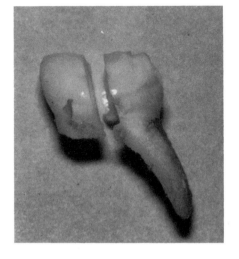

Figure 11–19 Over-retained second primary molar resulting from unresorbed distal root. This tooth was partially divided with a high-speed bur and then sectioned with a No. 301 elevator by rotating back and forth until the two segments broke apart. The two pieces were elevated separately and extracted (see Figure 11–20).

Figure 11–20 Second primary molar seen in Figure 11–19, after extraction. Note that the tooth was not entirely divided with the high-speed bur. Over-extension in this area may result in cutting into the underlying permanent tooth. Consequently, incomplete sectioning with the bur and final division of the segments with an elevator is suggested (see Figures 11–21 and 11–22).

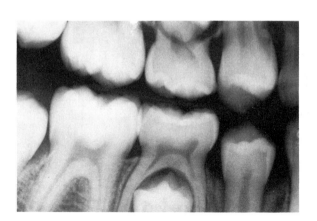

Figure 11–21 Bitewing radiograph of over-retained mandibular second primary molar at time of routine 6-month recall appointment. Prior to extracting this tooth, a periapical view was desirable to determine the extent and shape of roots (see Figure 11–22).

Figure 11–22 Periapical radiograph of patient seen in Figure 11–21. This tooth was obviously sectioned prior to extraction. However, the high-speed bur was used to *partially* divide the tooth, thereby avoiding cutting into the underlying permanent tooth. Final division of the segments was made with a No. 301 elevator as described in Figure 11–19.

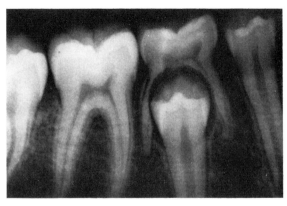

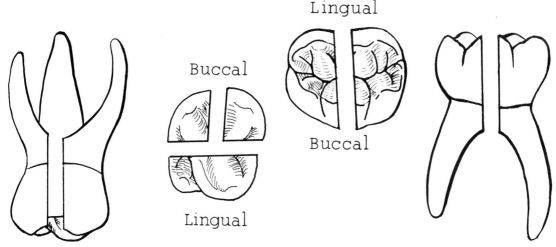

Figure 11–23 Three-part division of maxillary primary molar. Penetration of the bur into the trifurcation should be avoided unless the underlying permanent tooth is far enough away from possible cuts by the bur.

Figure 11–24 Two-part division of mandibular primary molar. Penetration of the bur into the bifurcation should be avoided unless the underlying permanent tooth is far enough away from possible cuts by the bur.

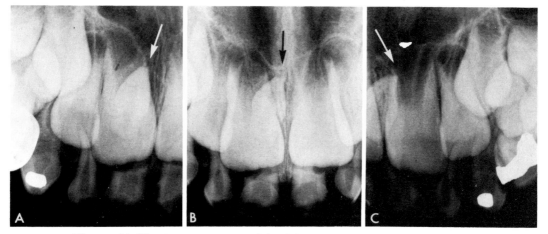

Figure 11–25 Determination of the labial or lingual position of a mesiodens can be frustrating unless several radiographs are taken. Whenever the mesiodens follows the direction of the movement of the x-ray head, it is located lingually to the other teeth. However, if it appears to have traveled in the opposite direction of the movement of the x-ray head, it is located labially to the other teeth. Note position of mesiodens in A, B, and C and how it has followed the direction of the x-ray head. This lingual impaction of a mesiodens was removed after a small palatal flap was reflected in this area (see Chapter 12, Pediatric Oral Surgery).

REFERENCE

Baldwin, D. C. Jr.: An investigation of psychological and behavioral responses to dental extraction in children. J. Dent. Res. 45:1637–1651, 1966.

PEDIATRIC ORAL
SURGERY

Chapter 12 _____

ROGER A. MEYER

Pediatric patients are subject to a wide range of surgical problems in the oral and maxillofacial area. Fortunately, because the dentist examines children at frequent intervals, he or she often sees these problems at their inception, and appropriate management is thereby facilitated. Most minor oral surgical procedures on children can be performed on an outpatient basis. The decision to hospitalize the child for oral surgery is based upon the patient's physical status, the length of the operation, the expected blood loss, the need for skilled postoperative nursing care, the potential for complications, and the need for endotracheal anesthesia to secure the airway. Patients should be admitted to the hospital for surgery when there is a co-existing medical problem whose management requires a degree of participation by the physician or by skilled nursing staff that cannot be provided to the outpatient. Operations which require general anesthesia and last longer than thirty minutes should be done with an endotracheal tube in place to ensure a good airway for the duration of the anesthesia. Note that the irritating effects of the endotracheal tube and cuff can cause significant edema of the larynx and vocal cords. Moreover, minor narrowing of the laryngeal aperature, which rarely produces ill effects in an adult, can produce partial or complete airway closure in a child. Thus, observation in management of the child after endotracheal anesthesia is mandatory and is best done in the hospital.

This chapter is divided into 10 sections:

I.	Examination	VI.	Salivary Gland Problems
II.	Surgical Technique	VII.	Frenum Problems
III.	Infections	VIII.	Trauma
IV.	Impacted Teeth	IX.	Tooth Transplantation
V.	Tumors and Biopsies	X.	Developmental Deformities

Examination

The essential components of a thorough examination by the dentist include: (1) observation of both head shape and head size, as well as observation of the relationships of the facial bones; (2) palpation of the neck for abnormal masses or enlarged lymph nodes; (3) assessment of cranial nerve function; and (4) evaluation of the oral and pharyngeal soft tissues and the dentition (see Figures 12-1 to 12-9 and Table 12-1).

I. EXAMINATION

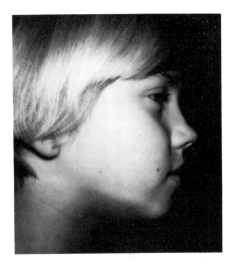

Figure 12–1 Check the profile for skeletal discrepancies (see Figure 12–8).

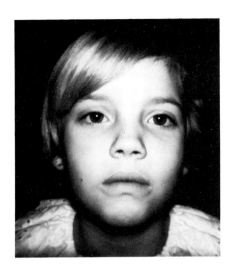

Figure 12–2 Examine the full face for asymmetry (see Figure 12–8).

I. EXAMINATION *Continued*

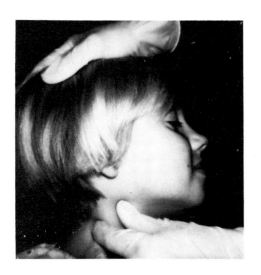

Figure 12–3 Palpate anterior cervical nodes (see Figure 12–8).

Figure 12–4 Palpate submental nodes (see Figure 12–8).

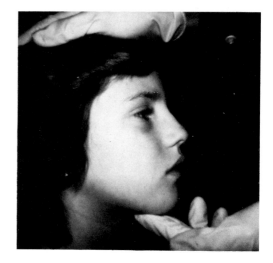

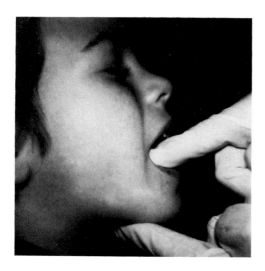

Figure 12–5 Palpate the submandibular area (see Figure 12–8).

I. EXAMINATION *Continued*

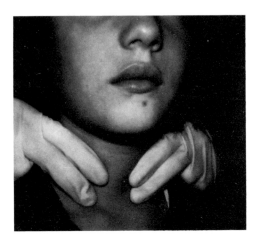

Figure 12–6   Examine the thyroid gland. Have the patient swallow in order to elevate the gland. A mass within the gland or a thyroglossal duct cyst may be felt.

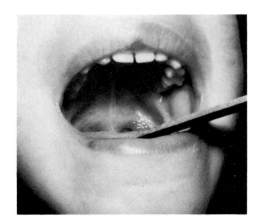

Figure 12–7   Examine the soft palate, tonsils, pharynx, and base of the tongue. Observe movement of the soft palate and uvula, note the size and appearance of the tonsils, and evaluate the state of the pharyngeal mucosa.

I. EXAMINATION *Continued*

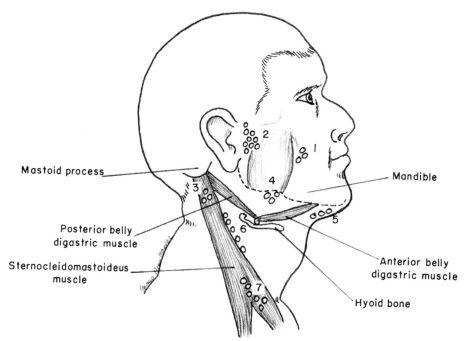

Figure 12–8 Important lymph nodes in the maxillofacial region: (1) facial nodes; (2) preauricular/parotid nodes; (3) superior deep cervical nodes (beneath sternocleidomastoideus muscle); (4) submandibular nodes; (5) submental nodes; (6) jugulodigastric nodes; (7) inferior deep cervical nodes (beneath sternocleidomastoideus muscle). Cervical lymph nodes may become enlarged secondary to acute bacterial odontogenic infections, chronic infections (e.g., tuberculosis, actinomycosis, cat scratch disease), or neoplastic processes (e.g., lymphoma).

Nodes	Maxillofacial involvement
Facial (1)	Maxilla
Preauricular/parotid (2)	Parotid gland
Superior deep cervical (3)	Adenoids
Submandibular (4)	Upper lip Maxillary sinus Mandible Submandibular gland Floor of mouth
Submental (5)	Lower lip Anterior floor of mouth
Jugulodigastric (6)	Tonsils Pharynx

All nodes drain into inferior deep cervical nodes (7).

I. EXAMINATION *Continued*

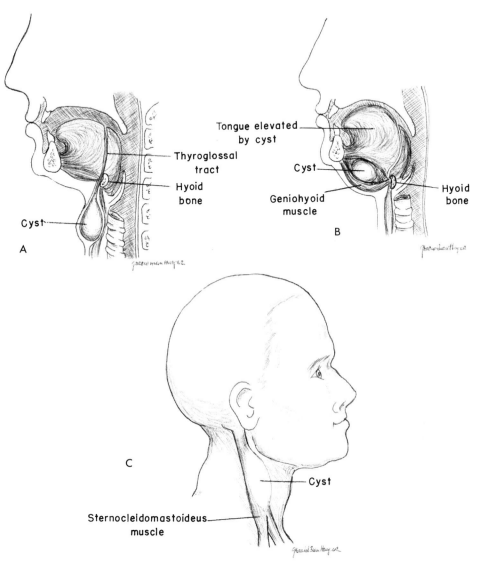

Figure 12–9 Developmental cysts that can present as swellings in the cervical region. A. The thyroglossal duct cyst develops from retained remnants of the thyroglossal tract and may be found at any site between the foramen cecum of the tongue and the thyroid gland. B. The dermoid cyst contains epithelium and skin appendages (hair, sebaceous glands, sweat glands). Both A and B are midline cysts. C. The branchial cleft cyst presents as a deep mass along the anterior border of the sternocleidomastoideus muscle. It develops from retained remnants of the first or second branchial cleft. Since these cysts may become infected or develop external fistulae, excision is the treatment of choice.

I. EXAMINATION *Continued*

TABLE 12-1   CLINICAL ASSESSMENT OF CRANIAL NERVE FUNCTION

CRANIAL NERVE	SIMPLE TEST OF FUNCTION	DEFICIT
I — Olfactory	Test sense of smell with familiar substance (coffee, peppermint) one nostril at a time.	Anosmia (loss of sense of smell)
II — Optic	Visual acuity — Snellen eye chart Visual fields — perimetry	Myopia (nearsightedness) Visual field defect
III — Oculomotor	All eye movements, except infero-lateral and lateral eye movements	Disconjugate gaze
IV — Trochlear	Inferolateral eye movement	Disconjugate gaze
V — Trigeminal	Sensory — pain, temperature, touch on forehead and upper and lower lips Motor — strength of contraction of masseter muscle	Anesthesia, paresthesia Weakness
VI — Abducens	Lateral eye movement	Disconjugate gaze
VII — Facial	Smile, wrinkle forehead Close eyelids tightly	Weakness Bell's sign (incomplete closure of eyelids)
VIII — Auditory	Cochlear — whispered voice Vestibular — stand with eyes closed, feet together, arms extended anteriorly	Impaired hearing Vertigo, inability to maintain position
IX — Glossopharyngeal	Sensory — gag reflex Special sense — taste on posterior third of tongue	Diminished or lost gag reflex Loss of taste (ageusia)
X — Vagus	Normal speech Motor limb — gag reflex	Hoarseness (weakness or paralysis of vocal cords) Diminished or lost gag reflex
XI — Spinal Accessory	Shrug shoulder — trapezius muscle	Weakness
XII — Hypoglossal	Protrude tongue	Fasiculations, deviation to affected (weak) side

Surgical Technique

Those performing surgery within the oral cavity should have expertise in certain basic surgical procedures. Correct placement of incisions, gentle handling of tissues, proper design and use of mucoperiosteal flaps, careful selection of methods of obtaining hemostasis, judicious drainage of infections, and meticulous suturing are all surgical fundamentals, regardless of which part of the body is being operated upon.

Clark has advocated "seven minimum essentials" in performing oral operations. Adherence to his principles assists in developing a systematic approach to surgery within the oral cavity. The seven minimum essentials are:

1. *Radiograph(s)* — one or more clear, recent x-rays of the operative site.

2. *Anesthetic* — an agent suitable for the patient and the operation.

3. *Forceps, elevators, and other instruments* — instruments appropriate to the operation.

4. *Flap tray* — additional instruments, sterile and ready, required in raising a mucoperiosteal flap.

5. *Light* — adequate illumination of the operative site 100 per cent of the time.

6. *Adequate assistance* — one or more trained assistants.

7. *Suction* — sufficient measures to keep the surgical field clear.

Certain of the elements in the above list — and some technical concerns not directly cited above — merit a few comments here. Specifically, the areas of instrumentation, mucoperiosteal flap procedures, drainage, and suture and needle selection require discussion.

Instruments. Among the instruments essential to oral surgery are scalpel blades, retractors, and bite blocks.

SCALPEL BLADES.   The No. 15 scalpel blade is used for most mucosal or gingival incisions. Drainage incisions are generally made with a No. 11 blade. The No. 12 blade is sometimes preferable for incising the gingival attachments around the teeth.

RETRACTORS.   Various types of retractors have been designed to protect the lips and mucosa during surgery. One or more of these should be available for every oral procedure.

BITE BLOCKS.   Bite blocks are useful in maintaining jaw position and in preventing transmission of force to the temporomandibular joints.

Mucoperiosteal Flaps.   Skill in designing and raising a mucoperiosteal flap is required of any dentist who performs an oral surgical procedure. Fashioning a mucoperiosteal flap is indicated whenever: (1) more adequate exposure of the operative field is required; (2) removal of bone is necessary; or (3) soft tissue may be injured by the contemplated surgery on teeth or bone. Thus mucoperiosteal flaps are used in cases involving (for example) removal or exposure of impacted teeth, recovery of fractured root tips, and biopsies of bone. Mastery of the basic technique of designing and raising a mucoperiosteal flap will enable the dentist to successfully conclude most minor oral operations. Of course, additional trauma occurs with the flap operation. The expected sequelae (pain, edema, ecchymosis) should be explained to the patient and parents, who should be provided also with appropriate instructions on postoperative care (application of ice, preparation of a soft or liquid diet, oral hygiene, use of analgesics).

Several important criteria must be met in the design of a mucoperiosteal flap:

1.   It must be large enough to give good exposure to all parts of the bony wound.

2.   Its base must be at least as wide as its free margin to ensure an adequate blood supply.

3.   The mucoperiosteum must be raised as a single layer, not split.

4.   Incisions must be placed over intact bone for adequate support during healing.

5.   The interproximal papilla must be included in vertical incisions placed near teeth.

Appropriate instruments for mucoperiosteal flap surgery should be readily available in sterilized pre-set packets or trays.

Although bleeding from oral incisions usually comes from capillaries or small vessels, large vessels in the tongue, cheek, lips, mandible, and palate are occasionally encountered. Bleeding from these vessels may be brisk and will require active management to minimize blood loss and prevent hematoma formation. Large soft tissue vessels should be clamped with a hemostat and tied with absorbable gut or silk sutures or coagulated with electrocautery. Nutrient vessels within bone can be occluded by crushing adjacent bone or by placement of absorbable gelatin sponges (gelfoam), oxidized cellulose packs (surgicel), or bone wax.

Drainage.   Evacuation of pus is possible when, as mentioned, a No. 11 scalpel blade is used to make an incision for drainage. Pain in overlying tissue is reduced with a local anesthetic, injected to form a wheal. If an abscess is "pointing" on the skin of the face, sterile skin preparation and draping are necessary. A ¼-inch Penrose drain is "feathered" and inserted into the abscess cavity to maintain drainage. The drain is held in place with a single suture.

Sutures and Needles.   A number of suture materials are available for oral surgery. Within the oral cavity, black silk and chromic catgut are commonly used in sizes 3–0 and 4–0. Black silk maintains a knot well and causes minimal reaction. Chromic catgut may come untied if squared "surgeons' knots" are not used, and it produces an inflammatory response. However, as chromic catgut resorbs or falls out in 1 to 3 weeks, it need not be removed — an advantage in uncooperative children.

Sutures that are swaged on to needles are easier to pass through the tissues than are un-swaged sutures. The preferred needles for suturing oral tissues are atraumatic cutting needles. Besides learning types of sutures and needles, the dentist should become familiar with various kinds of suturing techniques, including interrupted and continuous suture patterns.

II. SURGICAL TECHNIQUE

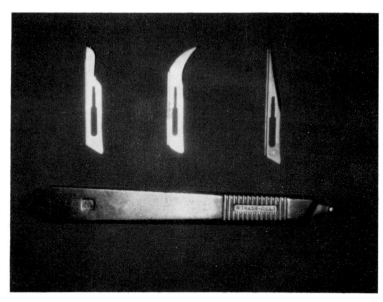

Figure 12–10 Scalpel blades Nos. 11, 12, and 15, and blade handle No. 3, used for various operations.

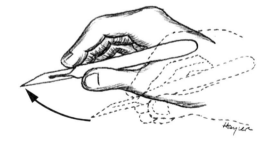

Figure 12–11 No. 11 blade, used for incision and drainage.

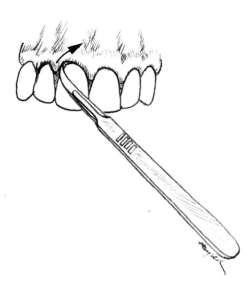

Figure 12–12 No. 12 blade, used to incise gingival attachment.

II.   SURGICAL TECHNIQUE *Continued*

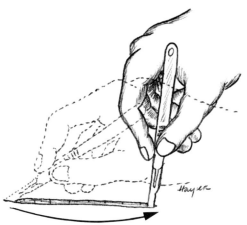

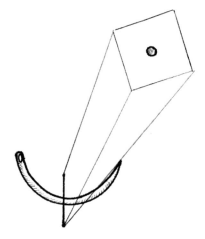

Figure 12–13   No. 15 blade, used for most muscosal or gingival incisions.

Figure 12–14   The type of suture needle shown here, a non-cutting (or "G.I.") needle, has a round configuration in cross section. It is difficult to pass through oral mucosa and gingiva and is unsuitable for oral suturing.

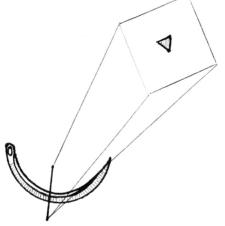

Figure 12–15   The cutting suture needle has a triangular shape in cross section and cuts oral tissue, facilitating passage of suture.

Figure 12–16   The eyelet needle requires that suture material be knotted for attachment. Knot circumference is greater than needle circumference, making passage of suture through tissues difficult.

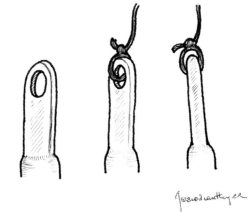

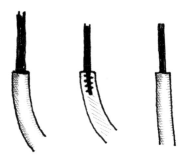

Figure 12–17   The "atraumatic" needle has suture material swaged into the needle shaft, making this needle preferable for oral suturing procedures.

II. SURGICAL TECHNIQUE *Continued*

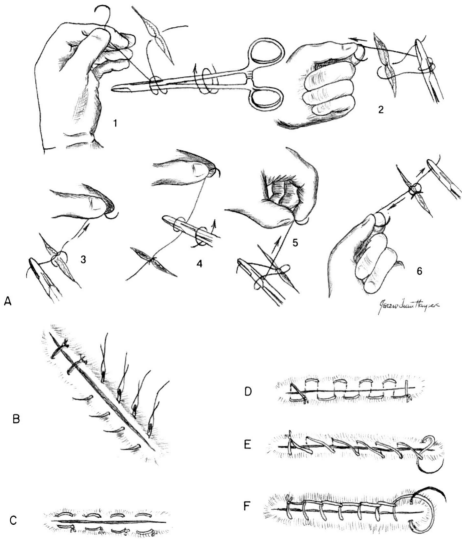

Figure 12–18   Suturing techniques. A. The instrument tie can be used for all suturing in the oral cavity. Technique: 1, The needle on the long end of the suture is held in the left hand while the needle holder makes two clockwise turns around it to form a loop. 2, The needle holder has crossed over to grasp the short end of the suture. 3, The hand and the needle holder have reversed positions to tighten the knot. The knot should lie to one side of the wound. 4, The needle holder makes one counterclockwise turn around the long end of the suture. 5. The instrument grasps the short end of the suture on the other side of the wound. 6, The knot is "squared" and tightened on the same side of the wound. B. Interrupted suture. C. Horizontal mattress suture, used to evert wound edges. D. Continuous horizontal mattress suture, which can be placed faster than other sutures because fewer knots are required in a long incision. E. Continuous suture. F. Continuous interlocking suture, useful in controlling bleeding from edges of an incision.

II. SURGICAL TECHNIQUE *Continued*

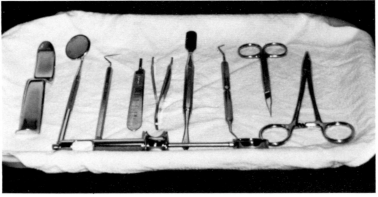

Figure 12–19 Instruments for a mucoperiosteal flap. Left to right: retractor, mirror, explorer, scalpel and blade, tissue forceps, periosteal elevator, double-ended curette, scissors, and needle holder. Bottom: anesthetic syringe.

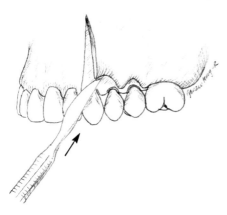

Figure 12–20 Use of the pointed end of the periosteal elevator to raise the interdental papilla.

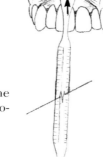

Figure 12–21 The rounded end of the periosteal elevator raises the remainder of the mucoperiosteum.

Figure 12–22 A "hockey-stick" flap for removal of a second premolar. The vertical limb is based on intact bone and the base of the flap is wider than the free margin.

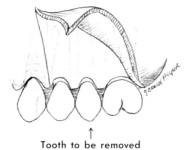

Tooth to be removed

Figure 12–23 An "envelope" type of flap for surgical removal of a mandibular first permanent molar.

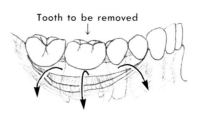

Tooth to be removed

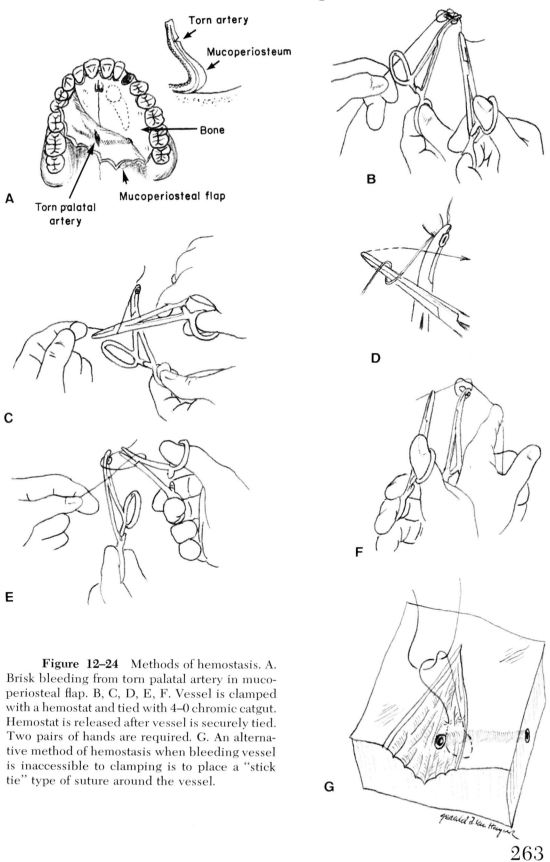

Figure 12–24 Methods of hemostasis. A. Brisk bleeding from torn palatal artery in mucoperiosteal flap. B, C, D, E, F. Vessel is clamped with a hemostat and tied with 4–0 chromic catgut. Hemostat is released after vessel is securely tied. Two pairs of hands are required. G. An alternative method of hemostasis when bleeding vessel is inaccessible to clamping is to place a "stick tie" type of suture around the vessel.

263

II.   SURGICAL TECHNIQUE *Continued*

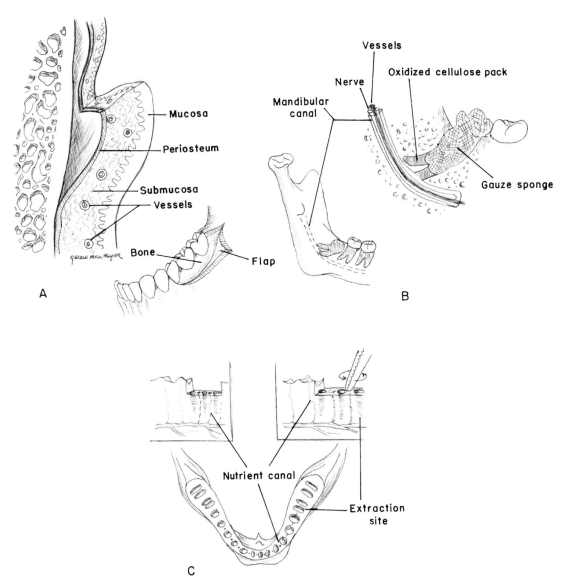

Figure 12–25   Further methods of hemostasis. A. Position of vessels within a mucoperiosteal flap. A suitable retractor prevents trauma. B. Hemorrhage when removal of mandibular molar root tears inferior alveolar vessels. Oxidized cellulose (Gelfoam, Surgicel) is packed against the bleeding vessel. C. Crushing, cauterization, or insertion of oxidized cellulose or bone wax will arrest the bleeding from nutrient vessels in bone.

Infections

Acute infections of the oral cavity are generally the result of neglected dental caries. If such infections spread beyond the confines of the periodontal membrane, an acute dento-alveolar infection develops. Unfortunately, children all too often present for their first dental care with the signs of such an infection — a toothache and swollen jaw. Affected children are irritable, frightened, and difficult to manage. Local anesthesia acts minimally, if at all, in the presence of infection. General anesthesia may be required if the dentist is to provide painless treatment. Whatever approach is taken, it is the dentist's clear responsibility to minimize any traumatic experiences the child may encounter.

An acute dento-alveolar infection, if untreated, can progress to facial cellulitis and systemic toxicity. The direction in which dental abscesses "point" (facially or orally) is largely determined by the relationship of the apices of the infected tooth roots to muscle attachments to the maxilla and mandible. Infection spreads first to adjacent fascial spaces; then, by fascial planes or blood vessels, infection spreads to the mediastinum or cranial cavity, with the potential for a fatal outcome.

Treatment of oral infections must be vigorous and prompt. Children usually mount a brisk response to infection and can appear quite ill. An evaluation of the blood pressure, pulse, temperature, state of hydration, condition of regional lymph nodes, ability to open the jaws and swallow, and status of the airway is essential. Additional requirements include an oral examination, x-rays, and a white blood cell count. The last of these is useful in determining the patient's ability to mount an appropriate response to acute infection. One aspect of such a response is, of course, the formation of abscesses, which should be incised for drainage. As part of the drainage procedure, samples of pus should be collected for Gram staining and culture for identification of infectious organisms. Such identification aids in the selection of appropriate antibiotic therapy. The initial antibiotic chosen for therapy — usually penicillin or erythromycin — should be given in a dosage calculated on the basis of the child's weight. Only when the infection is under control can surgical removal of teeth or other extensive procedures be considered (simple removal of teeth need not be deferred, though). During the course of treatment, the patient should be encouraged to drink fluids, and analgesics can be given for sedation and pain relief. Rapid resolution should occur; the patient whose condition does *not* improve requires special attention. A persistent rise in temperature, difficulty in swallowing or breathing, swelling extending into the neck or around the eyes, severe pain not relieved by codeine, increasing trismus, nausea, vomiting, chest pain, and changes in the sensorium are all signs of spreading infection or poor response to treatment. Immediate consultation with an oral surgeon is indicated, and hospitalization is often necessary.

III.　INFECTIONS

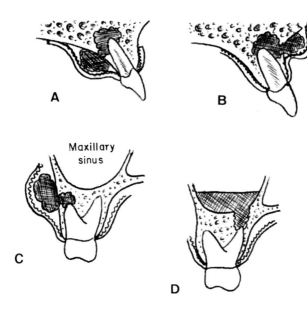

Figure 12–26 Pathways for spread of infection from the maxillary teeth. Infection can spread to the palate (A), to the labial space (B), to the buccal space (C), or to the maxillary sinus (D).

Figure 12–27 Spread of infection to the triangular area of the midface is potentially serious. The valveless angular vein in the infraorbital area may allow retrograde spread of the infection to the cavernous sinus.

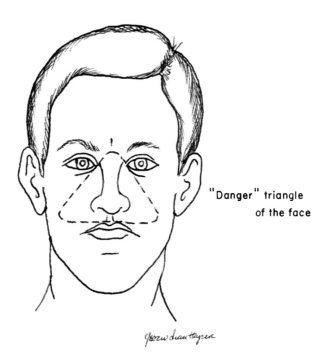

III.   INFECTIONS *Continued*

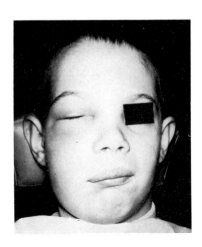

Figure 12–28   Clinical appearance of patient with infection in the "danger triangle" of the midface. Note fullness of the canine fossa with loss of perialar crease and periorbital edema.

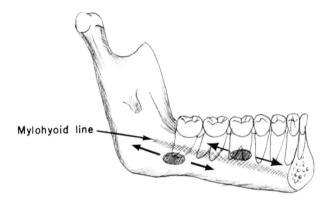

Mylohyoid line

Figure 12–29   Pathways for spread of infection from the mandibular teeth are governed by position of tooth root apices in relationship to muscle attachments.

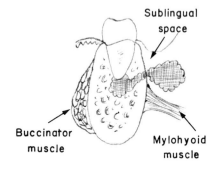

Sublingual space

Buccinator muscle

Mylohyoid muscle

Figure 12–30   Spread of infection from molar tooth root above the mylohyoid muscle attachment on lingual aspect of mandible involves the sublingual space and presents as a swelling in the floor of the mouth.

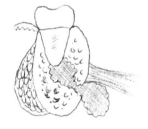

Figure 12–31   Infection of roots below mylohyoid line spreads to submandibular space with extraoral swelling (see Figure 12–33).

III.   INFECTIONS *Continued*

Figure 12–32 A and B. Buccal spread of infection from molar roots. A shows the spread of infection from molar roots below the buccinator muscle to the submandibular space, while B shows the spread from molar roots above the buccinator muscle to the buccal space (with oral presentation). C and D. Labial spread of infection from incisor roots. C shows the spread of infection from incisor root below the mentalis muscle attachment to the submental space, while D shows the spread from incisor root above the attachment to the labial space (with oral presentation).

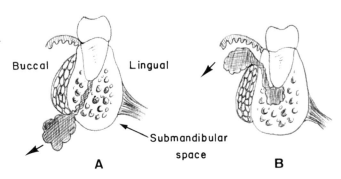

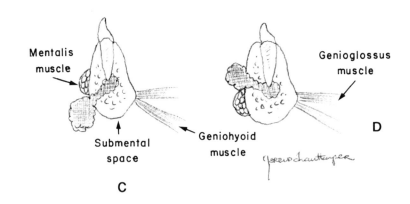

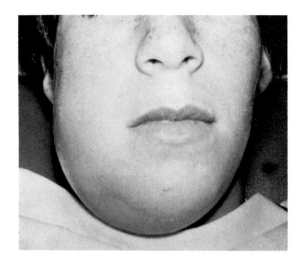

Figure 12–33 Patient with submandibular space infection (see page 265).

Impacted Teeth

A tooth is "impacted" when (1) it is still submerged beneath soft tissue or bone past its usual eruption time or (2) its normal path of eruption is blocked. Failure of a permanent tooth to erupt at the appropriate time may be due to lack of proper eruptive force, inadequate available space in the arch, or systemic conditions (e.g., hypothyroidism or cleidocrainial dysostosis). Early diagnosis is essential: if the tooth has functional significance, it can be guided into the dental arch; if not, it can be removed in order to prevent development of associated pathology. Therefore, x-rays should be taken of areas where permanent tooth eruption has been delayed past the normal time.

The maxillary incisors and canines and the maxillary and mandibular premolars are teeth which frequently have their eruption delayed. The maxillary incisors may be blocked by a supernumerary tooth. Removal of the extra tooth is often all that is required for the normal eruption of an underlying permanent tooth that has not completed its root development. Teeth with completed root development may lack sufficient eruptive force and this will require orthodontic assistance.

The maxillary canine often fails to erupt because of insufficient space. It may lie in either the labial or palatal aspect of the alveolus. Removal of an adjacent premolar and orthodontic assistance are often necessary to create adequate space in the arch. To facilitate eruption, surgical exposure of the canine is called for; to bring the tooth into the arch, orthodontic traction may be required.

Adequate space for permanent premolars is often lost if grossly decayed deciduous molars are removed before the normal shedding time and a space maintainer is not utilized (see Chapter 13, Space Maintenance). If collapse of teeth adjacent to a permanent premolar is not prevented prior to its eruption, the tooth will be impacted.

The third molar, or "wisdom tooth," is the most frequently impacted tooth in the human jaws. Most impacted third molars eventually become involved in a significant pathologic process necessitating their removal — often by extensive surgery, which increases morbidity. Among the pathologic processes associated with impaction of the third molar are:

1. Pericoronal infection with extension to adjacent fascial spaces.
2. Resorption of adjacent tooth roots.
3. Peridontal disease or caries of the adjacent tooth due to food-trapping.
4. Weakening of the angle of the mandible, making it more susceptible to fracture.
5. Formation of cysts or neoplasms in the follicular sac (e.g., dentigerous cyst, ameloblastoma, carcinoma).

The preventive approach — removing third molars as soon as it is determined that they are impacted — avoids these complications.

Inadequate space in the horizontal length of the mandible is the usual reason for third molar impaction. Since growth of the facial bones ceases at about the same time that growth of other bones in the body comes to a halt, a determination of whether adequate space exists between the second molar and the ascending ramus of the mandible can be made when the patient's growth is complete — i.e., after about 15 years of age in the female patient, and after about 18 years of age in the male patient. (Confirmation of growth cessation can be obtained from serial cephalometric x-rays or from wrist films to verify epiphyseal closure in the carpal bones.) Note that patients who have undergone removal of four premolars for orthodontic treatment are less likely than other patients to have impaction of the third molars.

Third molars are easiest to remove when one-half to two-thirds of root formation has occurred, which is usually at about the age of 17 to 20 in most patients. All four third molars are removed during a single operation, requiring only 15 to 30 minutes in skilled hands. Convalescence is neither longer nor more difficult when both sides are included in one procedure, and the patient is spared the discomfort and risk of a second procedure. Young patients heal faster and have fewer complications following wisdom tooth surgery than do adults. Clearly, most significant pathology is prevented by early diagnosis and removal of impacted third molars.

IV. IMPACTED TEETH

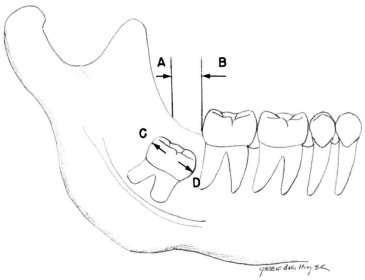

Figure 12–34 Making decisions about third molars. With the cessation of facial bone growth, at ages 14–15 in females and 18–20 in males, it is possible to determine if adequate space is available for eruption of third molars. In the mandible, the A–B distance must be equal to or greater than the width of the third molar crown (C–D) in order for there to be adequate space for normal molar eruption. If adequate space is not available, third molars become impacted.

IV. IMPACTED TEETH *Continued*

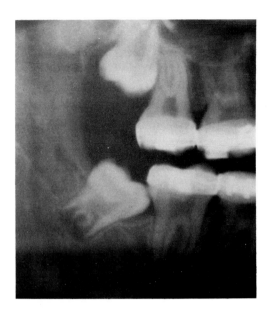

Figure 12–35 The optimal time for removal of impacted third molars is when root development is one-half to two-thirds completed, regardless of the amount of overlying bone.

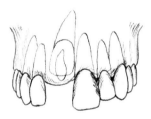

Figure 12–36 The maxillary central incisor region is often the site of a supernumerary tooth that prevents eruption of a permanent tooth. A radiographic evaluation will determine whether the supernumerary tooth is positioned palatally or labially (see Chapter 11, Figure 11–25).

Figure 12–37 Design of flap for removal of a supernumerary tooth from a labial approach.

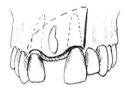

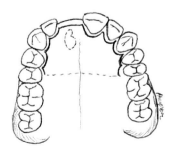

Figure 12–38 Flap design for removal of a palatally located supernumerary tooth. Contents of nasopalatine canal are sectioned to facilitate flap mobilization. Neither significant hemorrhage nor sensory deficit occurs.

IV.   IMPACTED TEETH *Continued*

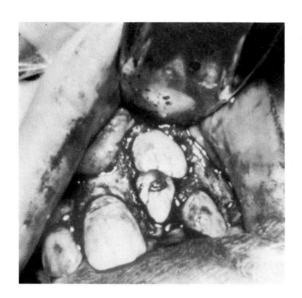

Figure 12–39 Labial mucoperiosteal flap design for exposure of a supernumerary tooth blocking the maxillary central incisor.

Figure 12–40 Removal of a supernumerary tooth (patient from Figure 12–39).

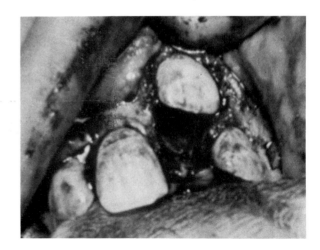

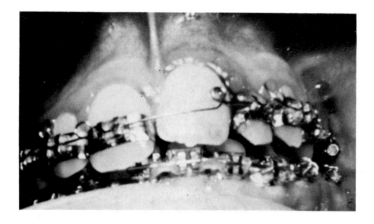

Figure 12–41   Patient from Figures 12–39 and 12–40 three months after the removal of the supernumerary tooth. Note that the central incisor has now erupted. Orthodontic therapy is frequently indicated in cases of this sort.

IV.   IMPACTED TEETH *Continued*

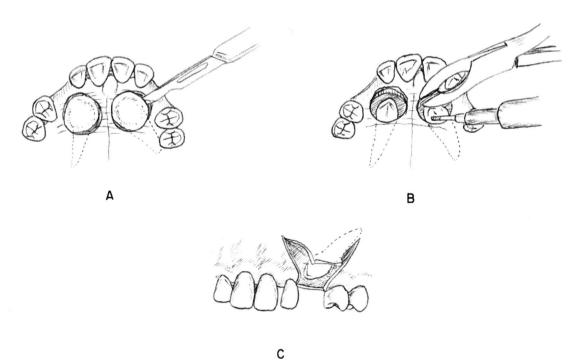

A   **B**

C

Figure 12–42 Exposure of the maxillary canine tooth. A. Excision of overlying mucoperiosteum. B. Removal of overlying bone and follicular sac. C. Modification of technique for labially located canine in order to (1) preserve attached gingiva around neck of tooth as it erupts and (2) prevent periodontal problems. A mucosal flap is raised, leaving periosteum attached to bone. Tooth is exposed by removal of periosteum and bone *only* over the crown. Flap containing attached gingiva is sutured to periosteum superior to crown.

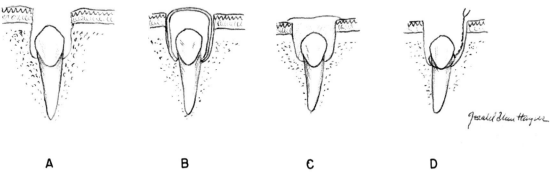

A   **B**   **C**   **D**

Figure 12–43 Adequate exposure of the crown of a tooth provides the best chance of the tooth erupting. A. All bone and soft tissue are removed to the level of the cervical line. B to D. Methods of management of exposed crown, including: placement of celluloid crown form filled with zinc oxide cement (B); filling the surgical defect with surgical cement (C); and placement of a wire ligature around the cervical line for orthodontic traction (D). Surgical packing or crown forms must be kept in place for at least two weeks; significant eruption of tooth often occurs during that time. Coordinating this care with that provided by an orthodontist is definitely indicated as the best form of treatment.

Tumors and Biopsies

Tumors in Children.   Squamous cell carcinoma is seldom found in the oral cavities of children. Most benign or malignant neoplasms in children, whether in soft tissue or bone, are of connective tissue origin rather than epithelial origin.

Vascular Lesions.   Hemangiomas in the soft tissue give a purplish hue to overlying skin or mucosa. Usually painless and easily compressible, hemangiomas blanch when subjected to pressure.

Central vascular lesions of bone are often accompanied by throbbing pain and loosening or extrusion of associated teeth. Radiographs demonstrate a radiolucent area, and palpation and auscultation frequently reveal a thrill and bruit, respectively.

Cysts.   Within the jaws, various types of cysts develop in association with teeth (e.g., dentigerous, primordial, and radicular cysts) or at areas of bony or epithelial fusion (e.g., globulomaxillary, naso-alveolar, incisive canal, and median palatine cysts). Other cysts may develop from branchial cleft or thyroglossal duct remnants and are found in the cervical region.

Biopsies.   Suspicious lesions, particularly those thought to be malignant, should be biopsied as soon as possible. Proper handling of the specimen for submission to the pathologist for diagnosis is outlined below:

1.   Avoid crushing tissue with instruments.

2.   Include normal tissue surrounding the specimen for comparison under the microscope.

3.   Use a scalpel rather than cautery.

4.   Tag tissue margins to orient the specimen position if indicated.

5.   Immediately fix the specimen in 10 per cent formalin solution.

6.   Submit along with the specimen a brief written history for use by the pathologist.

An *incisional* or *excisional* biopsy may be done, depending on the size and type of lesion. Biopsy of bony lesions requires raising a mucoperiosteal flap to gain access. Trauma to adjacent teeth, blood vessels, or nerves should be avoided. Vascular lesions should not be biopsied by the inexperienced surgeon.

V. TUMORS AND BIOPSIES

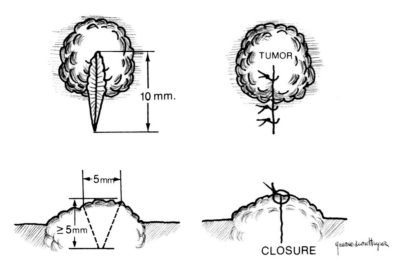

Figure 12-44 Incisional biopsy is generally called for when large lesions are present or when there is a question of malignancy. Surrounding normal tissue should be included with the specimen.

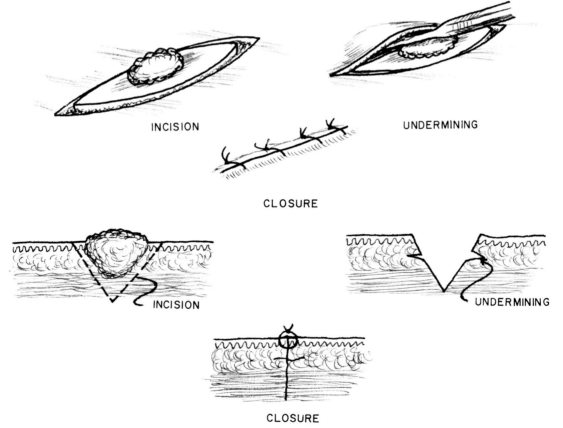

Figure 12-45 Excisional biopsy of a small, benign-appearing lesion. An adequate margin of normal tissue must be present on all sides of the specimen to insure complete removal.

Salivary Gland Problems

The structures responsible for the secretion of saliva include the major salivary glands — the parotid, submandibular, and sublingual glands — and collections of minor salivary tissue located principally in the lips and palate. Pedodontic interest in lesions of the salivary glands centers on infections, stone formation and obstruction, the mucus escape phenomenon, and tumors.

The most common salivary gland infection in children is probably viral parotitis ("mumps"). There is painful, diffuse, bilateral swelling of all the major salivary glands, accompanied by signs of systemic illness. Treatment by the pediatrician is primarily aimed at reducing the severity of symptoms. The disease is usually self-limiting, but occasionally encephalitis, orchitis, or pancreatitis may arise as a complication.

Stones (sialoliths) can form in salivary ducts, especially the submandibular (Wharton's) duct. Stones often become calcified and are visible on a mandibular occlusal x-ray. Obstruction of salivary flow causes swelling of the gland, especially during eating. Stasis within the salivary system may lead to secondary bacterial infection (sialadenitis) with purulent drainage from the salivary duct orifice. Surgery to remove stones obstructing Wharton's duct requires careful dissection to avoid injury to the lingual nerve.

The escape of secretions from the minor salivary glands of the lower lip into the surrounding tissues, evidenced by a *mucocele* in the lip, is common. Treatment for this problem, also known as the mucus escape phenomenon, requires total excision of the mucocele and removal of associated salivary tissue.

Salivary collection in the floor of the mouth (ranula) is usually due to escape from the sublingual gland. Removal of the mucosa overlying the ranula and marsupialization will often serve as adequate treatment. Recurrence of a ranula is usually treated by total excision of the sublingual gland.

Neoplasms of the salivary glands are uncommon in children under 16 years of age. When a neoplasm does arise, it may involve a major salivary gland — usually the parotid or submandibular gland — or minor salivary tissue — usually the salivary glands of the palate. A salivary gland tumor presents initially as a discrete, firm mass within the gland, rather than as a diffuse enlargement. Benign tumors are generally painless and grow slowly. In contrast, malignant tumors, which often are rock-hard in consistency, are painful and enlarge rapidly; in patients with malignant tumors of the parotid gland, weakness of the facial nerve is also common. Whenever a suspect growth of any type is found at a salivary gland, the affected patient should be referred to an oral surgeon.

VI. SALIVARY GLAND PROBLEMS

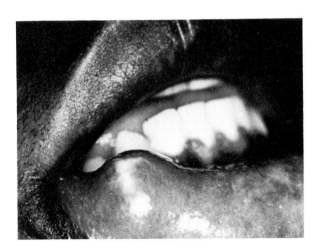

Figure 12–46 A mucocele in the lower lip results from the escape of salivary secretions into surrounding tissues.

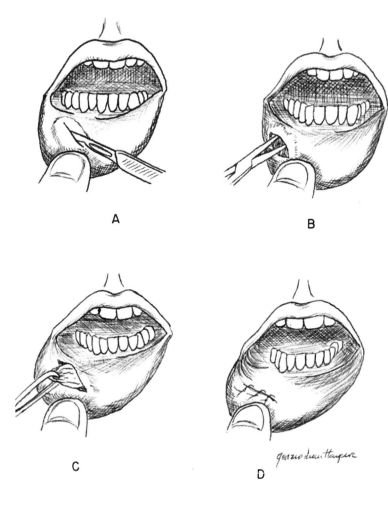

A

B

C

D

Figure 12–47 Removal of mucocele. A. Incision for removal of mucocele must be made just through the mucosa to avoid accidently decompressing the lesion. B. Mucosa is undermined, and the mucocele and associated salivary tissue are exposed. C. Mucocele and salivary tissue are excised en toto. D. Mucosa is closed with interrupted sutures.

VI.   SALIVARY GLAND PROBLEMS *Continued*

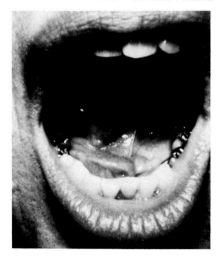

Figure 12–48 A ranula is due to the escape of salivary excretions (from the sublingual gland) in the floor of the mouth.

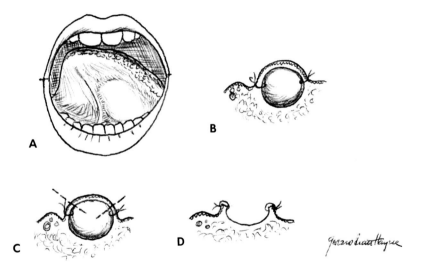

Figure 12–49   Treatment of a ranula. A. Ranula. B. Sutures are placed around the periphery of the lesion. C. The lesion is marsupulized by excision of the overlying mucosa. D. The exteriorized cavity should prevent recurrence.

Frenum Problems

A prominent maxillary labial frenum is often associated with a diastema between the primary or permanent central incisors. However, pressure from the permanent maxillary lateral incisors and canines as they erupt usually causes narrowing or closure of the space. If a diastema persists and the child's parents request treatment, consultation with an orthodontist is recommended. Generally the space is closed orthodontically first, followed by excision of the frenum. Gentle traction on the upper lip often causes blanching of the incisive papilla and shows the extent of the fibers of the frenum. These fibers should be incised during frenectomy.

The use of absorbable sutures (3–0 or 4–0 chromic catgut) is recommended (when necessary) in frenum surgery. Removal of silk or other nonabsorbable sutures from frenectomy sites is often painful.

Some children have an abnormally short lingual frenum (ankyloglossia, "tongue-tie"). The tongue may be bound down to the floor of the mouth, restricting its normal movement and interfering with speech and swallowing. The short lingual frenum may be irritated or ulcerated by the incisal edges of the lower incisors during forward tongue movement. Surgical correction of ankyloglossia should be deferred until a definite problem (lisping, frenum irritation, complaint of lack of tongue mobility) occurs. The practice of performing a frenectomy on every infant or young child with a short lingual frenum is to be condemned. Most patients either outgrow the problem or are never bothered by it. If after lingual frenectomy a speech impediment persists, consultation with a speech therapist should be sought.

VII.   FRENUM PROBLEMS

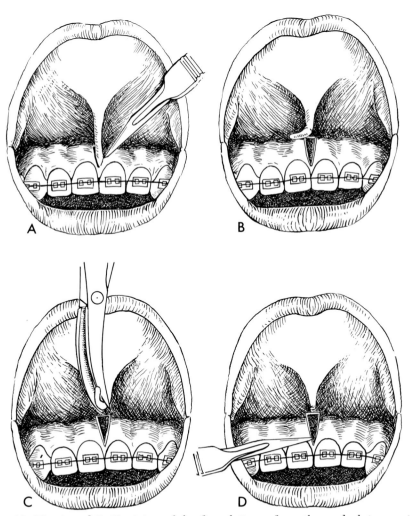

Figure 12–50   A and B. Excision of the frenal tissue from the underlying periosteum to a height approximately 3 mm. into the mucosal tissue. C. Removal of excised frenum from mucosal tissue. Extensive removal of mucosal tissue is not indicated. D. Denudation of alveolar bone by sharp excision of periosteum followed by destruction of transseptal fibers. (Modified from Edwards, J. G.: The diastema, the frenum, the frenectomy: A clinical study. Am. J. Orthod., 71:489, May, 1977.)

Trauma

Injuries involving the jaws and facial structures are not uncommon in active children. The incidence of such injuries can be minimized by the use of: (1) over-the-shoulder seat belts for automobile and school bus passengers; (2) helmets for motorcycle riders; and (3) protective headgear and mouth guards for participants in athletics.

Although the child with a facial injury usually is treated by an oral surgeon, the dentist may be called upon to evaluate the patient's dental or mouth injuries (see Chapters 16 and 17, on trauma in the primary and permanent dentitions). In such a case, the maxilla and mandible should be carefully checked for fractures. *Abnormal mobility* of the bones and *dental malocclusion* are hallmarks of fractures of the jaws. Radiographs confirm the presence of fractures.

Fracture treatment includes reduction into normal anatomical alignment and fixation for stability during the healing period, usually 4 to 6 weeks. Open reduction with direct bone wiring or bone plates or use of external pin fixation is seldom indicated in children and carries the risk of damage to permanent tooth buds. Re-establishment of *normal dental occlusion* is the key to fracture treatment, and it can often be accomplished with *intermaxillary fixation.* When attachment of dental arch bars to the teeth for intermaxillary fixation is difficult because of mixed dentition, *occlusal splints* attached by *circumferential* wires to the maxilla or mandible may be used. Alveolar fractures and loosened teeth are stabilized by application of an arch bar or an acrylic splint to a single dental arch.

Lacerations of the oral soft tissues should be thoroughly cleansed and closed primarily. Primary repair lowers the incidence of infection, reduces the formation of scar tissue, and lessens pain during healing.

All patients with orally compounded fractures require antibiotic medication, analgesics for pain relief, a full liquid diet with adequate protein and calories, and instruction in good oral hygiene.

Fractures of the mandibular condyle deserve special attention in the growing child because of their potential for complications. Condylar fractures should always be suspected in the child with chin injuries accompanied by preauricular pain (unilateral or bilateral) and open bite malocclusion. Treatment of the patient who exhibits these signs and in whom a diagnosis of condylar fracture is confirmed involves intermaxillary fixation, placed only to correct malocclusion. Early mobilization of the jaws — e.g., after 1 to 2 weeks — is advised so as to break up fibrous adhesions in the periarticular region and to re-establish normal mandibular opening and excursions. While the treated fracture may heal without incident, there still are potential problems that should be brought to the parents' attention. Fibrous or bony ankylosis of the temporomandibular joint may occur, leaving the jaw a limited capacity for opening and restricting access to areas of the mouth requiring dental care. Moreover, because the condyle is one of the growth areas of the mandible, the mandible on the injured side may not develop fully. Obviously, the child must be re-examined regularly during the growth period. Should ankylosis of the temporomandibular joint or a developmental deformity of the mandible arise, the child is referred to an oral and maxillofacial surgeon for correction of the abnormality.

Permanent teeth that have been avulsed completely out of the alveolus should be recovered for re-implantation, which can be successful in children if carried out soon after the accident (see also Chapter 17, Trauma to the Permanent Dentition). Even if re-implanted teeth are eventually lost to root resorption (a common occurrence), their presence during growth and eruption of other permanent teeth is a benefit that justifies use of this treatment in the child.

VIII.   TRAUMA

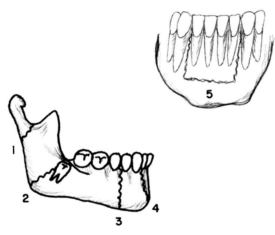

Figure 12–51 Common areas of fracture in the mandible: (1) subcondylar; (2) angle; (3) body; (4) symphysis; (5) alveolar. Mobility of mandibular segments, dental malocclusion, and anesthesia of the lower lip are common signs of mandibular fractures.

VIII.   TRAUMA *Continued*

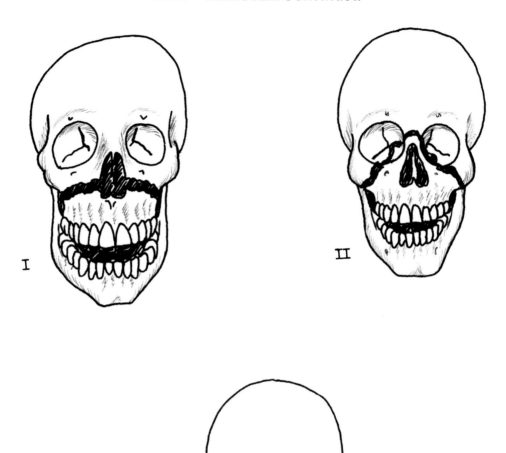

Figure 12–52 Fractures of the maxilla. LeFort's classification of maxillary fractures: I–horizontal; II–pyramidal; III–craniofacial dysjunction. Open bite malocclusion, maxillary mobility, and periorbital edema and ecchymosis are common signs of maxillary or midfacial fractures.

Tooth Transplantation

A developing tooth can be transplanted from one part of the mouth to another (an autologous transplant) with a high degree of success. Most often, use of this procedure is indicated when a grossly carious first or second permanent molar requires removal. The developing third molar in the same quadrant can be transplanted immediately into the fresh extraction socket. The patient is spared the need for prosthetic replacement or, if the tooth is not replaced, the problems associated with drifting or supra-eruption of other teeth in the area.

Careful selection of cases is the key to success. The patient should be a healthy, cooperative child with an otherwise adequate dentition. Acute infection and local cellulitis must be resolved, but chronic periapical infection does not contraindicate tooth transplantation. There must be adequate space in the recipient tooth socket for the donor tooth. Minor reduction of the interproximal enamel of the transplant can be done to facilitate its fit. The donor tooth roots should have completed one-half to two-thirds of their development and still have wide open apices. Adequate root length ensures stabilization in the socket, while open root apices permit revascularization of the pulpal tissue. The ideal time for tooth transplantation depends not upon the patient's age but upon the stage of development of the donor tooth.

The procedure can be performed under local anesthesia in a cooperative patient. A mucoperiosteal flap is raised to expose the donor and recipient sites. The carious tooth is removed atraumatically and buccal alveolar bone is preserved (sectioning may be necessary). The donor tooth is uncovered and gently removed, and follicular sac tissue is discarded. The donor tooth is "tried in" at the recipient socket. Alveolar bone is removed or the donor tooth is shaped as needed to achieve adequate space. The donor tooth is fitted snugly into the recipient socket with its occlusal level below that of the other teeth. The soft tissues are repositioned and sutured. Lower third molar transplants require no splinting or packing. Upper third molar transplants are supported by criss-crossing sutures over their occlusal surfaces.

Postoperative care requires use of an antibiotic (penicillin or erythromycin) for 7 to 10 days. Diet is restricted to liquids or soft foods, and participation in contact sports is forbidden for three weeks. The tooth should be firm by the end of the third week.

A success rate of more than 90 per cent is expected in autologous tooth transplants, success being defined as a transplant that is firm and functional after 5 years with no radiographic evidence of resorption. The single most important factor in transplants that fail to re-attach is *traumatic occlusion* during the healing period.

Some successfully transplanted teeth undergo ankylosis (about 5 per cent), and others never become responsive to vitalometer testing (15 per cent).

IX.   TOOTH TRANSPLANTATION

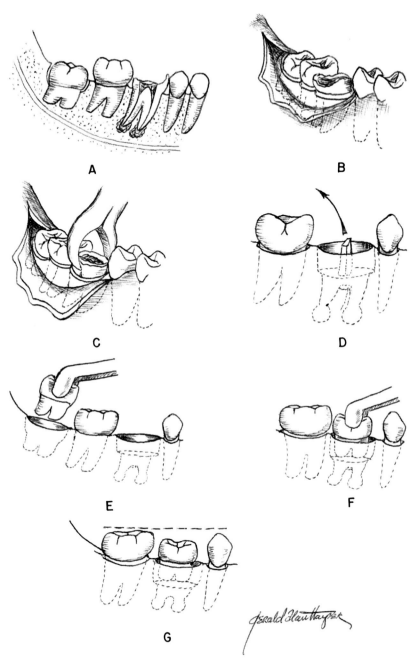

Figure 12–53   Autotransplantation of a tooth. A. Mandibular first molar must be removed because of unrestorable caries and periapical infection. Third molar has completed one-half of its root development. B. Incision for envelope-type mucoperiosteal flap to expose first and third molars. C. After exposure of third molar, first molar is removed with forceps technique to preserve buccal and lingual alveolar bone. D. Interseptal bone is removed and first molar socket is enlarged if necessary to receive transplant. E. Third molar is removed gently from its socket. F. Third molar is placed in recipient socket. Interproximal enamel may be shaped or reduced slightly to allow fit of third molar; a snug fit is desirable. G. Transplanted tooth is placed below level of occlusal plane to eliminate trauma during healing period; the soft tissues are closed with interrupted sutures. A splint or surgical packing is usually not necessary.

X. DEVELOPMENTAL DEFORMITIES

Developmental Deformities

The patient with a dentofacial deformity must deal with the significant functional problems that arise with dental malocclusion: periodontal breakdown, impaired mastication, tooth loss, transmission of abnormal forces to the temporomandibular joints, altered speech and swallowing patterns, and incompetent lip posture. In addition, the patient must cope with compelling esthetic concerns (a possible unpleasant smile and unappealing facial and profile characteristics) and psychological stress (the effect of peer ridicule and loss of self-confidence).

The patient with a dentofacial deformity should be seen initially for evaluation by consultants in both orthodontics *and* oral surgery as soon as the diagnosis is suspected by the dentist. Early recognition is important. Selection and timing of orthodontic and surgical treatment should be coordinated with growth for optimal results. Patients with severe skeletal disproportion between the maxilla and mandible cannot be treated by orthodontics alone. Moving the teeth orthodontically into a stable, functional occlusion may not be possible without treatment of the underlying skeletal deformity. If the teeth are able to be moved into occlusion but an underlying skeletal deformity is left untreated, facial esthetics often will be seriously compromised. Treatment goals include not only the restoration of a normal functional occlusion but also the alignment of the facial skeleton into normal position for enhanced facial esthetics, improved function, and better patient self-image.

A classification of dentofacial deformities is given below. Two or more deformities may occur in the same patient.

- A. Mandibular deformities
    - Prognathism
    - Retrognathia (micrognathia)
    - Chin deformities (macrogenia, microgenia)
    - Laterognathia (asymmetry)
    - Alveolar deformities
- B. Maxillary deformities
    - Protrusion
    - Retrusion
    - Vertical hyperplasia
    - Alveolar deformities
    - Cleft lip and palate
- C. Interocclusal deformities
    - Apertognathia (open bite)
    - Horizontal tilting of occlusal plane
    - Malocclusions (Angle classes I, II, III)
- D. "Syndromes," e.g.:
    - Long-face syndrome
    - Treacher-Collins syndrome (mandibulofacial dysostosis)
    - Branchial arch syndromes (hemifacial microsomia)
    - Crouzon's disease (craniofacial dysostosis)

REFERENCES

1. Bernstein, M. L.: Biopsy techniques: the pathological considerations. J.A.D.A. 96:438, March, 1978.
2. Catone, G. A., Merrill, R. G., and Henny, F. A.: Sublingual gland mucus escape phenomenon: treatment by excision of the sublingual gland. J. Oral Surg. 27:774, Oct., 1969.
3. Clark, D.: The management of impacted canines: free physiologic eruption. J.A.D.A. 82:836, April, 1971.
4. Clark, H. B., Jr., and Clark, H. B.: Minimum essentials for tooth removal operations. J.A.D.A. 27:571, April, 1940.
5. Clark, H. B., Jr., Tam, J. C., and Mitchel, D. F.: Transplantation of developing teeth. J. Dent. Res. 34:322, June, 1955.
6. Edwards, J. G.: The diastema, the frenum, the frenectomy: A clinical study. Am. J. Orthod., 71:489, May, 1977.
7. Gabrielson, M. L., and Stroh, E.: Antibiotic efficacy in odontogenic infections. J. Oral Surg. 33:607, Aug., 1975.
8. Kaban, L. B., Mulliken, J. B., and Murray, J. E.: Facial fractures in children: an analysis of 122 fractures in 109 patients. Plast. Reconstr. Surg. 59:15, Jan., 1977.
9. Kaban, L. B., Mulliken, J. B., and Murray, J. E.: Sialadenitis in children. Amer. J. Surg. 135:570, April, 1978.
10. Kincaid, L. C.: Flap design for exposing a labially erupted canine. J. Oral Surg., 34:270, March, 1976.
11. Laskin, D. M.: Anatomic considerations in diagnosis and treatment of odontogenic infections. J.A.D.A. 69:308, Sept., 1964.
12. Macht, S. D., and Krizek, T. J.: Sutures and suturing. J. Oral Surg. 36:710, Sept., 1978.
13. Megquier, R. J.: Splint technique for dental-alveolar trauma. J.A.D.A. 85:634, Sept., 1972.
14. Meyer, R. A.: Modern concepts of third molar management. J. Alberta Dent. Assoc. 10:4, Dec., 1969.
15. Meyer, R. A.: Cephalometric projections in planning surgical correction of dentofacial deformities. J. Maxillofac. Surg., in press.
16. Olson, R. E., Mincey, D. L., and Graber, T. M.: Orthosurgical teamwork. J.A.D.A. 90:998, May, 1975.
17. Slagsvold, O., and Bjercke, B.: Indications for autotransplantation in cases of missing premolars. Amer. J. Orthodont. 74:241, Sept., 1978.
18. Stubley, R.: The influence of transseptal fibers on incisor position and diastema formation. Amer. J. Orthodont. 70:645, Dec., 1976.

SPACE MAINTENANCE

Chapter 13

The preservation of arch length is the function of a space maintainer. A fixed or removable appliance is usually placed following premature loss of a primary tooth resulting from caries or other causes. Since the child's dentition undergoes many changes in the process of growth and development, it is the responsibility of the dentist to be alert to any situation that lends itself to intermediate treatment to prevent more serious malocclusion. A good example is the extraction of a primary molar with an indeterminate time existing before the eruption of the bicuspid. Here, a simple appliance will maintain space; sometimes a second appliance is required. It is seldom good judgment to "watch" or "observe" such spaces, since too often time slips by and the patient is seen after collapse has occurred, creating a far more difficult problem than existed originally. Fixed appliances are preferred over removable appliances, since they minimize such problems as breakage and patient cooperation. In some cases, suitable abutment teeth are not present, and a removable appliance is the only recourse. Intensive parent and patient education is necessary in these cases if dissapointment and failure are to be avoided.

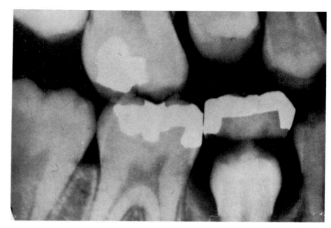

Figure 13-1 Radiograph demonstrating the most efficient space mainainer, the natural tooth.

287

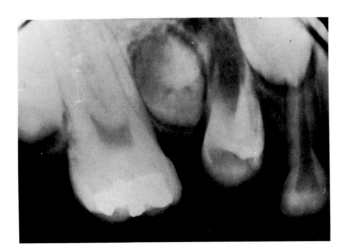

Figure 13-2 Radiograph showing effect of premature extraction of primary molar and failure to use a space maintainer. Maxillary second bicuspid is almost completely blocked out. It may lie dormant, become cystic, or erupt in a lingual position.

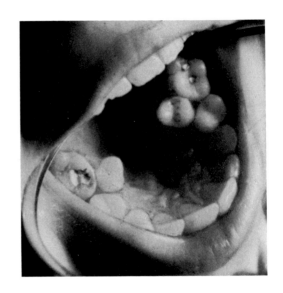

Figure 13-3 Mirror view of maxillary arch, showing right and left second bicuspids erupting in a lingual position as a result of premature extraction of both second primary molars. No provision was made for space maintenance.

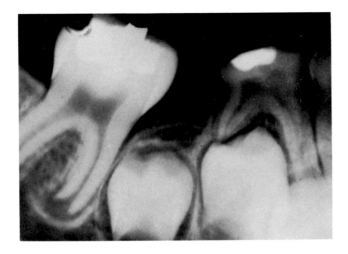

Figure 13-4 Radiograph showing premature loss of mandibular second primary molar. Note how the first permanent molar has tipped mesially, causing a loss in arch length: consequently the second bicuspid is blocked out from its natural path of eruption. A space maintainer should have been placed.

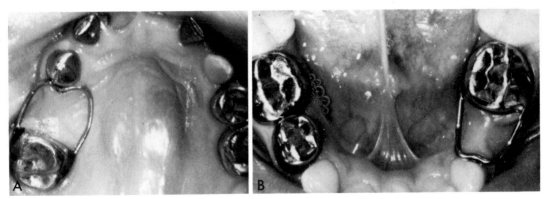

Figure 13–5 Stainless steel crown and loop unilateral space maintainers. These appliances are relatively inexpensive and may be completed in either one or two appointments, depending on the preference of the clinician.

Figure 13–6 Stainless steel unilateral space maintainer. Female unit is spot welded to crown in desired position. Male unit is then inserted and adjusted to desired length. Buccal and lingual female attachments are then crimped to secure position of male unit. Female unit is spot welded mesially to the crimp.

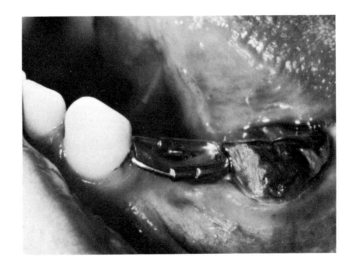

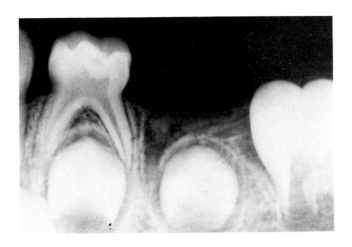

Figure 13–7 Radiograph of prematurely lost second primary molar. A space maintainer is necessary to prevent the first permanent molar from tipping over the underlying permanent tooth (see Figures 13–8 through 13–13).

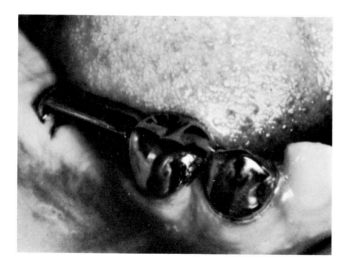

Figure 13–8 Unilateral stainless steel distal shoe appliance. Cuspid and molar crowns are soldered together with gold or silver. This appliance may be used when the first permanent molar has not erupted and the second primary molar is prematurely lost. It prevents the first permanent molar from drifting mesially into the space formerly occupied by the second primary molar. Appliance is seated after incision is made for distal extension.

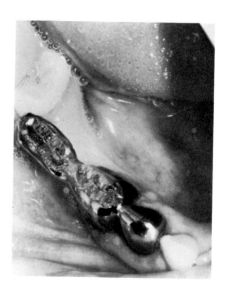

Figure 13–9 Failure of a mandibular distal shoe appliance. Any prosthetic appliance should be periodically checked for effectiveness.

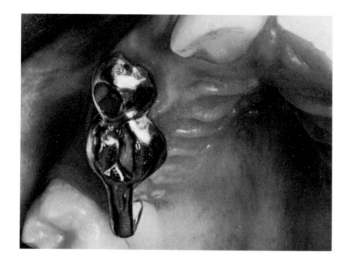

Figure 13–10 Failure of maxillary distal shoe appliance. This space loss could have been avoided if the child had been seen periodically by the dentist.

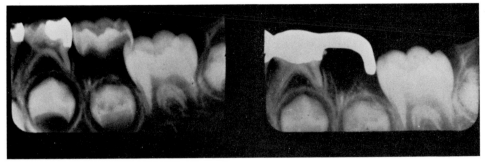

Figure 13–11 Radiograph on left shows an extopically erupting mandibular first permanent molar. Radiograph on right shows the first step in the correction of this situation. The mandibular second primary molar was extracted and a distal shoe appliance immediately cemented in place (see Figure 13–12).

Figure 13–12 Radiograph of distal shoe appliance after eruption of mandibular first permanent molar. Note how space has been maintained for erupting bicuspid. In this case, the distal extension of metal at the gingivae is too thick. It should have been tapered more. At the periodic check-up the dentist should be alert for signs that the appliance is blocking eruption of the second bicuspid.

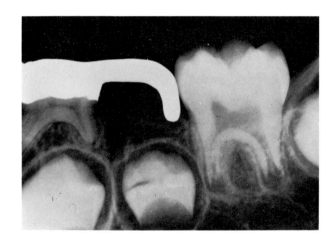

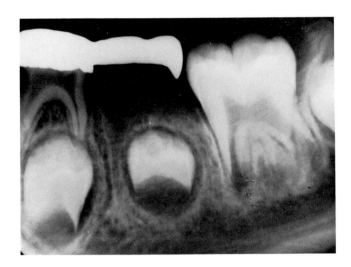

Figure 13–13 Radiograph of distal shoe space maintainer in position. Such a film is necessary prior to cementation in order to insure proper location of distal shoe. If adjustments are necessary, they may be conveniently made at this time.

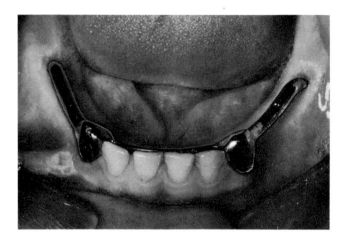

Figure 13–14 A bilateral distal shoe space maintainer with cuspids used as abutments and joined with a lingual bar.

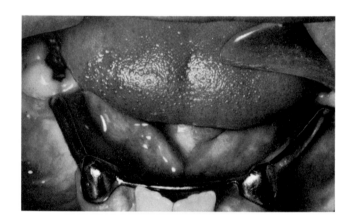

Figure 13–15 Patient seen in Figure 13–14, with first permanent molars erupting successfully into occlusion. At this stage, a new appliance should be considered — either a lingual arch space maintainer or a removable spacer.

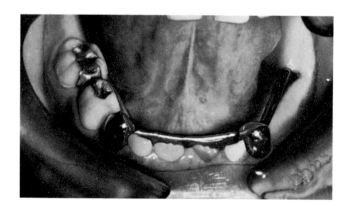

Figure 13–16 Unilateral distal shoe space maintainer. Note that both primary molars on the left side have been extracted. The distal extension reaching back to the unerupted left first permanent molar was cast with the left primary cuspid crown.

Figure 13–17 Mandibular lingual arch space maintainer. This is a convenient means of bilateral space maintenance when first permanent or second primary molars are present. However, whenever bands are placed on teeth, the patient must be *carefully* watched. Caries will progesss rapidly under a loose band. It is, therefore, *imperative* to check the patient frequently, and if a loose band is found it must be removed and recemented immediately.

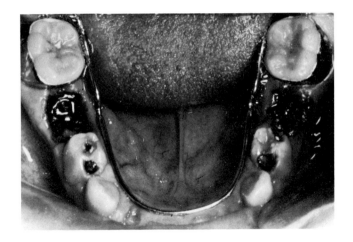

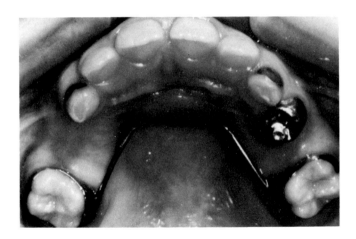

Figure 13–18 Maxillary lingual arch space maintainer using a button of acrylic to add stability and prevent the wire from traumatizing the palatal mucosa.

Figure 13–19 A 4½-year-old child with missing first primary molars. A lingual arch that rests on the primary incisors was placed. As the primary teeth exfoliate, the space must be watched closely to avoid eruption of the permanent incisors lingual to the wire. If this should start to occur, the spacer should be removed until the permanent incisors assume a more labial position. The lingual arch is then reinserted.

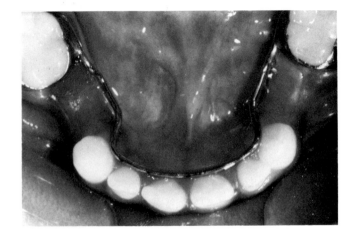

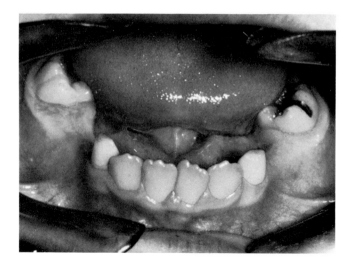

Figure 13–20 Child with bilaterally missing first and second primary molars (see Figures 13–21 and 13–22).

Figure 13–21 Removable acrylic spacer with teeth and wire clasps. This appliance will increase masticatory effectiveness for several years.

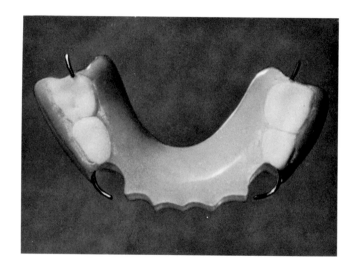

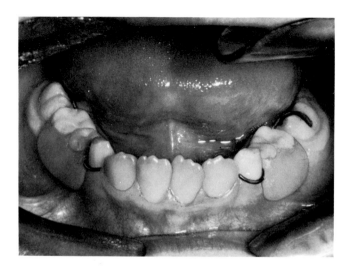

Figure 13–22 Removable acrylic spacer in place.

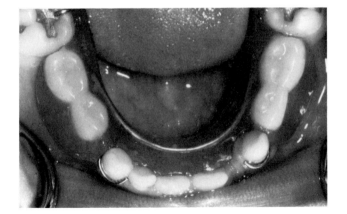

Figure 13-23 Removable acrylic space in place. Note wire clasp and rest.

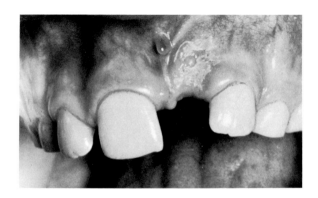

Figure 13-24 A case demonstrating mesial drifting of adjacent teeth after the maxillary permanent left central incisor was traumatically avulsed. There will invariably be a loss of space if an anterior tooth is lost during the mixed dentition period, unless a prosthetic appliance is used.

Figure 13-25 Temporary partial denture replacing a maxillary central incisor. This appliance prevents mesial migration of teeth into the area of the lost incisor and also restores esthetics for the patient. A fixed bridge will eventually be placed.

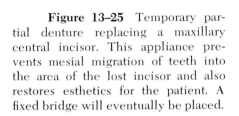
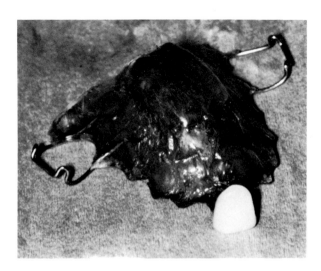

ORTHODONTIC DIAGNOSIS

Chapter 14 _____

MARC R. JOONDEPH

Comprehensive oral health care for the child and adolescent is a top priority in the quest for optimum health for all people. The family dentist is responsible for the recognition and identification of all oral and dental diseases including orthodontic diagnosis. The purpose of this chapter is to promote early recognition, diagnosis, education, prevention, and treatment of some orthodontic problems in the child and adolescent patient. A sequential system for the description and classification of malocclusion problems is presented so that one can identify patients with uncomplicated problems, treat those patients, and refer the others with more severe problems to a specialist. The habit of classifying all malocclusion problems into their respective categories culminates in a logical problem-oriented approach to their diagnosis and treatment. It is not the intent of this chapter to exhaustively treat the complete subject of orthodontics and appliance construction for active tooth movement. The more common orthodontic problems that may be conveniently managed by the family dentist are described.

The material is presented in the following order:

- I.   Description of malocclusion.
- II.   Cephalometric analysis.
- III.   Oral health.
- IV.   Facial patterns.
- V.   Evaluation of dental arch perimeter.
- VI.   Anterior-posterior relationships.
- VII.   Transverse relationships.
- VIII.   Vertical relationships.

I. DESCRIPTION OF MALOCCLUSION

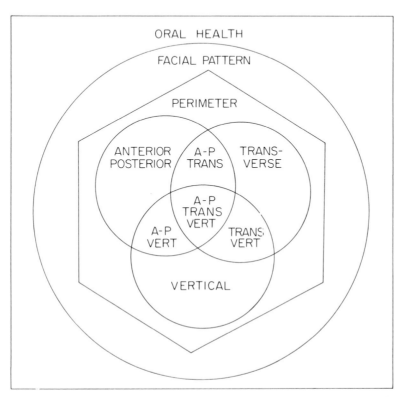

Figure 14–1 Oriented description-classification system of malocclusion. A modified Venn symbolic logic diagram is used as an organizing framework. Within the large universe of oral health, all malocclusion problems will exist. Oral health is considered first, since it is most important in any treatment plan. The facial pattern is the next category to consider in this classification of malocclusion, which becomes progressively more complex. Within this division are the characteristics of individual arch perimeter. All malocclusions will have some unique, individual tooth alignment problems that are considered within the category of perimeter. Within the division of perimeter, further malocclusion classification is indicated among the subsets: anterior-posterior, transverse, and vertical. A given patient may have malocclusion problems that involve none, one, two, or all three of these subsets. The subsets represent a three-dimensional assessment of the malocclusion in the corresponding planes of space. Each malocclusion should be classified following this organized system, in an orderly step-by-step fashion. (Modified from Graber, T. M.: *Orthodontic Principles and Practice*, 3rd ed. W. B. Saunders Co., Philadelphia, 1972, p. 251.)

I. DESCRIPTION OF MALOCCLUSION *Continued*

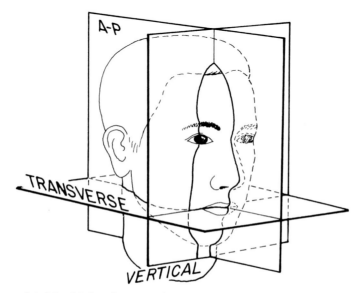

Figure 14–2A   Malocclusion subsets. This diagram graphically illustrates the description of malocclusion in three planes (subsets) of space. The anteroposterior (AP) plane should be thought of as a sagittal plane. The transverse subset should be considered a horizontal plane at the level of the occlusal table and encompasses malocclusion problems that are mediolateral — in configuration, as one would view a patient frontally. The vertical subset is used to classify malocclusion problems that are vertical in nature. The sagittal depth of this plane is variable, as vertical problems may exist anteriorly as well as posteriorly. (Modified from Simon, P., In Moyers, R. E.: *Handbook of Orthodontics*, 3rd ed., Year Book Medical Publishers, Chicago, 1973, p. 311.)

I. DESCRIPTION OF MALOCCLUSION *Continued*

PROBLEM LIST	SOLUTION LIST
ORAL HEALTH	
FACIAL PATTERN	
PERIMETER	
ANTERIOR-POSTERIOR	
TRANSVERSE	
VERTICAL	
INTERACTIONS	

Figure 14–2B   An oriented problem-solution list is used to record all malocclusion problems in their respective categories. This is done after patient records (clinical examination, radiographs, photographs, study casts) have been analyzed. By limiting one's point of view to each category individually and sequentially, one is able to organize and concentrate thoughts on that category. In this manner, a potential malocclusion problem is less likely to be overlooked. The potential solutions for each problem are listed opposite that problem, again considering each category on its own merit. The last section, *interactions,* is used to list problems that do not fit the categories listed, but nevertheless may influence treatment. Interactions to be considered may include growth potential, finances, emotional-psychological profile, attitude and behavior, pertinent medical and dental histories and so forth. The treatment plan is then generated from the solution list. For example, often a potential solution will appear more than once in different categories. Treatment planning from the solution list will follow a logical order. The remainder of this chapter will illustrate examples of malocclusion problems in each of the six categories. (From University of Washington, School of Dentistry: Dentistry 460/461 — Syllabus — Orthodontic Diagnosis. Department of Orthodontics, Seattle, 1979, p. 63.)

II. CEPHALOMETRIC ANALYSIS

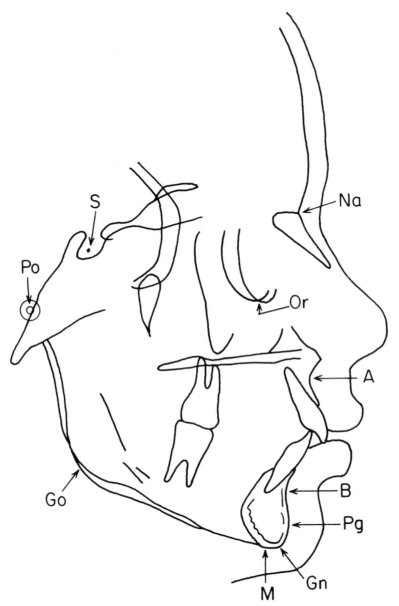

Figure 14–3 The most commonly used cephalometric landmarks. A landmark is a point used: (1) as a measuring point or (2) for constructing reference lines. Cephalometric landmarks are divided into two types: anatomic and derived. Anatomic landmarks (S, N, B, Pg, Gn, and M) are those representing actual anatomical structures of the skull. Derived landmarks (Or, Go, and Po) are points constructed from anatomical structures — for instance, the intersection of structural outlines. As long as these landmarks are located in the *mid-sagittal plane*, they can be drawn as one point. Bilateral structures, however, yield *bilateral* landmarks, which are seldom coincident. One single point can be derived by using the midpoint of the line connecting two bilateral landmarks. See opposite page for identification and definition of cephalometric landmarks, and see Figure 14–5 for cephalometric measurements and interpretation.

II. CEPHALOMETRIC ANALYSIS *Continued*

MID-SAGITTAL LANDMARKS

Sella (S):   The center of the hypophyseal fossa (sella turcica).

Nasion (Na):   The junction of the nasal and frontal bones at the most pos-
                    terior point on the curvature of the bridge of the nose (fronto-
                    nasal suture).

A-Point (A):   An arbitrary measure point on the innermost curvature from
                    the maxillary anterior nasal spine to the crest of the maxil-
                    lary alveolar process. The A-point is the most anterior point
                    of the maxillary apical base and usually is opposite the root
                    tip of the maxillary central incisor.

B-Point (B):   An arbitrary measure point on the anterior bony curvature of
                    the mandible. The B-point is on the innermost curvature
                    from the chin to the alveolar junction and usually is opposite
                    the root tip of the lower central incisor. The B-point repre-
                    sents the most anterior point of the mandibular apical base.

Pogonion (Pg):   The most anterior point on the contour of the chin.

Gnathion (Gn):   The most outward and everted point on the profile curvature
                    of the symphysis of the mandible. The gnathion is located
                    midway between the pogonion and menton.

Menton (M):   The lowest point on the symphysis. It is usually determined
                    by using a line tangential to the lower border of the mandi-
                    ble.

BILATERAL LANDMARKS

Orbitale (Or):   A point midway between the lowest points on the inferior
                    bony margins of the two orbits.

Gonion (Go):   A point midway between the points representing the middle
                    of the curvature at the left and right angles of the mandible.
                    The left and right gonions represent the junction of the
                    ramus and body of the mandible at its posterior inferior as-
                    pect.

Porion (Po):   A point midway between the top of the image of the left
                    ear-rod of the cephalometer and the top of the image of the
                    right ear-rod of the cephalometer.

II. CEPHALOMETRIC ANALYSIS *Continued*

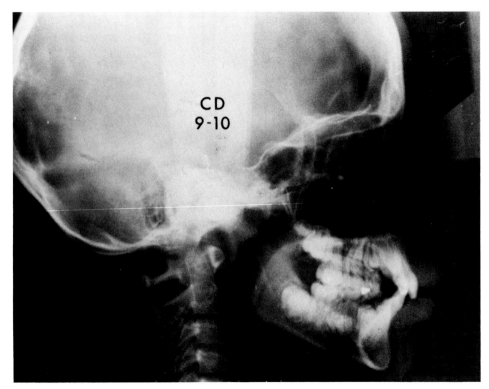

Figure 14–4 Cephalometric radiograph. An example of a lateral cephalometric radiograph, which is part of the diagnostic records for an orthodontic case analysis in the mixed dentition. The tracing and measurements of this radiograph appear in Figure 14–5.

II. CEPHALOMETRIC ANALYSIS *Continued*

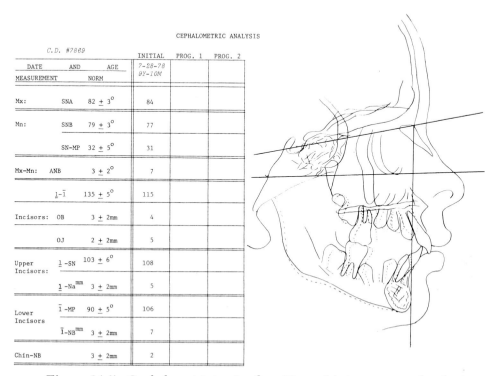

CEPHALOMETRIC ANALYSIS

C.D. #7869

DATE AND AGE MEASUREMENT NORM	INITIAL 7-28-78 9Y-10M	PROG. 1	PROG. 2
Mx: SNA 82 ± 3°	84		
Mn: SNB 79 ± 3°	77		
SN-MP 32 ± 5°	31		
Mx-Mn: ANB 3 ± 2°	7		
1-1̄ 135 ± 5°	115		
Incisors: OB 3 ± 2mm	4		
OJ 2 ± 2mm	5		
Upper Incisors: 1-SN 103 ± 6°	108		
1-Na^mm 3 ± 2mm	5		
Lower Incisors 1̄-MP 90 ± 5°	106		
1̄-NB^mm 3 ± 2mm	7		
Chin-NB 3 ± 2mm	2		

Figure 14–5 Cephalometric tracing from Figure 14–4, as measured and oriented on the analysis sheet. The reference planes drawn are Sella-Nasion, Frankfort Horizontal, and Facial Plane (Nasion-Pogonion). Note that primary teeth have not been traced and that all left-sided structures are traced as a solid outline and right-sided structures are traced as a dashed outline. A narrative cephalometric summary for this case would read as follows:

1. In relation to the cranial base, the maxilla (SNA) is slightly prognathic and the mandible (SNB) is slightly retrognathic.
2. The normal mandibular plane angle (SN-MP) indicates ideal facial proportions in the vertical plane.
3. The maxilla-to-mandible measurement (ANB) indicates a skeletal Class II relationship.
4. The maxillary and mandibular incisors are procumbent (1–1̄).
5. The overbite (OB) is slightly deep, and the overjet (OJ) is excessive.
6. The maxillary incisor is angular (1-SN) and bodily (1-Na) protrusive.
7. The mandibular incisor is also angularly (1̄-MP) and bodily (1̄-NB) protrusive.
8. There is an adequate chin button.

Cephalometric radiographic technique is illustrated in Figures 4–71 and 4–72. Tracing and interpretation techniques can also be found in orthodontic texts, and self-instructional texts are available (see references).

III. ORAL HEALTH

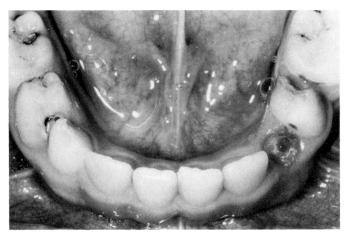

Figure 14–6   Multiple, untreated carious lesions in this lower arch could lead to the loss of arch length through mesial migration of posterior teeth. Failure to restore proximal caries in primary molars may make an extraction case out of what should have been a nonextraction case. See Figure 14–7 (radiograph) and Figure 14–46 (diagram).

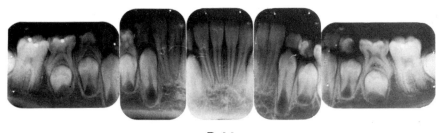

D M
10-2

Figure 14–7   Radiograph of patient shown in Figure 14–6, indicating multiple untreated carious lesions.

III. ORAL HEALTH *Continued*

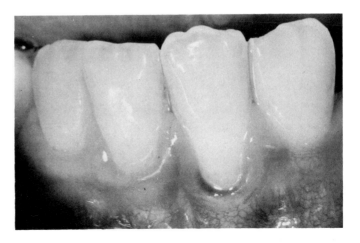

Figure 14–8 Gingival recession accompanied by an inadequate band of attached gingiva. The tissue is inflamed and hemorrhages spontaneously. This 10-year-old patient should be referred to a periodontist for evaluation and treatment.

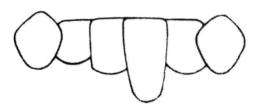

Figure 14–9 Diagrammatic illustration of periodontal problem illustrated in Figure 14–8. The gingival recession and lack of attached gingiva is often the result of incisor crowding. The treatment of choice is to eliminate the crowding and place a free gingival graft as illustrated in the following figure. (From Thurow, Raymond C.: *Atlas of Orthodontic Principles.* 2nd ed. The C. V. Mosby Co., St. Louis, 1977.)

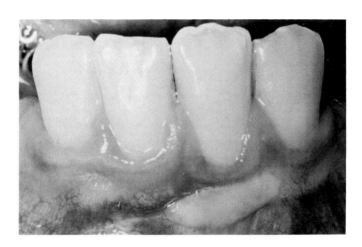

Figure 14–10 Same patient as in Figure 14–9, shown 3 months postoperatively after free gingival graft was placed and frenum was revised. Edema, inflammation, and recession are much improved. The graft is indicated prior to and whether or not orthodontic treatment is anticipated.

IV.   FACIAL PATTERN

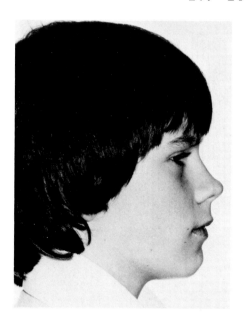

Figure 14-11   An example of an ideal orthodontic profile exhibiting excellent facial balance.

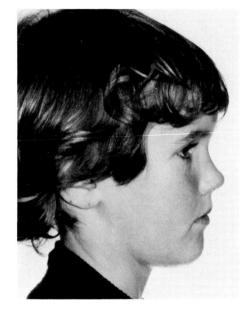

Figure 14-12   An example of a straight profile.

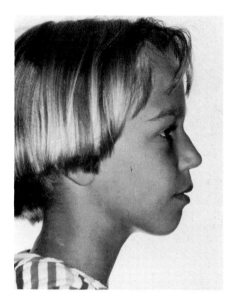

Figure 14-13   An example of a double protrusion type of facial profile. Both maxillary and
mandibular dentitions are protrusive, leading to an
overall convex facial profile.

IV. FACIAL PATTERN *Continued*

Figure 14–14 An example of a Class II facial pattern, exhibiting maxillary protrusion, mandibular retrusion, and lip incompetency. The overall facial profile is convex.

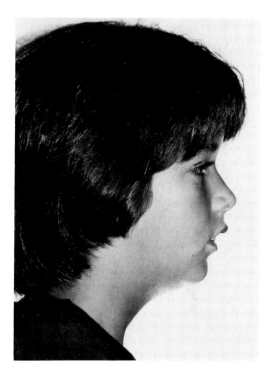

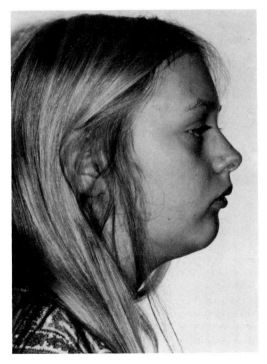

Figure 14–15 An example of a severe Class II facial pattern. There is concomitant maxillary protrusion and mandibular retrusion, giving an overall facial convexity as well as lip incompetency.

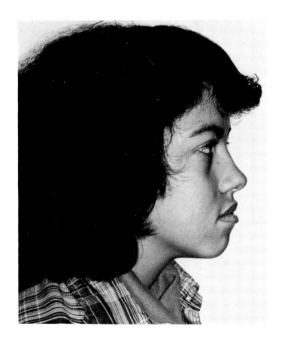

Figure 14–16 An example of a Class III prognathic facial profile. Mandibular prognathism accompanied by dental protrusion, leading to a concave facial profile.

V. DENTAL ARCH PERIMETER

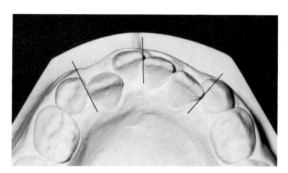

Figure 14–17 Mandibular arch length analysis. An evaluation of the space required for all the permanent teeth and of the space that is available in the arch for those teeth must be made. This is typically done with an anterior arch length assessment, an intermediate arch length assessment, and a posterior arch length assessment — combining all three to identify the arch length adequacy or inadequacy. The self-instructional material provided in the following pages will be of assistance in performing a rapid and accurate arch length assessment. The armamentarium consists of an orthodontic model, a metric ruler, periapical radiographs of unerupted mandibular teeth, and periapical or panoramic radiographs of mandibular posterior teeth. The following instructions can be followed to obtain a mandibular anterior arch length analysis: Choose an appropriate dental midline, either the contact point of the central incisors or the point at which the incisor overlap divides. Choose a point to represent the distal surface of the lateral incisors, or if malposed, project the distal surface in relation to the alveolar ridge. Measure the left and right incisor distances and compute the sum. (From Little, R. M., and Wallen, T. R.: *Continuing Education Syllabus — Systematic Mixed Dentition Assessment.* Department of Orthodontics, University of Washington, Seattle, 1976, pp. 5–12.)

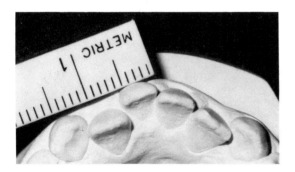

Figure 14–18 Measure the mesiodistal dimension of each incisor as viewed from the incisal edge. This illustrates the preferred method of measurement. (From Little, R. M., and Wallen, T. R.: *Continuing Education Syllabus — Systematic Mixed Dentition Assessment.* Department of Orthodontics, University of Washington, Seattle, 1976, pp. 5–12.)

Figure 14–19 This represents another acceptable method of measuring incisor dimension. Derive the sum of the mesiodistal dimension measurements of the incisors. If one or more incisors is unerupted, use the corresponding incisor dimension from the opposite side. (From Little, R. M., and Wallen, T. R.: *Continuing Education Syllabus — Systematic Mixed Dentition Assessment.* Department of Orthodontics, University of Washington, Seattle, 1976, pp. 5–12.)

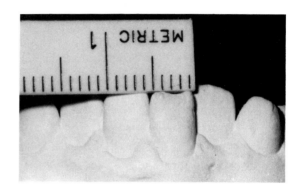

V. DENTAL ARCH PERIMETER *Continued*

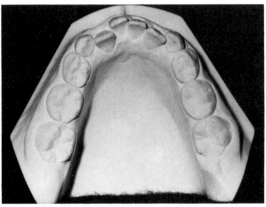

Figure 14-20   STEP 1   Measure space available
Left incisor segment _____ mm.
Right incisor segment _____ mm.
SPACE AVAILABLE _____ mm.

STEP 2   Measure space required
Left central incisor   _____ mm.
Right central incisor   _____ mm.
Left lateral incisor   _____ mm.
Right lateral incisor   _____ mm.
SPACE AVAILABLE _____ mm.

STEP 3   Compute the difference between space available and
space required and indicate deficiency (−) or excess (+)
NET ANTERIOR ARCH LENGTH _____ mm.

(From Little, R. M., and Wallen, T. R.: *Continuing Education Syllabus—Systematic Mixed Dentition Assessment.* Department of Orthodontics, University of Washington, Seattle, 1976, pp. 5–12.)

V. DENTAL ARCH PERIMETER *Continued*

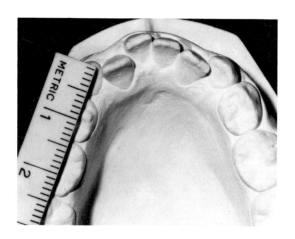

Figure 14–21 Mandibular interme-diate arch length. To determine space avail-able measure from the distal surface of the lateral incisors to the mesial surface of the first permanent molars. In cases in which the lateral incisor is blocked out of normal arch form, project the distal surface back to the patient's alveolar ridge. (From Little, R. M., and Wallen, T. R.: *Continuing Education Syllabus — Systematic Mixed Dentition As-sessment*. Department of Orthodontics, Uni-versity of Washington, Seattle, 1976, pp. 5–12.)

Figure 14–22 Mandibular arch length: To determine space required meas-ure the least distorted images of unerupted cuspids and bicuspids from periapical and bitewing radiographs. Measure the primary molars on the same films and compare them with model measurements. Reduce each x-ray measurement by the amount of radiographic enlargement. Compute left versus right quadrant space requirements.

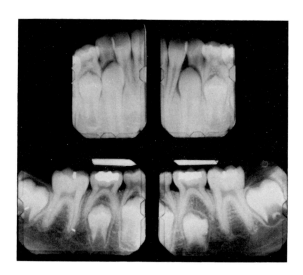

V. DENTAL ARCH PERIMETER *Continued*

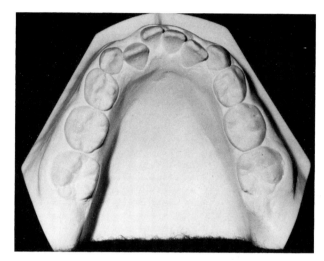

Figure 14–23 An example of a procedure for collecting data of use in analyzing arch length.

Step 1 Measure space available from models:
   Left buccal segment _____ mm.
   Right buccal segment _____ mm.

Step 2 Measure space required from models and radiographs:

| | X-RAY | | MODEL | | CORRECTED SIZE | |
	Lt	Rt	Lt	Rt	Lt	Rt
Cuspid	____	____			____	____
First Bicuspid	____	____			____	____
Second Bicuspid	____	____			____	____
Primary first molar	____	____	____	____		
Primary second molar	____	____	____	____		

Step 3 Compute the sum of the corrected sizes of cuspids and two bicuspids for each side:
   Left buccal segment _____ mm.
   Right buccal segment _____ mm.

Step 4 Compute the difference between space available and space required and indicate deficiency (−) or excess space (+):
   NET LEFT INTERMEDIATE ARCH LENGTH _____ mm.
   NET RIGHT INTERMEDIATE ARCH LENGTH _____ mm.

(From Little, R. M., and Wallen, T. R.: *Continuing Education Syllabus— Systematic Mixed Dentition Assessment.* Department of Orthodontics, University of Washinton, Seattle, 1976, pp. 5–12.)

V.   DENTAL ARCH PERIMETER *Continued*

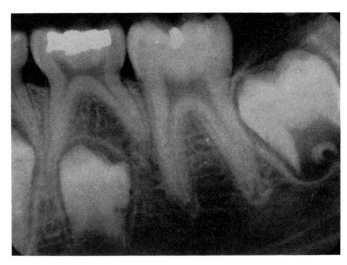

Figure 14–24   Position of erupting permanent second molars: Evaluate anteroposterior position of second molars. Are they crowded? Can they erupt? Is there space distal to the first permanent molar for eruption? (From Little, R. M., and Wallen, T. R.: *Continuing Education Syllabus — Systematic Mixed Dentition Assessment.* Department of Orthodontics, University of Washington, Seattle, 1976, pp. 5–12.)

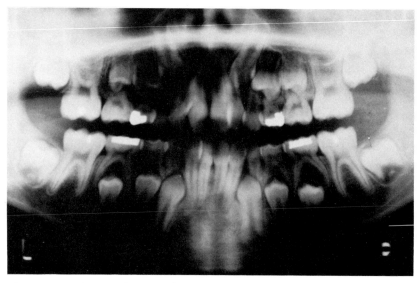

Figure 14-25   Angulation of erupting permanent second molars: Evaluate angular position of permanent second molars on periapical and panoramic radiographs as they relate to permanent first molars. Will they impact? Can they erupt? Subjectively rate *Position* and *Angulation* of the permanent second molars for this case:

Position   _____

Angulation _____

(From Little, R. M., and Wallen, T. R.: *Continuing Education Syllabus — Systematic Mixed Dentition Assessment.* Department of Orthodontics, University of Washington, Seattle, 1976, pp. 5–12.)

V. DENTAL ARCH PERIMETER *Continued*

Mandibular Arch Length

Anterior
> Space Available _____ mm.
> Space Required _____ mm.
> NET   _____ mm.

	Lt	Rt
Intermediate		
Space Available	____ mm.	____ mm.
Space Required	____ mm.	____ mm.
NET	____ mm.	____ mm.

Posterior
> Left second molar—position-angulation _____
> Right second molar—position-angulation _____

Decide if: The case definitely has excess arch length
> The case definitely has deficient arch length
> The case has a borderline arch length situation

Decide where the arch length problem is located:
> Anterior?   Intermediate?   Posterior?

V. DENTAL ARCH PERIMETER *Continued*

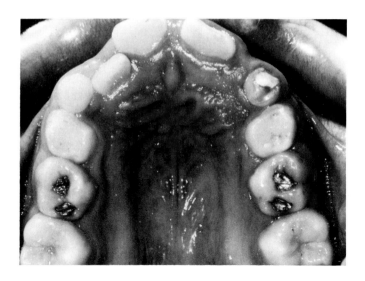

Figure 14–26 Maxillary occlusal view of a 7½-year-old patient showing anterior crowding and the presence of three permanent incisors. There is inadequate space available for the eruption of all four permanent incisor teeth.

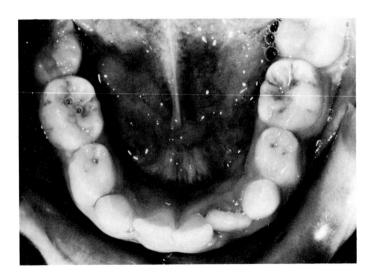

Figure 14–27 Mandibular occlusal view of same patient as in Figure 14–26 illustrates inadequate space for even three permanent incisors. The mandibular right lateral incisor is completely blocked out of the arch and is unable to erupt at this point (see Figure 14–28 for radiographs). This case illustrates an ideal indication for the family dentist to proceed with the extraction of the four primary cuspid teeth. This will at least allow the four permanent incisors, in each arch, a chance to erupt into better alignment. This is an obvious extraction case and must be referred to the orthodontist at the appropriate time for the decision to be made concerning extraction of permanent teeth.

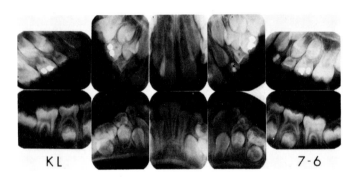

Figure 14–28 Periapical radiographic survey of the patient seen in Figures 14–26 and 14–27. This illustrates the severity of incisor crowding in maxillary and mandibular segments. This degree of arch length deficiency should initially be managed by extraction of the four primary cuspids.

V. DENTAL ARCH PERIMETER *Continued*

Figure 14–29 This frontal view shows multiple open contacts between each tooth. See Figures 14–30 and 14–31.

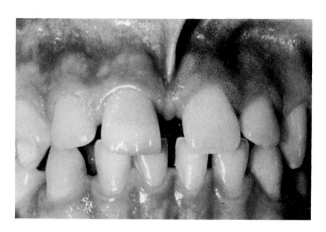

Figure 14–30 Mandibular arch of patient in Figure 14–29 showing multiple spaces between all the teeth. With this pattern of spacing, one must consider possible etiologies for this condition. (See Figure 14–31.)

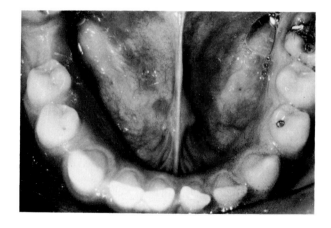

Figure 14–31 In this case the etiology was macroglossia. The scalloped, lateral borders of the tongue fit precisely between the teeth. This patient is a trumpet player.

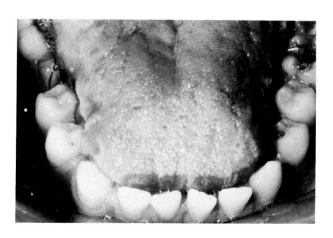

V. DENTAL ARCH PERIMETER *Continued*

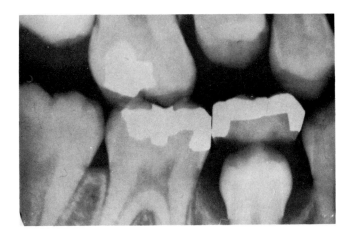

Figure 14–32 This radiograph demonstrates the most efficient space maintainer available; the existing primary tooth.

Figure 14–33 Nance type of maxillary holding arch that was fabricated by the indirect technique. The acrylic button adds stability and will prevent the wire from traumatizing the palatal mucosa.

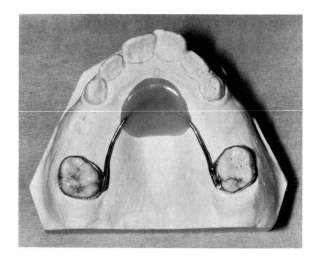

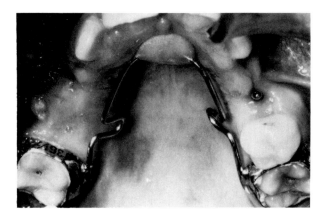

Figure 14–34 Nance type of maxillary holding arch that was constructed by the indirect technique using molar bands and .036-inch arch wire. Vertical adjustment loops have been provided as well as an anterior acrylic button to prevent impingement of the arch wire upon tissue. This appliance is adjustable and fixed. It is being used in this case to maintain molar symmetry following premature loss of primary molars on the patient's right side.

V. DENTAL ARCH PERIMETER *Continued*

Figure 14–35 An example of a removable mandibular lingual arch space maintainer. This is a convenient means of bilateral space maintenance. However, whenever bands are placed on teeth, the patient must be carefully monitored on a periodic recall basis. Caries will progress rapidly under a loose band. Therefore, it is imperative to check the patient frequently, and if a loose band is detected it must be removed and recemented immediately.

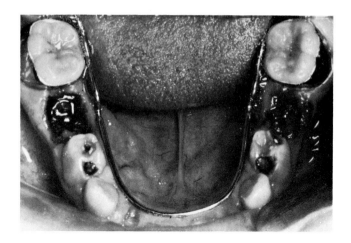

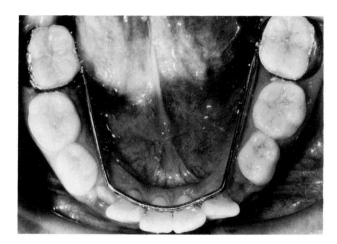

Figure 14–36 An example of a soldered (fixed) lingual arch space maintainer. This appliance is constructed using an indirect technique with orthodontic bands cemented to both first permanent molar teeth. A .036-inch arch wire is contoured and adapted to ideal arch form and soldered to the lingual surface of both molar bands. This type of lingual arch is constructed to be passive and nonadjustable. See Figure 14–37.

Figure 14–37 Diagrammatic view of fixed lower lingual arch space maintainer (see Figure 14–36). (Modified from Thurow, Raymond C.: *Atlas of Orthodontic Principles.* 2nd ed. The C. V. Mosby Co., St. Louis, 1977.)

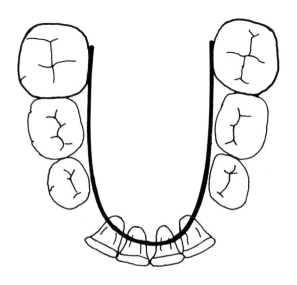

V. DENTAL ARCH PERIMETER *Continued*

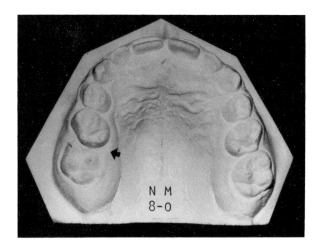

Figure 14–38 Ectopic eruption of the maxillary right first permanent molar. Before a particular method of treatment is chosen, a radiograph of the ectopically erupting molar should be carefully evaluated. If the entire distal root of the primary second molar has been resorbed and the first permanent molar occupies this area, use of the brass wire technique will likely be unsuccessful. See Figures 14–39 to 14–43.

Figure 14–39 Diagrammatic illustration of condition shown in Figure 14–38. Radiographic investigation is indicated prior to any treatment planning. Other malocclusion problems, such as arch length deficiency or congenital premolar absence, must also be considered before formulation of a treatment plan. (From Thurow, Raymond C.: *Atlas of Orthodontic Principles*. 2nd ed. The C. V. Mosby Co., St. Louis, 1977.)

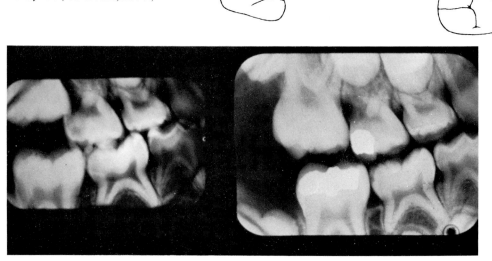

Figure 14–40 Radiograph (left) of an ectopically erupting maxillary first permanent molar. Radiograph (right) of the maxillary first permanent molar, following correction of the eruptive path with a twisted interproximal brass wire. The wire was placed between the maxillary second primary molar and the maxillary first permanent molar (see following figures).

V. DENTAL ARCH PERIMETER *Continued*

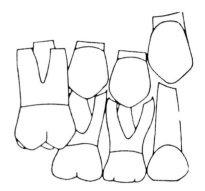

Figure 14–41 Diagrammatic illustration of the pretreatment radiograph seen in Figure 14–40. Radiographic evaluation will also rule out congenital absence of the second premolar, which may result in the same type of impaction. (From Thurow, Raymond C.: *Atlas of Orthodontic Principles*. 2nd ed. The C. V. Mosby Co., St. Louis, 1977.)

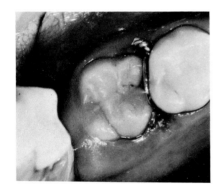

Figure 14–42 Use of a soft brass wire (.020 inch) to correct an ectopically erupting maxillary first permanent molar. The wire is inserted around the contact area and tightened on a weekly basis until the eruptive path is normalized.

Figure 14–43 Diagrammatic illustration of brass wire placement shown in Figure 14–42. If it is impossible to intercept the ectopically erupting first molar in a timely fashion, it will most likely result in exfoliation or extraction of the primary molar (as in Figures 14–44 and 14–45), requiring more extensive orthodontic intervention. This should be undertaken by or in consultation with an orthodontic specialist. (From Thurow, Raymond C.: *Atlas of Orthodontic Principles*. 2nd ed. St. Louis, The C. V. Mosby Co., 1977.)

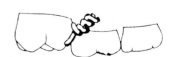

V. DENTAL ARCH PERIMETER *Continued*

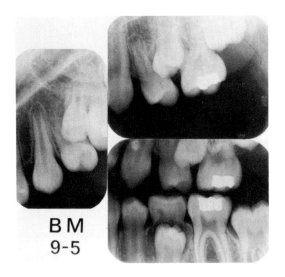

Figure 14–44 Periapical radiograph exhibiting impaction of maxillary left second bicuspid. Comparison of multiple radiographic views shows the impacted tooth is located on the palatal side of the alveolus. This confirms the location of the crown, which is palpable in the oral cavity upon digital examination. The etiology of this condition is the premature loss of a second primary molar without provisions for space maintenance. This has also resulted in a molar asymmetry in the maxillary arch and a subdivision type of malocclusion (see Figures 14–109 to 14–112).

Figure 14–45 Diagrammatic illustration of bicuspid impaction shown in Figure 14–44. Mesial migration of the first permanent molar may become severe enough to create a space deficiency for later eruption of even the first bicuspid. (From Thurow, Raymond C.: *Atlas of Orthodontic Principles.* 2nd ed. The C. V. Mosby Co., St. Louis, 1977.)

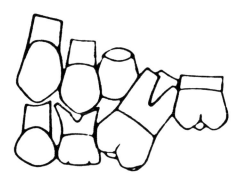

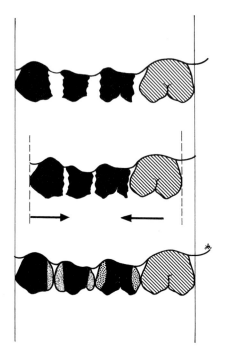

Figure 14–46 Diagrammatic view of how arch length may be lost because of extensive untreated proximal caries in the primary dentition. This amount of arch length loss may create an extraction situation in what otherwise should be a nonextraction situation (see Figures 14–6 and 14–7). (From Graber, T. M.: *Orthodontic Principles and Practice*, 3rd ed., W. B. Saunders Co., Philadelphia, 1972, p. 393.)

V. DENTAL ARCH PERIMETER *Continued*

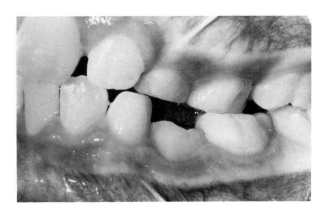

Figure 14–47 Patient with an ankylosed mandibular left first primary molar. This is confirmed by percussion testing and by observing the occlusal step and marginal ridge discrepancies between this and adjacent teeth.

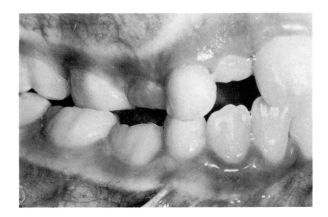

Figure 14–48 Right lateral view of same patient as in Figure 14–47, indicating a similar condition on this side. These ankylosed teeth must be observed very closely to prevent a subsequent arch length problem, such as impaction of the first bicuspid (see Figure 14–49).

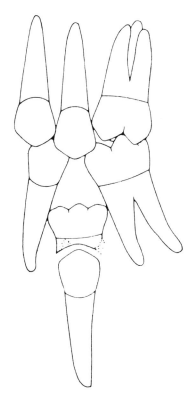

Figure 14–49 Diagrammatic illustration of primary molar ankylosis. Ankylosis will prevent the normal physiological eruption that occurs as teeth keep pace with vertical growth of the alveolar process and face. Any primary tooth not in occlusal contact with the opposing arch must be suspected of ankylosis. The severity of clinical problems resulting from ankylosis depends upon the growth that occurs between the time of ankylosis and the normal exfoliation time for that tooth. Thus, ankylosis occurring near the normal exfoliation time can be safely ignored. Ankylosis over a long period can produce the impaction illustrated in this figure. The primary molar is completely submerged, and the space has been almost completely lost. This situation may occur with or without congenital absence of the bicuspid. An ankylosed tooth should not be allowed to cause this degree of impaction. In cases of long-term ankylosis affected teeth should ordinarily be extracted (see Figures 3–149 through 3–152). (From Thurow, Raymond C.: *Atlas of Orthodontic Principles.* 2nd ed. The C. V. Mosby Co., St. Louis, 1977.)

V. DENTAL ARCH PERIMETER *Continued*

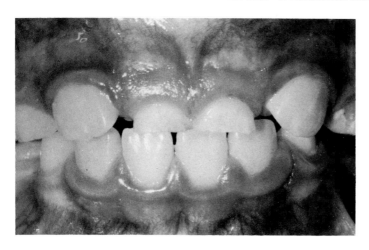

Figure 14–50 Frontal view of an 8½-year-old patient shows over-retained maxillary primary central incisors with eruption of permanent lateral incisors (see radiographs in Figures 14–51 and 14–52 for interpretation). The over-retention of these maxillary primary central incisors may have been due to a traumatic injury to these teeth at an early age.

Figure 14–51 Panoramic radiograph of patient shown in Figure 14–50 illustrates that diagnosis of supernumerary teeth in the anterior segment is impossible from a panoramic radiograph alone (see Figure 14–52 for periapical views).

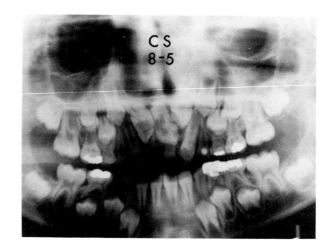

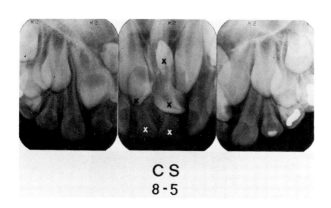

Figure 14–52 Radiograph corresponding to Figure 14–50. Note the presence of two retained primary maxillary central incisors (white "Xs"). There is also a mesiodens and two supernumerary maxillary permanent central incisors (black "Xs").

V. DENTAL ARCH PERIMETER *Continued*

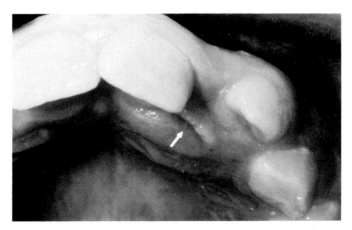

Figure 14–53 Maxillary anterior occlusal view showing the presence of two permanent left lateral incisors. Tooth size measurements revealed that the most palatally placed lateral incisor (arrow) was more nearly equivalent in mesiodistal width to the right lateral incisor. Thus, the tooth to be extracted was the most labially positioned lateral incisor (see Figure 14–54 for radiograph).

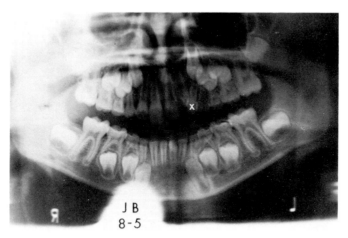

Figure 14–54 Panoramic radiograph of patient seen in Figure 14–53 showing presence of supernumerary maxillary left lateral incisor (X).

V. DENTAL ARCH PERIMETER *Continued*

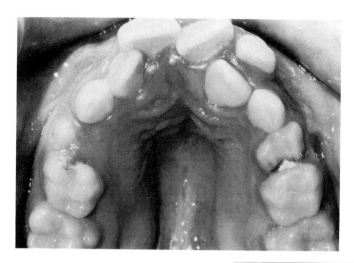

Figure 14–55 Maxillary occlusal view of patient showing extreme crowding of the anterior segment and presence of a supernumerary left lateral incisor (see Figure 14–56 for radiograph).

Figure 14–56 Radiograph of patient seen in Figure 14–55 showing presence of two supernumerary teeth: maxillary left lateral incisor and mesiodens.

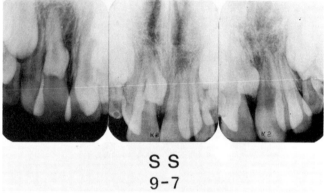

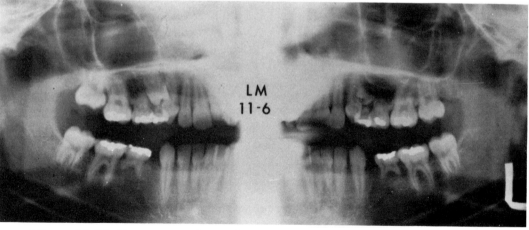

Figure 14–57 Panoramic radiograph exhibiting extreme case of multiple congenitally absent teeth. In the mandibular arch, both first and second bicuspids are missing, whereas there are retained second primary molars. In the maxillary arch, second bicuspids are absent. Note that the only third molar developing at this time is in the lower left quadrant. Note also the developmental difference between the maxillary first bicuspids: on the right side, 50 per cent of the root has formed, whereas on the left side only 50 per cent of the *crown* has formed. There is a chance that this maxillary left first bicuspid may not form completely or erupt as an adequate tooth in that quadrant.

V. DENTAL ARCH PERIMETER *Continued*

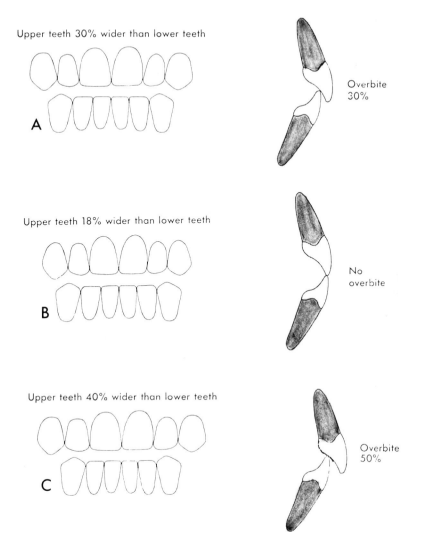

Upper teeth 30% wider than lower teeth

A

Overbite 30%

Upper teeth 18% wider than lower teeth

B

No overbite

Upper teeth 40% wider than lower teeth

C

Overbite 50%

Figure 14–58   Anterior tooth size versus overbite-overjet. This figure illustrates the inter-relationships of individual anterior tooth size between the arches and the resultant overbite-overjet relationship.

A, The ideal anterior relationship will occur when there is 30 per cent overbite. In order to achieve this relationship, the maxillary anterior teeth must measure 30 per cent wider than the mandibular anterior teeth. *B,* A minimal overbite or an edge-to-edge incisor relationship will exist when the maxillary teeth measure only 18 per cent wider than the mandibular teeth. *C,* An excessive overbite will be present when the maxillary anterior teeth measure 40 per cent wider than the mandibular anterior teeth. (From Thurow, Raymond C.: *Atlas of Orthodontic Principles.* 2nd ed. The C. V. Mosby Co., St. Louis, 1977.)

V. DENTAL ARCH PERIMETER *Continued*

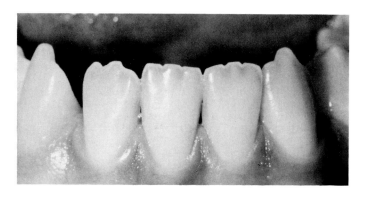

Figure 14–59 This patient is congenitally missing one mandibular left lateral incisor. The space has been allowed to close and this creates an anterior tooth size discrepancy.

Figure 14–60 Frontal view of a patient showing mesiodistal width discrepancy in tooth size between the maxillary central incisors. This case also illustrates an unusual anterior crossbite situation, a malformed lower incisor, and a concomitant periodontal problem involving this incisor.

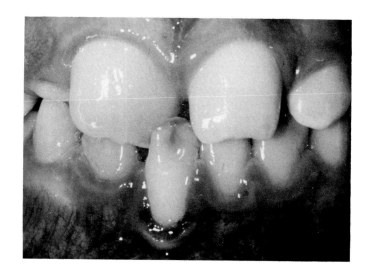

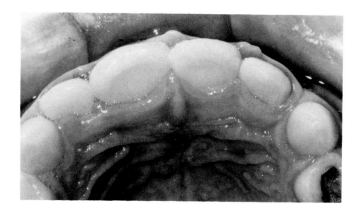

Figure 14–61 Maxillary occlusal view of anterior segment (from previous figure) showing right central incisor 2 mm. larger in mesiodistal width than left central incisor.

V. DENTAL ARCH PERIMETER *Continued*

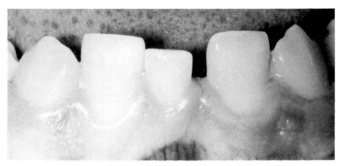

Figure 14–62 This case illustrates congenital absence of both mandibular permanent central incisors. Note also the presence of one retained primary central incisor. This patient was first seen by the orthodontist at age 9¼ years; by that time the arch perimeter had closed sufficiently to allow space for only one of the missing incisors. The combination of four mandibular anterior teeth functioning against six maxillary anterior teeth creates a significant anterior tooth size discrepancy. At this point it is impossible to open sufficient space for two adequately sized mandibular incisor pontics for bridgework. Eventual orthodontic management of this case will be as if the two mandibular central incisor teeth had been extracted. The primary incisor will be removed, the space closed, and the lateral incisors will then function as central incisors. The cuspids will be recontoured and substituted as lateral incisors, and the first bicuspids will function as cuspids. The maxillary arch will be managed with first bicuspid extractions (see Figure 14–63 for radiograph).

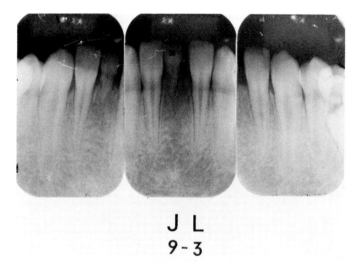

Figure 14–63 Radiographic survey of patient seen in Figure 14–62. Note that the retained primary incisor has inadequate root length. The two permanent central incisors are congenitally absent.

V. DENTAL ARCH PERIMETER *Continued*

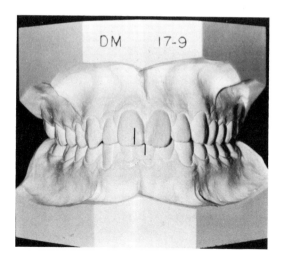

Figure 14–64 Frontal view of a patient 17¾ years of age illustrating a dentist-created anterior tooth size discrepancy. Note the mandibular midline is shifted 3 mm. to the right.

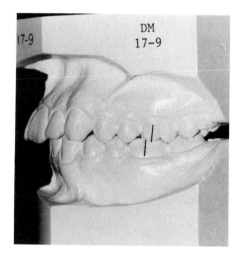

Figure 14–65 Left lateral view shows an ideal Class I buccal occlusion with excessive overjet.

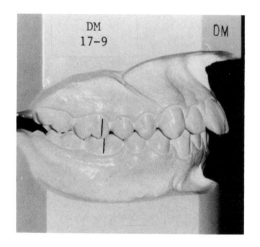

Figure 14–66 Right lateral view also shows an ideal Class I buccal occlusion.

V. DENTAL ARCH PERIMETER *Continued*

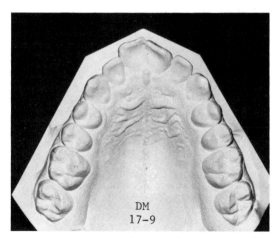

Figure 14–67   Maxillary occlusal view showing crowding and rotation in the anterior segment.

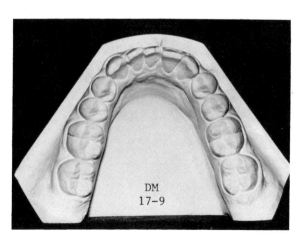

Figure 14–68   Mandibular occlusal view showing the presence of three mandibular incisor teeth. Comparison of tooth sizes indicates that the right central incisor had apparently been removed at some earlier age as a treatment for crowding. Although this treatment has resolved crowding in the mandibular arch, it has done nothing for the anterior occlusal relationship. This treatment has left the patient with excessive overbite and overjet in the anterior segment. These features are very typical of a tooth size discrepancy that would best be described as a mandibular anterior deficiency. The patient has been done a disservice by this type of treatment. At this point about the only orthodontic treatment that can be offered is to reduce maxillary anterior tooth size by interproximal enamel reduction in an attempt to decrease overbite and overjet. That treatment, of course, is a compromise and is severely limited by interproximal enamel thickness and esthetic considerations.

V. DENTAL ARCH PERIMETER *Continued*

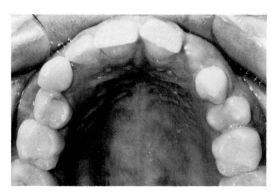

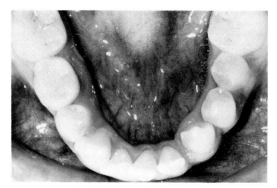

Figure 14–69 Maxillary view of a patient with a congenitally missing left lateral incisor. Both primary cuspids are present.

Figure 14–70 Mandibular view of patient in Figure 14–69 showing congenital absence of a mandibular left lateral incisor as well. This very unusual pattern of missing teeth creates quite an occlusal problem due to the anterior tooth size discrepancy in both arches (see Figure 14–71 for radiograph).

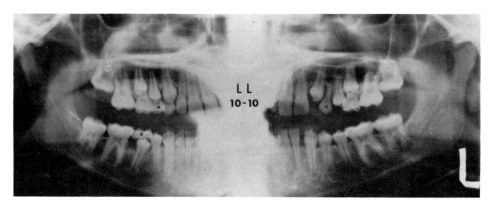

Figure 14–71 Panoramic radiograph of patient seen in Figures 14–69 and 14–70. Both maxillary and mandibular left lateral incisors are congenitally absent. Apparently, third molars are also absent.

V. DENTAL ARCH PERIMETER *Continued*

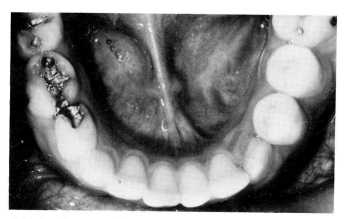

Figure 14–72 This mandibular occlusal view is included in order to point out the large discrepancies that may exist between dental and chronological ages. Note that on the left side, both bicuspids and cuspid are fully erupted, whereas on the right side three primary teeth are present. A panoramic radiograph of this patient appears in a subsequent figure. Some clinicians would state that they could predict the patient's chronologic age from these records. Actually this patient's age is 10 years 7 months. This case presents a problem in managing arch length and arch perimeter during the transition from primary to permanent dentition, resulting from an asymmetric eruption pattern.

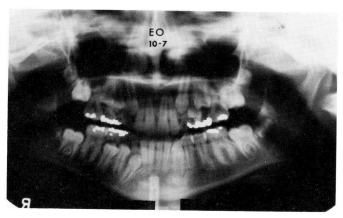

Figure 14–73 Panoramic radiograph of Figure 14–72. This case was managed with a fixed lingual arch space maintainer and subsequent extraction of the primary teeth in the left quadrant. The lingual arch was maintained until the permanent teeth had fully erupted.

V. DENTAL ARCH PERIMETER *Continued*

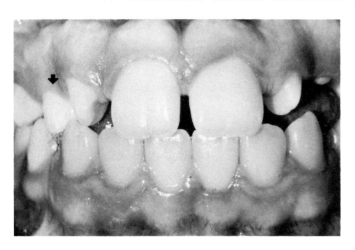

Figure 14–74 Frontal view of patient 12¼ years of age illustrating retained maxillary right primary cuspid (arrow) (see Figures 14–75–14–79).

Figure 14–75 Occlusal view illustrating retained primary cuspid and emergence of a newly erupting left permanent cuspid. Note that both lateral incisors are narrow in mesiodistal width and are rotated 90 degrees. Close inspection of palatal contours (arrow), indicates the possibility of a palatal impaction on the right side; however, a radiographic survey is mandatory.

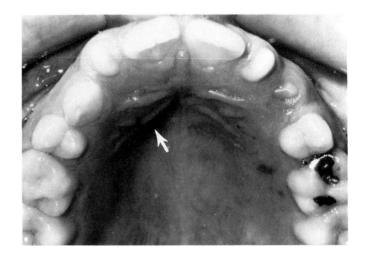

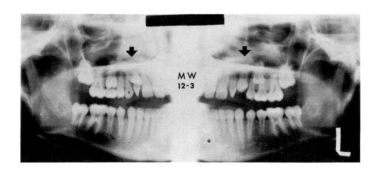

Figure 14–76 Panoramic radiograph illustrating normal eruption of maxillary left cuspid and apparent impaction of maxillary right cuspid (arrows).

V.   DENTAL ARCH PERIMETER *Continued*

Figure 14–77 Periapical survey of impacted maxillary right cuspid illustrates overlapping of the cuspid crown with the lateral incisor root. Comparison of the three images taken at differing angulations reveals that this tooth is impacted on the palatal side of the alveolus.

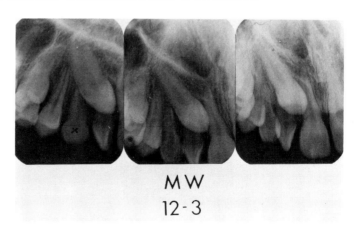

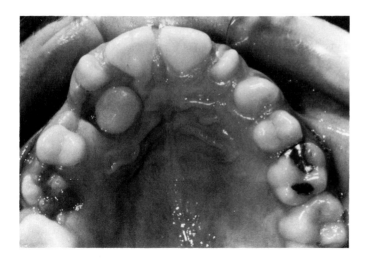

Figure 14–78 The treatment of choice in this case was to extract the primary cuspid, surgically expose the impacted cuspid, and allow for any remaining eruptive potential to bring this tooth closer to normal arch alignment. This occlusal view illustrates the palatal position of the impacted cuspid at the 1-month postoperative visit (see Figure 14–79).

Figure 14–79 Diagrammatic illustration of palatal impaction of the maxillary right permanent cuspid. This illustrates the proximity between the cuspid crown and lateral incisor root. A series of periapical views (Figure 14–77) is necessary to determine the correct location of the impacted tooth. (From Thurow, Raymond C.: *Atlas of Orthodontic Principles.* 2nd ed. The C. V. Mosby Co., St. Louis, 1977.)

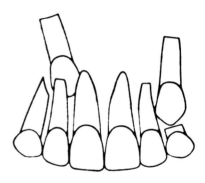

V.   DENTAL ARCH PERIMETER *Continued*

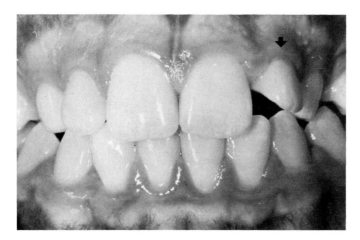

Figure 14–80 Frontal view of a patient 11¾ years of age showing eruption of all permanent anterior teeth with the exception of maxillary cuspids. Note the discrepancy in crown angulation of the maxillary left lateral incisor (arrow) (see Figures 14–81–14–86).

Figure 14–81 Occlusal view illustrates the retained primary cuspids and proclination of the left lateral incisor.

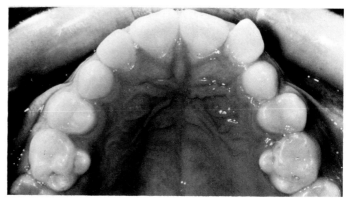

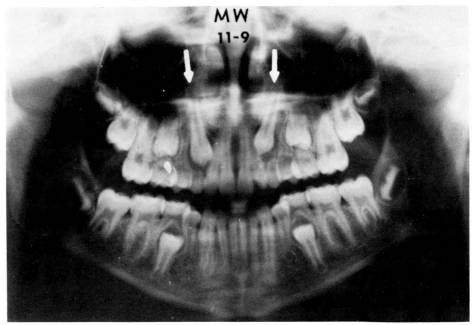

Figure 14–82 Panoramic radiograph illustrating position of the maxillary cuspids (arrows) (see Figures 14–83 and 14–84 for periapical survey).

V. DENTAL ARCH PERIMETER *Continued*

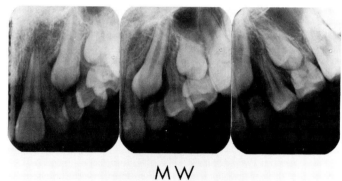

Figure 14–83 Periapical survey of unerupted maxillary left cuspid illustrates the proximity of the cuspid crown to the lateral incisor root. Comparison of the different films reveals the impacted tooth to be on the labial side of the alveolus.

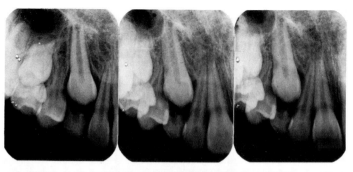

Figure 14–84 Periapical survey of unerupted right maxillary cuspid shows that a normal eruption pattern can be expected for this tooth.

Figure 14–85 Diagrammatic illustration of labial impaction of the maxillary left permanent cuspid. This illustrates the proximity between the cuspid crown and lateral incisor root. A series of periapical views (Figure 14–83) is necessary to determine the correct location of the impacted tooth. (From Thurow, Raymond C.: *Atlas of Orthodontic Principles.* 2nd ed. The C. V. Mosby Co., St. Louis, 1977.)

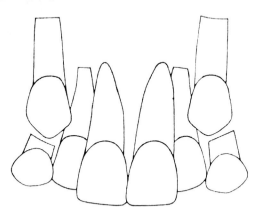

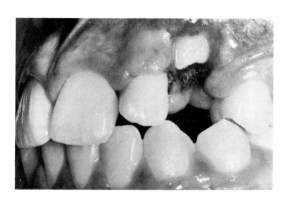

Figure 14–86 The treatment of choice was to extract both primary cuspids, surgically expose the impacted left cuspid, and allow for any remaining eruptive potential to bring this tooth closer to normal arch alignment. This view of the area shows healing at the 2-week postoperative visit. The left cuspid will be allowed to erupt as far as possible on its own before intervention with orthodontic appliances is considered.

VI. ANTERIOR-POSTERIOR RELATIONSHIPS

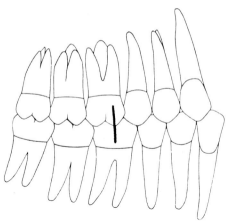

Figure 14-87   Angle Class I. Normal molar relationship, with mesial buccal cusp of maxillary first molar placed over the buccal groove of the mandibular first molar. In addition, the maxillary cuspid is placed in the embrasure between the mandibular cuspid and the first bicuspid. With normal molar and cuspid relationships, most angle Class I malocclusions result from perimeter problems. (From Thurow, Raymond C.: *Atlas of Orthodontic Principles*. 2nd ed. St. Louis, The C. V. Mosby Co., 1977.)

Figure 14-88   Angle Class II. The maxillary arch is positioned mesially, with the mesial buccal cusp above or approaching the embrasure between the mandibular first molar and second bicuspid. In addition, the maxillary cuspid is seated anterior to the mandibular cuspid. Class II occlusions are further classified by their anterior relationships (see Figure 14-90). (From Thurow, Raymond C.: *Atlas of Orthodontic Principles*. 2nd ed. The C. V. Mosby Co., St. Louis, 1977.)

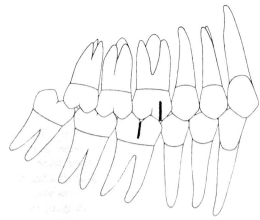

Figure 14-89   Angle Class III. Mandibular arch is displaced mesially or maxillary arch is displaced distally, with mesiobuccal cusp of the maxillary first molar occluding distal to the buccal groove of the mandibular first molar. (From Thurow, Raymond C.: *Atlas of Orthodontic Principles*. 2nd ed. The C. V. Mosby Co., St. Louis, 1977.)

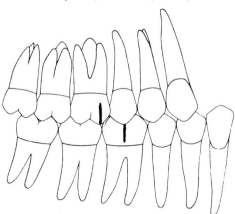

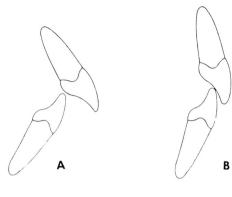

Figure 14-90   Angle Class II anterior relationships. Division 1 incisors (A) normally display excessive anterior overjet. Division 2 incisors (B) are generally more upright and have less anterior overjet but a deeper vertical overbite. Many Class II, Division 2 malocclusions are characterized by retroclined central incisors and proclined lateral incisors (C). This results in lateral incisors that are more labially positioned. (From Thurow, Raymond C.: *Atlas of Orthodontic Principles*. 2nd ed. The C. V. Mosby Co., St. Louis, 1977.)

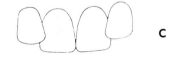

VI. ANTERIOR-POSTERIOR RELATIONSHIPS *Continued*

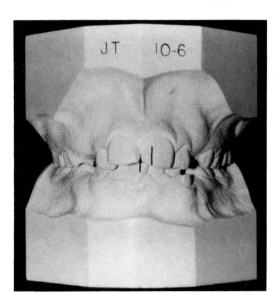

Figure 14–91   Angle Class II, Division 1 malocclusion. This type of pattern exhibits proclined maxillary incisors with excessive anterior overjet (see Figures 14–88 and 14–90 to 14–92).

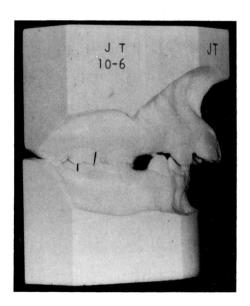

Figure 14–92   Right side Class II molar relationship. Note excessive overjet (9 mm).

Figure 14–93   Left side Class II molar relationship.

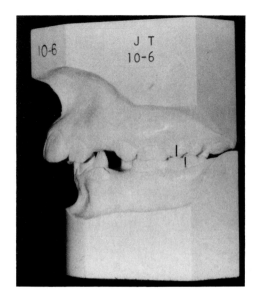

VI.   ANTERIOR-POSTERIOR RELATIONSHIPS *Continued*

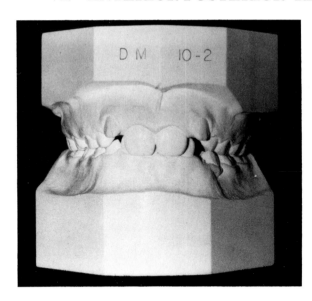

Figure 14–94 Angle Class II, Division 2 malocclusion. Typical Division II incisor configuration with retroclined central incisors and proclined lateral incisors, along with deep overbite (see Figures 14–88, 14–90 and 14–95 to 14–97).

Figure 14–95 Maxillary occlusal view showing classic Division 2 incisor configuration.

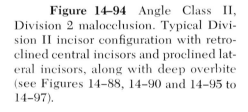

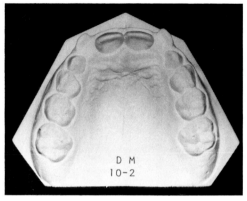

Figure 14–96 Right side Class II molar relationship.

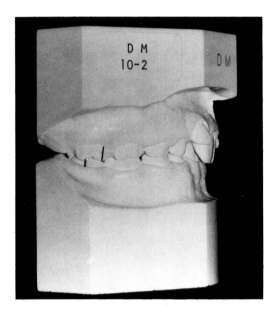

Figure 14–97 Left side Class II molar relationship.

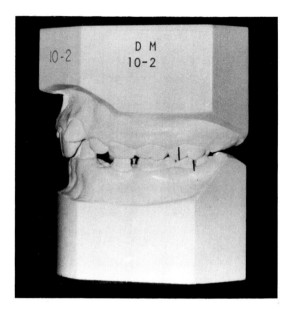

VI. ANTERIOR-POSTERIOR RELATIONSHIPS *Continued*

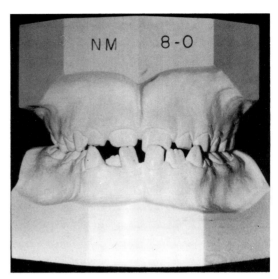

Figure 14–98 Angle Class III malocclusion. Apparent Class III malocclusion with anterior crossbite is more closely termed "pseudo-Class III." This patient actually had a Class I molar relationship with a 2 mm. anterior shift from centric relation (CR) to centric occlusion (CO) position. Casts are shown in CO position.

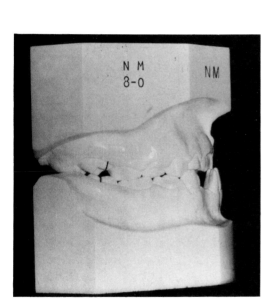

Figure 14–99 Right side molar relationship appears to be Class I because of mesial migration of maxillary first permanent molar (see Figure 14–38).

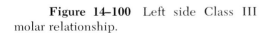

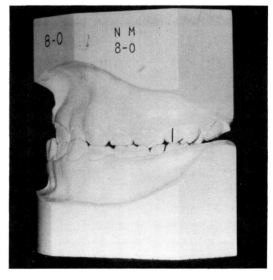

Figure 14–100 Left side Class III molar relationship.

VI. ANTERIOR-POSTERIOR RELATIONSHIPS *Continued*

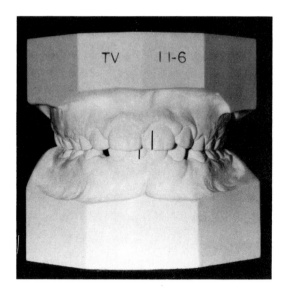

Figure 14–101   Angle Class II, Division 1, subdivision (right) malocclusion. A typical subdivision type of malocclusion normally also has a deviated mandibular midline. This midline is most often deviated to the side opposite the Class I molar relationship. This is due to the anterior-posterior molar asymmetry in the mandibular arch. This frontal view shows a mandibular midline deviated 2 mm to the patient's left. When describing a subdivision malocclusion, the Class I side is indicated as noted above in parentheses.

Figure 14–102   Mandibular   occlusal view indicates anterior-posterior molar asymmetry: the right first permanent molar is displaced 2 mm anterior to the left.

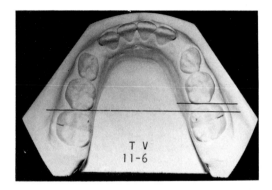

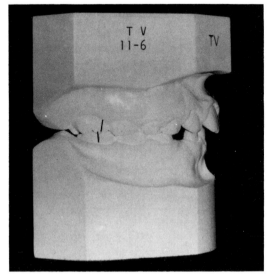

Figure 14–103   Right side Class I relationship.

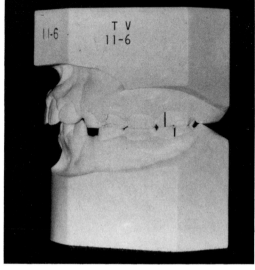

Figure 14–104   Left side Class II relationship.

VI. ANTERIOR-POSTERIOR RELATIONSHIPS *Continued*

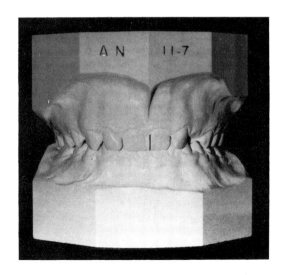

Figure 14–105 Angle Class II, Division 2 subdivision (right) malocclusion. Typical Division 2 incisor configuration is illustrated along with a midline discrepancy. The mandibular midline has shifted 1 mm to the patient's left.

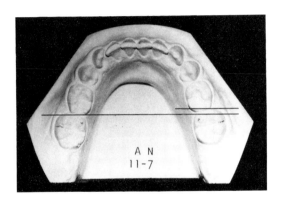

Figure 14–106 Mandibular occlusal view illustrating anterior-posterior molar asymmetry. The right first permanent molar is displaced 1.5 mm anteriorly to the left.

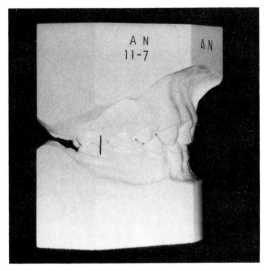

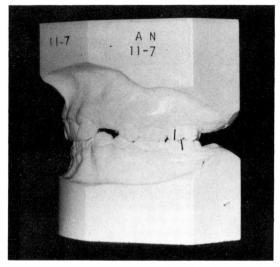

Figure 14–107 Right side Class I relationship.

Figure 14–108 Left side Class II relationship.

VI. ANTERIOR-POSTERIOR RELATIONSHIPS *Continued*

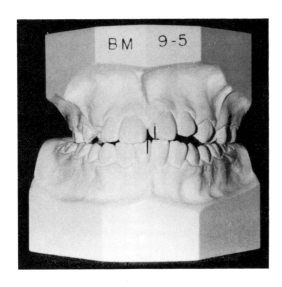

Figure 14–109 Angle Class II, Division 1 subdivision (right) malocclusion. The mandibular midline is deviated 2 mm. to the patient's left.

Figure 14–110 Maxillary occlusal view displaying anterior-posterior molar asymmetry. The left first molar is displaced 2 mm. anterior to the right first molar. Both the left first bicuspid and molar have rotated toward each other. The etiology in this case was premature loss of the left second primary molar with no provisions for space maintenance. This, in turn, lead to impaction of the left second bicuspid (see radiograph, Figure 14–44).

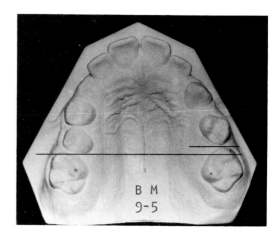

Figure 14–111 Right side Class I relationship.

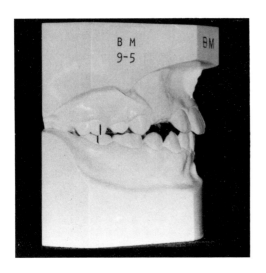

Figure 14–112 Left side Class II relationship.

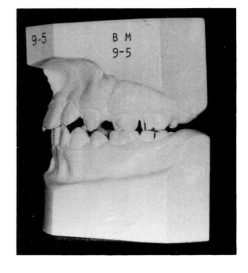

VI. ANTERIOR-POSTERIOR RELATIONSHIPS *Continued*

ANTERIOR CROSSBITE

DIFFERENTIAL DIAGNOSIS

ETIOLOGY → CHARACTERISTICS	SIMPLE DENTAL MALPOSITION ECTOPIC ERUPTION	FUNCTIONAL CENTRIC PREMATURITY ANTERIOR CR - CO SHIFT	SKELETAL MAXILLARY HYPOPLASIA MANDIBULAR HYPERPLASIA
MOLAR CR	I	I	III
MOLAR CO	I	III	III
CHIN CR	MESOGNATHIC	MESOGNATHIC	PROGNATHIC
CHIN CO	MESOGNATHIC	PROGNATHIC OR MESOGNATHIC	PROGNATHIC
MANDIBULAR CLOSURE	SMOOTH ARC	ANTERIOR SHIFT	SMOOTH ARC
TREATMENT	ORTHODONTIC TOOTH MOVEMENT (TIPPING)	ORTHODONTIC TOOTH MOVEMENT (TIPPING)	ORTHODONTIC TREATMENT ORTHOGNATHIC SURGERY

```
CHIN          RETROGNATHIC =   POSTERIOR DIVERGENT
POSITION      MESOGNATHIC  =   NORMAL
              PROGNATHIC   =   ANTERIOR DIVERGENT
```

Figure 14–113 Differential diagnosis of anterior crossbite. This chart is used to identify the characteristics, etiology, and recommended treatment for anterior crossbite. Please note that molar CR is centric relation and molar CO is centric occlusion. Angle class is represented by a roman numeral.

VI. ANTERIOR-POSTERIOR RELATIONSHIPS *Continued*

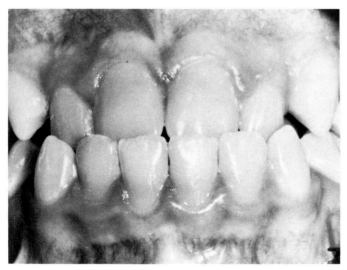

Figure 14–114 A patient displaying an anterior crossbite must be checked for occlusal function. This frontal view reveals an apparent Class III incisor relationship in CO position.

Figure 14–115 Frontal view of the same patient guided into CR position. Note the end-to-end incisor relationship.

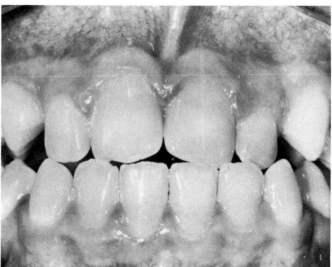

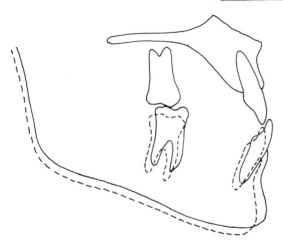

Figure 14–116 Cephalometric tracing illustrating this patient's anterior and vertical mandibular shift from CR to CO. The mandible in CR position is a dashed outline, whereas the CO position is a solid outline. Treatment of this problem is illustrated in Figures 14–119 to 14–128 and should be completed as soon as possible during the mixed dentition period in order to restore normal mandibular function.

VI.   ANTERIOR-POSTERIOR RELATIONSHIPS *Continued*

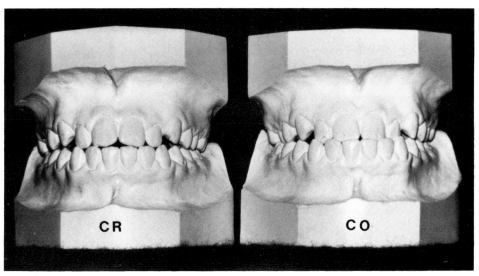

Figure 14–117   Frontal model view of the same case illustrating CR position on the left side and CO position on the right side.

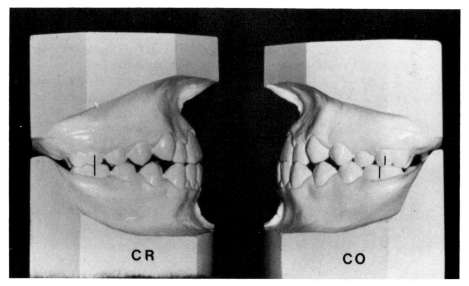

Figure 14–118   Lateral model view illustrating CR position on the left and CO position on the right. Note that in the CR position this patient has edge-to-edge incisors and a Class I molar relationship, whereas in CO position both the incisor and molar relationships appear to be Class III. This patient is demonstrating an anterior mandibular shift from CR to CO, resulting in a "pseudo-Class III" relationship.

VI.   ANTERIOR-POSTERIOR RELATIONSHIPS *Continued*

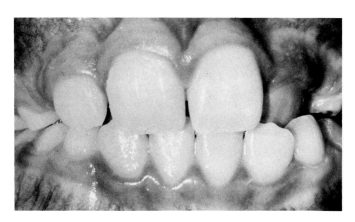

Figure 14-119   This case fulfills the two criteria for anterior crossbite correction: a Class I molar relationship, and sufficient space in the arch for the tooth (maxillary left lateral incisor) in crossbite.

Figure 14-120   Close-up of area in Figure 14-119.

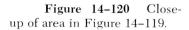
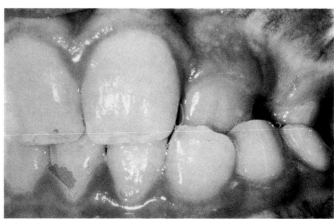

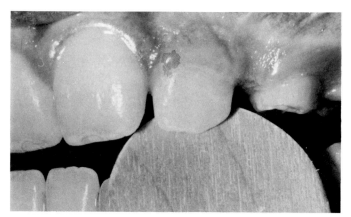

Figure 14-121   Tongue blade or popsicle stick used to correct anterior crossbite of patient shown in Figure 14-120. This technique is usually successful when the vertical overbite is not more than 3 to 5 mm. and the patient is conscientious in the use of the tongue blade. Pressure, causing slight blanching of the labial mucosa of the tooth in crossbite, is applied in the direction that is 90 degrees to the long axis of the tooth. The mandibular incisors are used as a fulcrum. Pressure must be applied for 5 to 10 minutes at a time, at least 6 times per day. Success with this treatment method depends upon a highly motivated patient, and will usually require 2 to 3 weeks of effort.

VI. ANTERIOR-POSTERIOR RELATIONSHIPS *Continued*

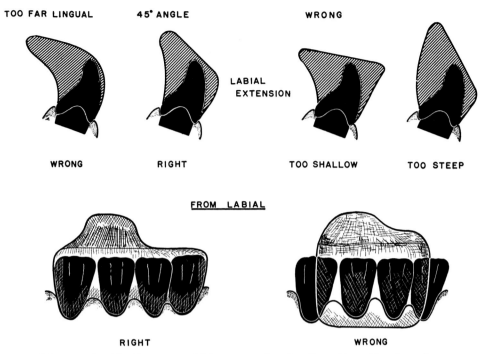

Figure 14–122   Design and fabrication details of acrylic guide plane for correction of anterior crossbite. Relationship of tooth in crossbite to the inclined plane is illustrated. Only the tooth in crossbite contacts the guide plane (see Figures 14–123–14–126). (From Graber, T. M.: *Orthodontic Principles and Practice*, 3rd ed., W. B. Saunders Co., Philadelphia, 1972, p. 836.)

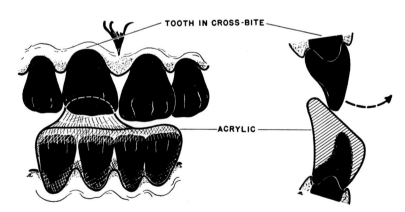

Figure 14–123   Design, coverage, and inclination of guide plane are important. A plane that is too shallow is as likely to cause failure as a plane that is too steep. (From Graber, T. M.: *Orthodontic Principles and Practice*, 3rd ed. W. B. Saunders Co., Philadelphia, 1972, p. 836.)

VI. ANTERIOR-POSTERIOR RELATIONSHIPS *Continued*

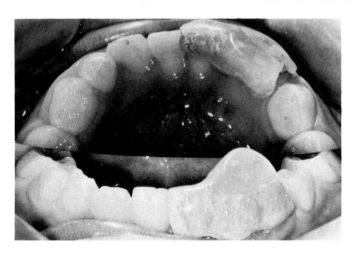

Figure 14–124 Labial and lingual views of acrylic guide plane after cementation.

Figure 14–125 Close-up of cemented guide plane.

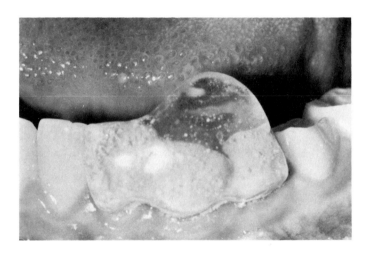

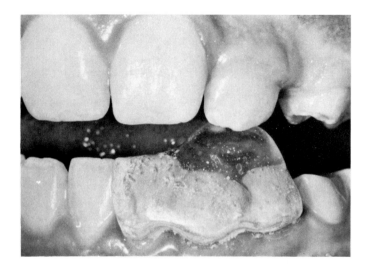

Figure 14–126 Acrylic guide plane cemented in place over mandibular incisors with zinc phosphate cement. Note how the maxillary incisor contacts the guide plane. The bite should not be opened more than 4 to 5 mm. The appliance should be checked in 1 week, and the crossbite should be corrected in 7 to 14 days. This treatment method is usually quite effective as long as the applicance remains cemented. It does, however, interfere with speech and occlusion, and this must be taken into consideration in treatment planning.

VI.   ANTERIOR-POSTERIOR RELATIONSHIPS *Continued*

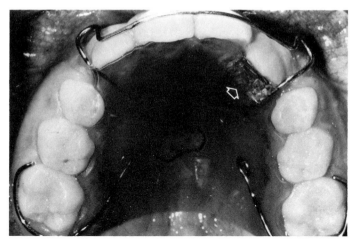

Figure 14–127   Use of a removable Hawley design bite plate with finger spring to correct anterior crossbite. The finger spring is covered by an acrylic shelf (arrow) to prevent its deflection down the lingual surface of the incisor during activation. The labial bow has been adjusted to provide retention on the three incisors in normal occlusion, and yet allow space for correction of the crossbite. Circumferential clasps retain the appliance to the first permanent molars. The cold-cure acrylic has been built up in the incisor region to form a bite plane. The use of "snoopy" in the palatal acrylic leads to improved patient cooperation. The spring is reactivated at 2-week intervals, and correction usually takes 6 to 10 weeks. This appliance must be worn fulltime; it is only removed to brush and floss. Removable appliances are seldom lost or broken when worn correctly. Again, this requires good patient cooperation.

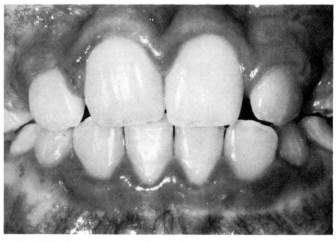

Figure 14–128   Anterior crossbite shown after correction. The correction should be retained approximately 3 to 6 months, using the removable appliance as a retainer. The bite plane must be reduced at this point to prevent further bite opening.

VII. TRANSVERSE RELATIONSHIPS

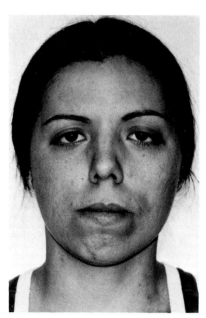

Figure 14–129   Facial symmetry must be the first item checked when examining problems in the transverse plane of space. Frontal view of this patient indicates a mandibular asymmetry with deviation of the chin to the patient's right.

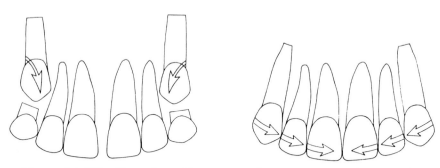

Figure 14–130   Normal maxillary incisor diastema. During the period of mixed dentition, it is quite normal to have maxillary incisor spacing. This is commonly referred to as the "ugly duckling stage." Often, the parent must be reassured that there is little advantage in early closure of such moderate spacing. A normal cuspid eruption follows a path close to the lateral incisor root, applying a mesial vector of force to the lateral incisors. This tends to close any spaces that may remain at that time. Closure of midline diastemas prior to cuspid eruption usually requires some form of retention device until these teeth erupt, in order to maintain control over subsequent incisor drifting. Tooth movement attempted during root formation can cause serious root deformity (dilaceration). Therefore, an unusually wide incisor diastema should not be closed until root development is almost completed. Closure will then allow the adjacent teeth to erupt into more normal positions (see Figures 14–131 to 14–135). (From Thurow, Raymond C.: *Atlas of Orthodontic Principles*. 2nd ed. The C. V. Mosby Co., St. Louis, 1977.)

VII. TRANSVERSE RELATIONSHIPS *Continued*

Figure 14–131 Frontal view of maxillary diastema, which measures 10 mm. Note position of the lateral incisors directly lingual to the central incisors.

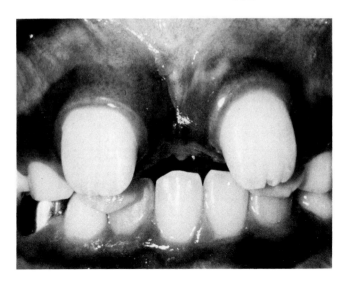

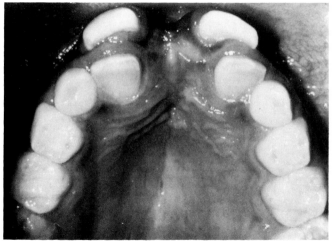

Figure 14–132 Maxillary occlusal view of patient seen in Figure 14–131. Note the size of diastema as well as the malalignment of all four incisors.

Figure 14–133 Treatment of the diastema accomplished with bonded edgewise brackets, a sectional round arch wire, and elastic traction (see Figure 14–134).

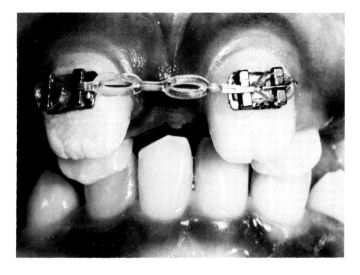

VII.   TRANSVERSE RELATIONSHIPS *Continued*

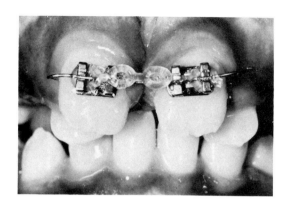

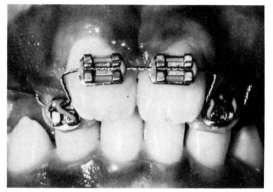

Figure 14–134   This patient is seen at 2-week intervals, at which time the traction force is renewed and the arch wire shortened appropriately. The time interval between this figure and Figure 14–133 was approximately 2 months (see Figure 14–135).

Figure 14–135   The   diastema   was closed after 6 months of treatment.

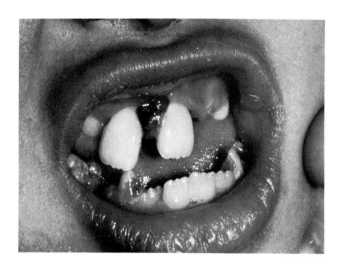

Figure 14–136   Appearance of maxillary central incisors following an attempt to correct a diastema between the incisors by stretching a rubber elastic band around them. The elastic slipped apically and stripped the periodontal membrane almost entirely from the roots (see Figure 14–137).

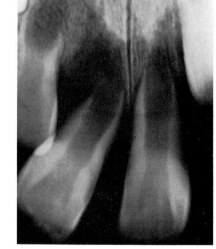

Figure 14–137   Radiographic   appearance   of maxillary central incisors following rubber elastic band therapy (patient from Figure 14–136). This poorly designed treatment was supposed to correct the diastema. Unfortunately, the central incisors were exfoliated because of destruction of the supporting structures.

VII.   TRANSVERSE RELATIONSHIPS *Continued*

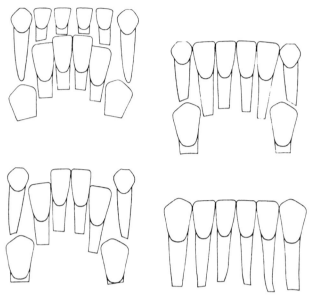

Figure 14–138   Diagrammatic view of the normal course of mandibular anterior eruption. The earliest indicator of space availability for these permanent teeth is the primary incisors, which should be well spaced. Lateral incisors normally develop in a position lingual to the central incisors and cuspids, moving into the arch perimeter as they erupt. (From Thurow, Raymond C.: *Atlas of Orthodontic Principles*. 2nd ed. The C. V. Mosby Co., St. Louis, 1977.)

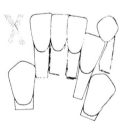

Figure 14–139   Mandibular anterior crowding can lead to lateral incisor impaction. On the patient's left side, the incisor has been crowded laterally so that it has caused some resorption of the primary cuspid root. A lateral incisor erupting partially under the primary cuspid may eventually bypass the cuspid and erupt lingually. It may also remain impacted indefinitely, or it may cause the early loss of the primary cuspid as shown on the patient's right side in this figure. (From Thurow, Raymond C.: *Atlas of Orthodontic Principles*. The C. V. Mosby Co., St. Louis, 1970.)

VII. TRANSVERSE RELATIONSHIPS *Continued*

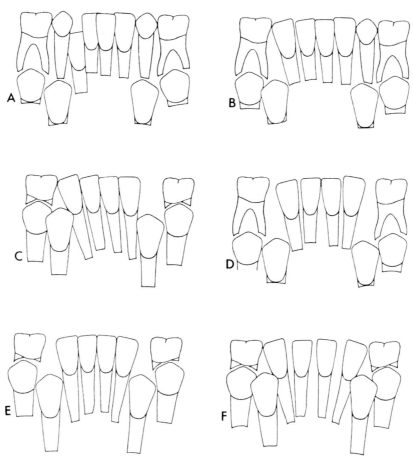

Figure 14–140 Primary cuspid loss, natural or by extraction, alters the relationships in the mandibular anterior region in several ways. Asymmetric primary cuspid loss is often the most disruptive. *A* shows an asymmetric crowded relationship that is relatively stable and in many cases may be safely left undisturbed until later. Attempting to solve this problem by removal of the right cuspid will result in aggravation of the asymmetry, as shown in *B* and *C*, a much more difficult treatment situation than the original condition. The same changes occur with spontaneous early exfoliation of the cuspid as seen in Figure 14–139. Removing both primary cuspids, or removing the remaining one after early spontaneous loss on one side, will result in partially predictable success. *D* shows what we would like to happen — some incisor improvement (realignment and midline correction) with the remaining space available for the permanent cuspids. *E* shows further permanent cuspid eruption that condenses the incisors and may crowd them as the cuspids erupt. Cuspid space is usually inadequate at this stage, but their eruption is not greatly impeded, as these teeth usually erupt in a more labial position than the adjacent teeth. *F* shows what often happens instead of the desirable response described previously (*D*, and *E*). The incisors flare laterally and use all the available space — impeding permanent cuspid eruption or forcing cuspids to erupt completely labially to the other teeth. Once again, this is a more difficult treatment situation than most cases of incisor crowding. Where one cuspid is lost spontaneously, the risk of this response may be justified, but it should be considered carefully before removing both cuspids to relieve moderate crowding. (From Thurow, Raymond C.: *Atlas of Orthodontic Principles.* 2nd ed. The C. V. Mosby Co., St. Louis, 1977.)

VII. TRANSVERSE RELATIONSHIPS *Continued*

POSTERIOR CROSSBITE

DIFFERENTIAL DIAGNOSIS

ETIOLOGY → CHARACTERISTICS	SIMPLE ECTOPIC ERUPTION DENTAL MALPOSITION ARCH LENGTH DISCREPANCY	FUNCTIONAL CENTRIC PREMATURITY LATERAL CR - CO SHIFT ARCH WIDTH DISCREPANCY	SKELETAL ASYMMETRICAL GROWTH ARCH WIDTH DISCREPANCY NARROW MAXILLA / WIDE MANDIBLE
MIDLINE CR			
MIDLINE CO			
MOLAR CR			
MOLAR CO			
MANDIBULAR CLOSURE	SMOOTH ARC	LATERAL SHIFT	SMOOTH ARC
TREATMENT	ORTHODONTIC TOOTH MOVEMENT (TIPPING)	PALATAL EXPANSION DENTAL EXPANSION	PALATAL EXPANSION ORTHOGNATHIC SURGERY

Figure 14–141 Differential diagnosis of posterior crossbite. This chart is used to identify the characteristics, etiology, and recommended treatment for posterior crossbite. The dental midline configuration is as it would appear from a frontal view. The transverse molar relationships are also viewed in a frontal plane. For example, the functional crossbite illustrated has dental midlines that are coincident in CR, but in CO the mandibular midline is deviated to the patient's right. In CR the transverse molar relationship is edge-to-edge, but in CO the patient's left molars are in a normal overjet relationship, whereas the right molars are in crossbite. This is caused by a lateral mandibular shift to the patient's right and is usually treated by palatal expansion.

VII. TRANSVERSE RELATIONSHIPS *Continued*

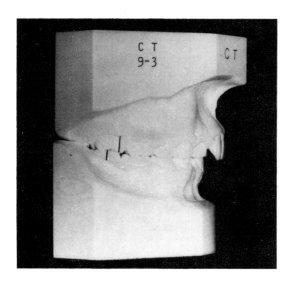

Figure 14–142 On this patient's right side there is a Class II, Division 1 relationship with no posterior crossbite.

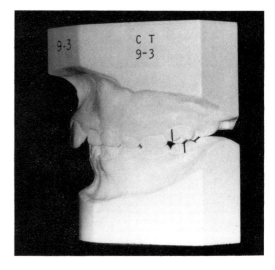

Figure 14–143 On the patient's left side there is a posterior dental crossbite involving the first permanent molars.

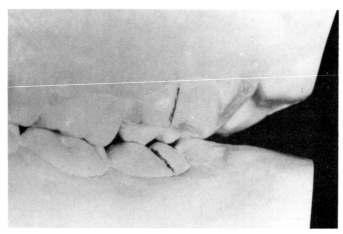

Figure 14–144 Close-up view shows a maxillary buccal crossbite.

VII. TRANSVERSE RELATIONSHIPS *Continued*

Figure 14-145 Maxillary arch view shows left first permanent molar displaced buccally. The appropriate treatment for correction of this crossbite involves the use of cross elastics, as diagramed in Figure 14-147. Since the mandibular molar is in an ideal transverse position, the correction should involve lingual tooth movement of the maxillary molar only. To achieve this, a passive mandibular lingual arch is constructed in order to prevent buccal movement of the mandibular molar during the crossbite correction.

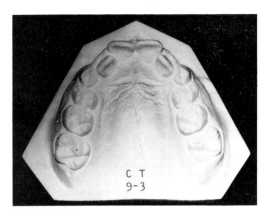

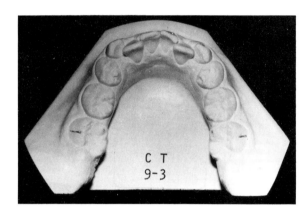

Figure 14-146 Mandibular arch shows left first permanent molar in ideal transverse position.

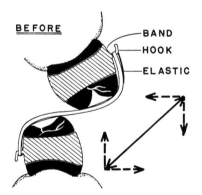
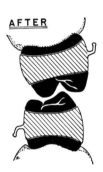

Figure 14-147 Diagrammatic illustration of unilateral dental posterior crossbite correction using cross elastics. The involved teeth are banded with hook attachments appropriately placed to facilitate the attachment of rubber elastics. The patient is instructed to wear the elastics fulltime, removing them only for eating, brushing, and flossing. The patient should carry a small package of elastics with him at all times. This will ensure that spare elastics are always available in case one should break. Whenever the elastic is removed it should be discarded and replaced by a fresh one. This will ensure that the elastic is changed at least 6 times daily. This treatment depends on patient cooperation, and may require 4 to 8 weeks to complete. Once corrected, occlusal intercuspation is usually sufficient to retain the correction. (From Graber, T. M.: *Orthodontic Principles and Practice*, 3rd ed., W. B. Saunders Co., Philadelphia, 1972, p. 849.)

VII.   TRANSVERSE RELATIONSHIPS *Continued*

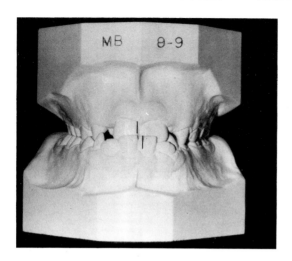

Figure 14–148 The frontal view of this patient displays unilateral posterior crossbite (right side). Any "apparent" unilateral posterior crossbite must be viewed with suspicion. More often than not it is actually a bilateral crossbite with a lateral mandibular shift from CR to CO position (see Figure 14–152). This patient also displays an anterior crossbite that is an anterior-posterior problem. Note the midline discrepancy caused by a mandibular shift to the right.

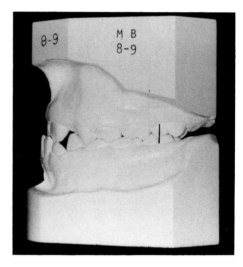

Figure 14–149 Left buccal view showing an apparently ideal transverse relationship. The models were trimmed in centric occlusion position.

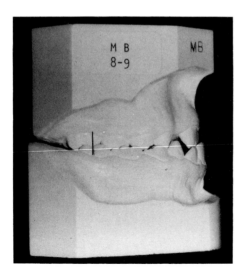

Figure 14–150 Right buccal view showing posterior crossbite.

VII.   TRANSVERSE RELATIONSHIPS *Continued*

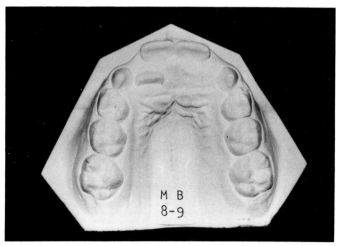

Figure 14–151   Maxillary occlusal view showing transversely constricted arch. This type of posterior crossbite should be referred to an orthodontist for palatal suture expansion.

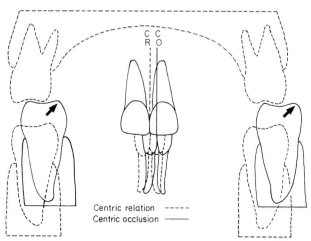

Figure 14–152   Diagnosis of functional posterior crossbite. In centric relation position dental midlines are coincident, but maxillary and mandibular molars function in an end-to-end relationship. As the mandible closes, it shifts laterally (left) into centric occlusion position. Thus, in CO the mandibular midline is deviated to the left, and there is an apparent unilateral left posterior crossbite. Actually, there is a bilateral posterior crossbite. See Figure 14–141. (Modified from Chaconas, S. J.: Preventive orthodontics: when and why. J. Preventive Dentistry 5:30, 1978, p. 33.)

VIII. VERTICAL RELATIONSHIPS

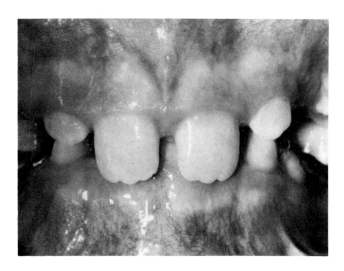

Figure 14–153 This patient displays a very deep overbite for the mixed dentition. The mandibular incisors impinge on palatal mucosa and are completely hidden from view by the overerupted maxillary incisors. An overbite of this severity should have been referred earlier to a specialist.

Figute 14–154 Anterior open bite in the mixed dentition. Note that mammelons are still present on incisal edges. These teeth have yet to function normally.

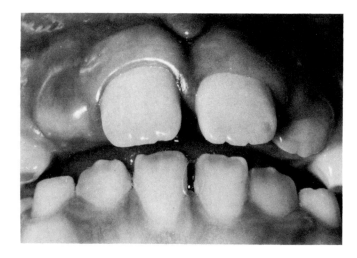

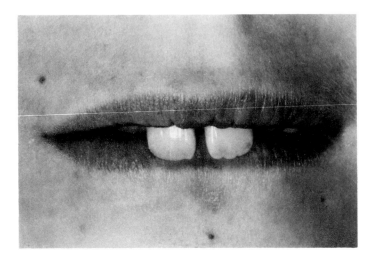

Figure 14–155 Same patient as in Figure 14–154. A lip-biting habit was the cause of the anterior open bite (see Figure 14–156).

VIII. VERTICAL RELATIONSHIPS *Continued*

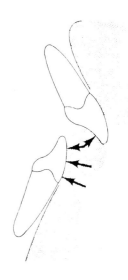

Figure 14–156   Diagrammatic illustration of how a lip-biting habit can contribute to an anterior open bite. (From Thurow, Raymond C.: *Atlas of Orthodontic Principles*. 2nd ed. The C. V. Mosby Co., St. Louis, 1977.)

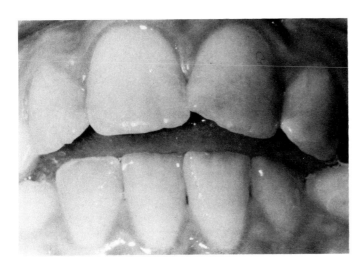

Figure 14–157   Anterior open bite caused by a tongue thrust habit. See Figure 14–158.

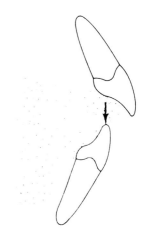

Figure 14–158   Diagrammatic illustration demonstrating how a tongue thrust habit can be the cause of an anterior open bite. (From Thurow, Raymond C.: *Atlas of Orthodontic Principles*. 2nd ed. The C. V. Mosby Co., St. Louis, 1977.)

VIII.   VERTICAL RELATIONSHIPS *Continued*

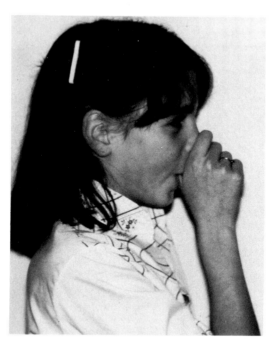

Figure 14–159   One of the most common causes of anterior open bite during the mixed dentition period is thumb sucking. Although thumb or finger sucking is a normal physiological function during infancy, the family dentist should devote serious attention to any sucking habit that persists during the eruption of permanent incisors, from roughly 4 to 7 years of age. This is a good time to approach the habit because it is the best time to solve the dental problems related to thumb sucking. One of the most conservative and successful approaches is counseling the child. This begins with a calm, friendly discussion, with no threats or shame, in order to identify the problem and educate the child about it. When questioning a child, it is best to avoid questions that may be answered by a simple "yes" or "no." For example, instead of asking "Do you suck your thumb?", one should ask, "Which thumb do you suck?". This child realizes unconsciously that the dentist is aware of his habit and will be very responsive to the dentist's concern. It is most important to be gentle, for this is probably the first friendly discussion he has ever had concerning his habit. It is also important that parents be informed that the subject should not be a matter for family discussion, because the dentist and the child will take care of the problem between them. Within this relaxed, tension-free setting, almost any habit reminder technique will be successful. Reminders range from having the child keep a written daily record of his efforts at habit control, prescribing bandages to be placed on the thumb each night by the child, constructing a tongue blade or popsicle stick splint for the thumb (many children enjoy pretending they have a broken thumb), or wearing a sock over the hand during sleep. A thumb habit that does not respond to these suggestions within 2 or 3 months may require more specific treatment in the form of an appliance. At this stage the child should be referred to a specialist (orthodontist or pedodontist) for design and management of the appliance. Occasionally the specialist may recommend further consultation with a clinical psychologist or psychiatrist.

VIII. VERTICAL RELATIONSHIPS *Continued*

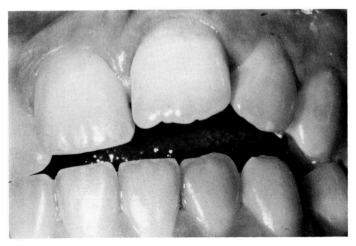

Figure 14–160 Note asymmetric open bite, which is secondary to a thumb-sucking habit. This 14-year-old patient was a thumb-sucker until 13½ years of age.

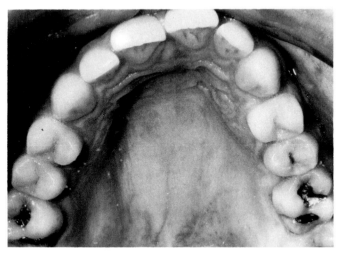

Figure 14–161 Maxillary occlusal view of patient in Figure 1–160. Note the degree of distortion in the alveolar arch form caused by the habit.

TABLE 14-1 MIXED DENTITION MALOCCLUSION GUIDELINES

PLANE OF SPACE	PROBLEM LIST	WHAT TO DO	WHEN?
Facial Pattern	1. Profile convexity (dental protrusion in both arches)	ortho°	as soon as permanent incisors erupt
	2. Maxillary prognathism/mandibular retrognathism—Class II (may also be convex profile)	ortho°	female: 8–9 years male: 11–12 years
	3. Maxillary retrognathism/mandibular prognathism—Class III (usually concave profile)	ortho°	as soon as recognized
Anterior-Posterior	1. Class I skeletal relationship with anterior crossbite	*treat*	as soon as recognized when maxillary permanent incisors erupt
	2. Class II (mandibular retrognathism, maxillary prognathism, i.e., positive overjet)	ortho°	female: 8–9 years male: 11–12 years
	3. Class III (mandibular prognathism maxillary retrognathism, i.e. negative overjet)	ortho°	as soon as recognized
Vertical	1. Deep bite (greater than 50% of lower incisor covered)	ortho°	as soon as recognized
	2. Open bite (lack of incisor contact, mammelons)	ortho°	as soon as recognized (not younger than 6–7 yrs.)
Transverse	1. Bilateral posterior functional crossbite (lateral mandibular CR-CO shift w/ midline deviation)	ortho°	as soon as recognized in primary or mixed dentition
	2. Midline deviation	ortho°	as soon as recognized
	3. Unilateral crossbite	*treat*	as soon as recognized
	4. Maxillary midline diastema	*treat*	after eruption of maxillary permanent cuspids
Perimeter	1. Arch length deficiency	ortho°	as soon as recognized when mandibular permanent incisors are erupting
	2. Tooth size discrepancy (peg laterals, missing teeth, supernumeraries, etc.)	ortho°	as soon as recognized
	3. Abnormal eruption pattern (early, late, ectopic, impaction, etc.)	ortho°	as soon as recognized
	4. Critical arch length requirement (for space maintenance)	*treat*	as soon as recognized

°These malocclusion problems are usually managed by the orthodontic specialist due to their inherent severity and their tendency to appear concurrently with other severe malocclusion problems.

TABLE 14-1   MIXED DENTITION MALOCCLUSION GUIDELINES — (*Continued*)

WHY?	REQUIREMENT FOR TREATMENT	HOW TREATED
treatment must be timed & oriented toward maximum incisor retraction		
requires growth-related correction (headgear)		
observation for possible surgical correction		
eliminate function interferences	Class I molar, adequate space, limited to 1 or 2 teeth	guide plane: tongue blade, acrylic splint, hawley w/springs, equilibrate/ extract primary cuspids
requires growth-related correction (headgear)		
observation for possible surgical correction		
usually indicates a developing Class II		
usually habit related (thumb, tongue, etc.)		
allow for normal transverse and A-P growth of maxilla, eliminate functional interference (treatment involves maxillary sutural expansion) usually indicates an arch length deficiency (see perimeter) eliminate functional interferences	no lateral mandibular CR-CO shift, limited to 1st permanent molar	cross elastics
improve esthetics, eliminate need for frenectomy or over-contoured restorations	adequate over bite/overjet to accommodate correction	bond or band w/elastic traction, retention (fixed or removable)
to plan eruption guidance (timed selective extraction) program		
to plan eruption guidance program		
to plan eruption guidance program		
to prevent loss of arch length, maintain arch symmetry	critical arch length requirement	lingual arch, band & loop, properly contoured restorations, etc.

REFERENCES

1. Bolton, W. A.: Disharmony in tooth size and its relation to the analysis and treatment of malocclusion. Angle Orthodont. 28:113–130, 1958.
2. Chaconas, S. J.: Preventive orthodontics: when and why. J. Preventive Dentistry 5:30, 1978.
3. Graber, T. M.: *Orthodontic Principles and Practice,* 3rd ed., W. B. Saunders Co., Philadelphia, 1972.
4. Law, D. B., Lewis, T. M., and Davis, J. M.: *An Atlas of Pedodontics,* 1st ed., W. B. Saunders Co., Philadelphia, 1969.
5. Little, R. M.: *Roentgenographic Cephalometry — An Individualized Learning Program — Measurement of Tooth and Jaw Position.* Department of Orthodontics, University of Washington, Seattle, 1976.
6. Little, R. M., and Wallen, T. R.: *Continuing Education Syllabus — Systematic Mixed Dentition Assessment.* Department of Orthodontics, University of Washington, Seattle, 1976.
7. Moyers, R. E.: *Handbook of Orthodontics,* 3rd ed., Year Book Medical Publishers, Chicago, 1973.
8. Thurow, Raymond C.: *Atlas of Orthodontic Principles.* 2nd ed. The C. V. Mosby Co., St. Louis, 1977.
9. University of Washington, School of Dentistry: Dentistry 460/461 — Syllabus — Orthodontic Diagnosis. Department of Orthodontics, Seattle, 1979.

PROSTHODONTICS

Chapter 15 _____

Full and partial dentures are the chief topics of discussion in this chapter.

Complete dentures are occasionally required in order to provide esthetics and function in a preschool child. There may be anodontia as a result of hereditary ectodermal dysplasia, or multiple extraction of teeth may have been performed because of rampant caries. In general, small children tolerate dentures very well. Their tissues are healthy and resistant, and their mental attitude is one of lack of concern over small irritations. They usually start eating immediately upon being fitted with dentures and seldom complain afterward. No inhibition of oral growth and development will be caused by dentures. In time, as changes occur, the dentures will simply no longer fit properly, and it will be obvious that alterations or a complete remake is required. The same procedures that are employed in preparing dentures for the adult should be followed in treating the child. In general, it is inadvisable to attempt to make complete dentures for a child under the age of 4 years because of his or her lack of comprehension and understanding at this young age.

The chief problems with complete dentures in children arise during the period of the eruption of the maxillary and mandibular incisors. The dentures must be cut away and relieved to allow room for the new teeth. This in turn destroys the seal of the denture flange, and poor retention results. Even if the child continues to wear the denture there is usually the problem of cleanliness and food retention around the cut-away areas.

Partial dentures are quite successful in children of all ages and are usually well tolerated. If at all possible, partial dentures rather than complete dentures should be constructed. Frequently, in planning treatment for a badly broken down mouth in a preschool child, the dentist can save a few teeth by heroic measures. It is worth crowning two cuspids and perhaps a primary molar if they can be retained and used as abutments for a removable denture.

367

During the transition period of the anterior teeth the partial denture can be successfully retained, whereas full dentures offer many problems.

In most clinical cases the choice of partial denture material will be acrylic resin. However, in cases that involve long-term use of the appliance, such as complete loss of permanent anteriors at an early age, the use of cast chrome-cobalt alloy partial dentures should be considered.

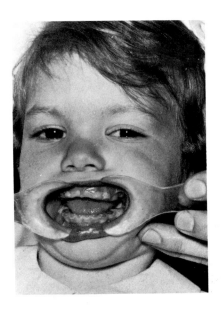

Figure 15-1   Patient J. B., a 3½-year-old girl with hereditary dentinogenesis imperfecta. Rapid wearing away of enamel and dentin is common with this condition. Prostheses are necessary for both function and esthetics. Management of this case will be illustrated through age 21 (Figures 15-1 to 15-22).

Figure 15-2 Maxillary arch. Mote abrasion of teeth and chronic abscess formation. Pulpal exposures may occur in these cases because of the wearing away of enamel and dentin, and extractions become necessary.

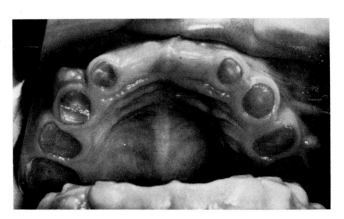

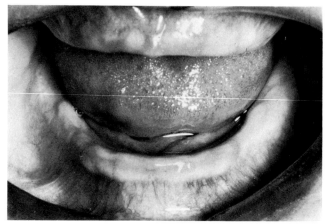

Figure 15-3 Age 4 years. All primary teeth have been extracted because of development of pulpal abscesses. Full dentures are now indicated for the health of this patient.

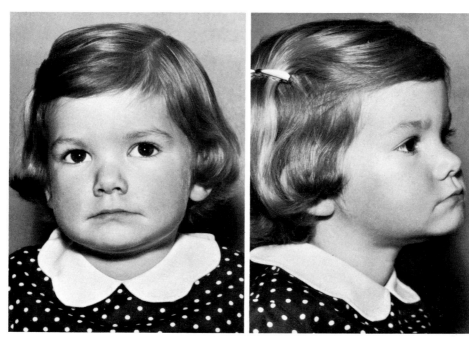

Figure 15-4 Profile and full face view. Patient is 4 years old. Extraction of all primary teeth has resulted in loss of vertical dimension.

Figure 15-5 Full dentures in place. Note shape, size, color, and spacing of the denture teeth to resemble those of natural primary teeth. The same steps in fabrication of full dentures for adults should be used in the child patient.

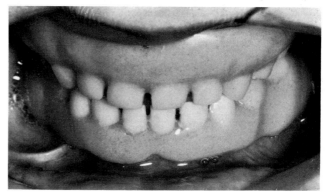

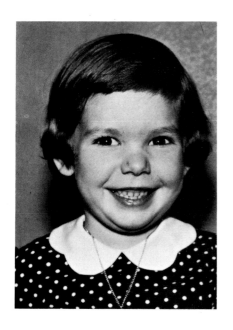

Figure 15-6 Full face view. Note the improvement in appearance and personality. Small children adapt very quickly to prosthetic appliances, and very few adjustments are usually necessary.

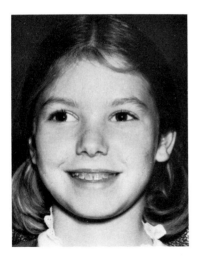

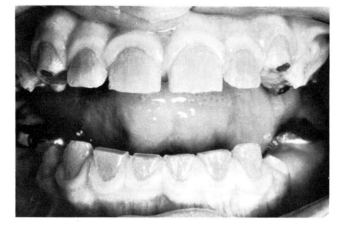

Figure 15-7 Patient is now 11 years of age. Permanent teeth have typical brown-opalescent color and are beginning to show abrasion and wear.

Figure 15-8 Anterior view. Mandibular incisors appear more worn than do the maxillary teeth.

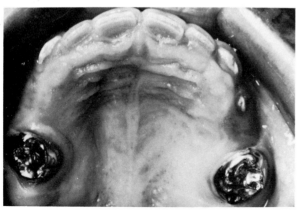

Figure 15-9 Maxillary arch. First permanent molars have been protected with stainless steel crowns. A simple acrylic palatal space maintainer was used as a temporary space holding appliance during this age period.

Figure 15-10 Mandibular arch. Permanent molars protected with stainless steel crowns. A simple acrylic space maintainer was also constructed for this arch.

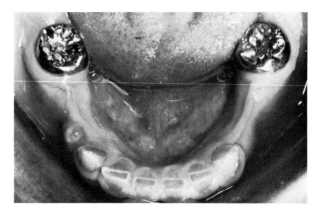

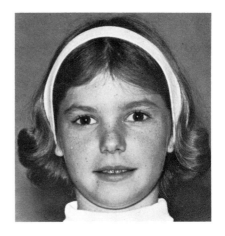

Figure 15-11 Age 13 years. The problem of esthetics is increasingly important during the patient's adolescent years.

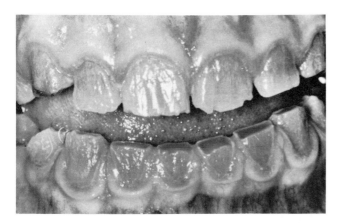

Figure 15-12 Anterior view. Chipping and abrasion are evident on the incisors.

Figure 15-13 Maxillary arch. Patient is 13 years old.

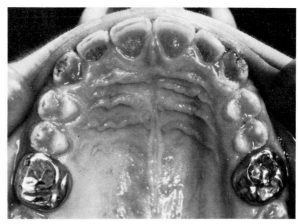

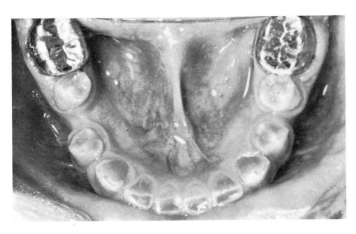

Figure 15-14 Mandibular arch. Patient is 13 years old. A decision as to further treatment must be made before significant loss of tooth structure occurs. For posterior teeth, stainless steel crowns are considered adequate interim restorations until definitive permanent restorations may be placed (see Figures 15-15 through 15-22).

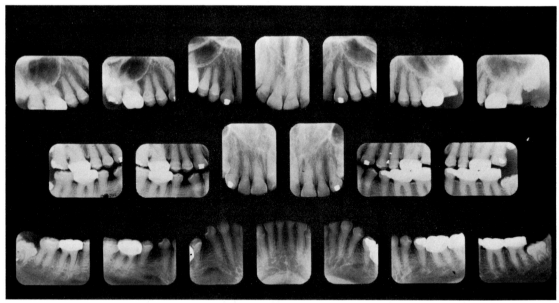

Figure 15-15   Radiographs of patient J. B. at age 14. Note typical appearance of dentino-genesis imperfecta with obliteration of pulp canals.

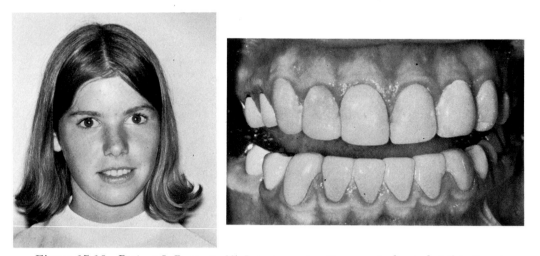

Figure 15-16   Patient J. B. at age 15. Interim restorations are indicated at this time to protect the teeth and restore esthetics until porcelain-fused-to-gold restorations may be placed on all teeth (see Figures 15–17 through 15–22).

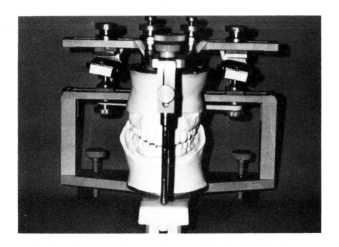

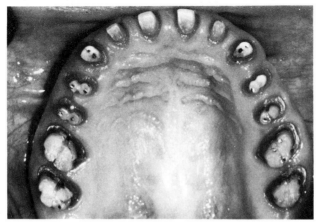

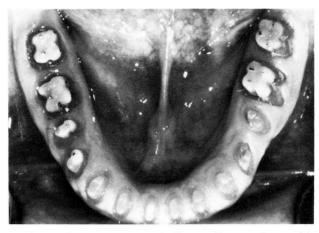

Figure 15-17   Models and preparations of all maxillary and mandibular teeth of patient J. B. at age 21 prior to placement of porcelain-fused-to-gold restorations. Only after careful diagnosis and treatment planning, combined with mounted study models and pre-planned restorative therapy, should extensive restoration of multiple teeth be undertaken. More time is required in the planning and coordination of therapy in order that the final result is both a functional and an esthetic success. See Figures 15-18 to 15-22 for this patient's full mouth restoration. (Photos courtesy of Dr. Roger Harper.)

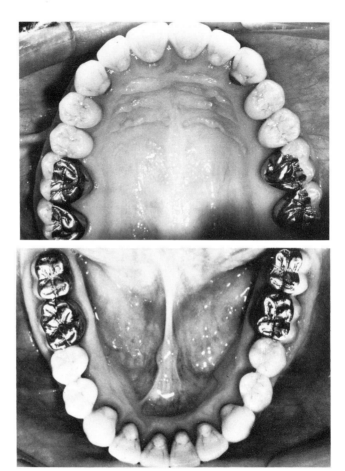

Figure 15-18   Patient J. B. at age 21. Placement of maxillary and mandibular porcelain-fused-to-gold restorations. (Photos courtesy of Dr. Roger Harper.)

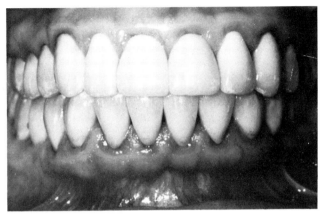

Figure 15-19 Patient J. B. at age 21. Anterior view of maxillary and mandibular porcelain-fused-to-gold restorations. (Photo courtesy of Dr. Roger Harper.)

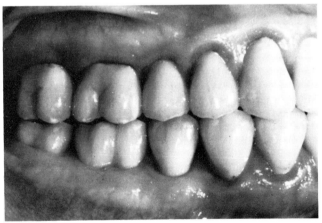

Figure 15-20 Patient J. B. at age 21. Right posterior view of maxillary and mandibular porcelain-fused-to-gold restorations. (Photo courtesy of Dr. Roger Harper.)

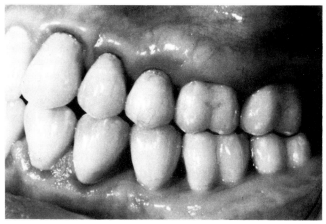

Figure 15-21   Patient J. B. at age 21. Left posterior view of maxillary and mandibular porcelain-fused-to-gold restorations. (Photo courtesy of Dr. Roger Harper.)

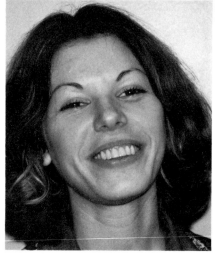

Figure 15-22   Full face view of patient J. B. at age 21, after final restorations were placed. (Photo courtesy of Dr. Roger Harper.)

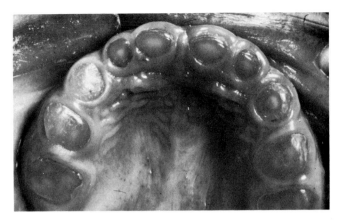

Figure 15-23 Maxillary arch of a 5-year-old girl, D. C., with dentinogenesis imperfecta. No tendency to develop pulpal abscesses was observed and it was decided to retain the teeth and construct the maxillary denture over them. Figures 15-21 to 15-28 illustrate this case.

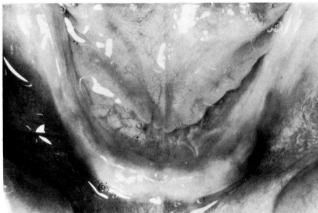

Figure 15-24 Mandibular arch. Teeth had previously been extracted when patient was first seen by authors.

Figure 15-25 Tissue side of maxillary and mandibular dentures. Note impressions of maxillary crowns in the upper denture.

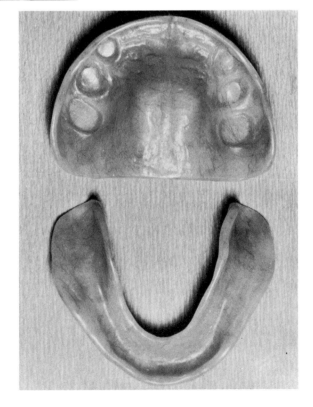

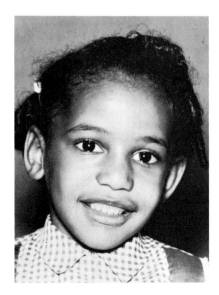

Figure 15-26   Dentures in place. No problem was encountered in retention of the maxillary denture.

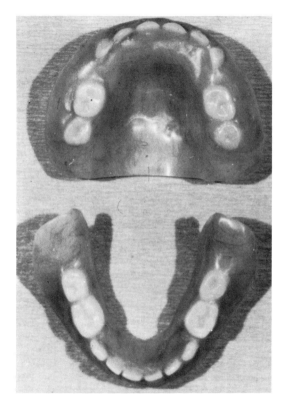

Figure 15-27   Occlusal view of dentures.

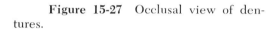

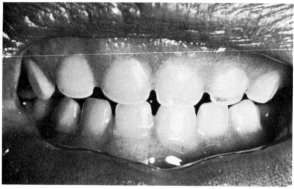

Figure 15-28 Anterior view, showing properly spaced and shaped denture teeth for a preschool child.

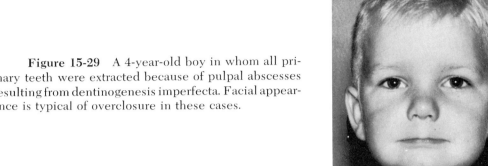

Figure 15-29   A 4-year-old boy in whom all primary teeth were extracted because of pulpal abscesses resulting from dentinogenesis imperfecta. Facial appearance is typical of overclosure in these cases.

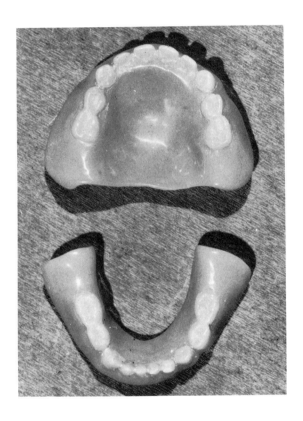

Figure 15-30   Maxillary and mandibular dentures fabricated for boy shown in Figure 15-29. Note distal extensions of denture to gain maximum stability.

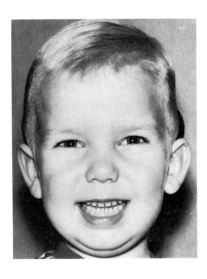

Figure 15-31   Same boy as seen in Figure 15-29 with maxillary and mandibular dentures in place. Note improved appearance. The spacing of denture teeth is important when making dentures for children.

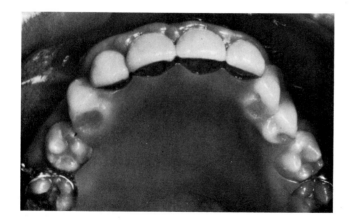

Figure 15-32 Maxillary acrylic partial dentures constructed for a child with ectodermal dysplasia. Anterior teeth were conical and were restored with porcelain bonded to gold crowns.

Figure 15-33 A mandibular acrylic bridge constructed for a child with missing mandibular incisors.

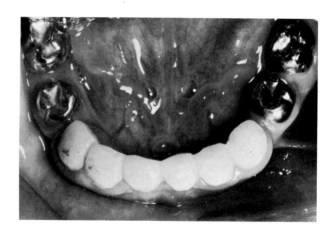

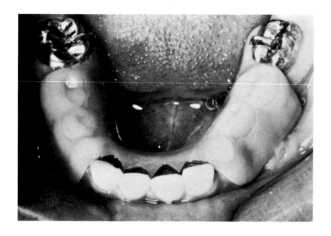

Figure 15-34 Mandibular acrylic partial denture for a child with ectodermal dysplasia. Conical incisors have been restored with porcelain bonded to gold crowns.

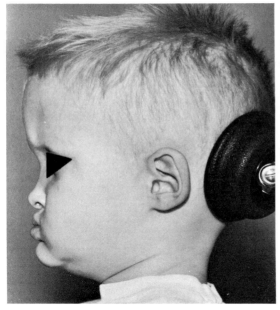
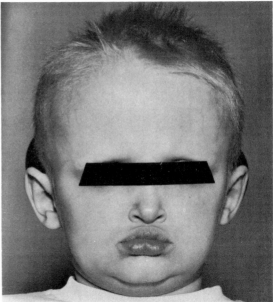

Figure 15-35   **Figure 15-36**

Figure 15-35   Profile of J. W., 4½-year-old boy with hereditary ectodermal dysplasia. Note typical appearance of saddle nose, everted lips, and absence of eyebrows. Lack of teeth causes overclosure. (From Bolender, C. L., Law, D. B., and Austin, L. B.: Prosthodontic treatment of ectodermal dysplasia. J. Pros. Dent. *14*[2]:317-325, March–April, 1964.) Figures 15-35 to 15-45 illustrate this case.

Figure 15-36   Anterior view. Affected patients require full or partial dentures to restore function as well as esthetics.

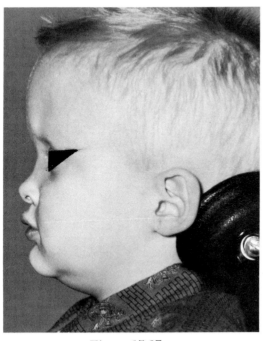
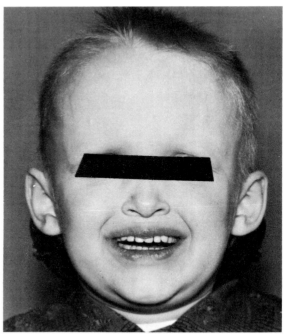

Figure 15-37   **Figure 15-38**

Figure 15-37   Complete prosthetic rehabilitation. Note improved profile.

Figure 15-38   Anterior view, showing natural appearance after treatment has been completed.

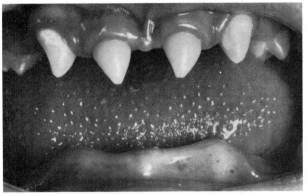

Figure 15-39 Intraoral view, before treatment. There is complete absence of erupted teeth in the mandibular arch. The maxillary arch has two erupted molars and four anteriors.

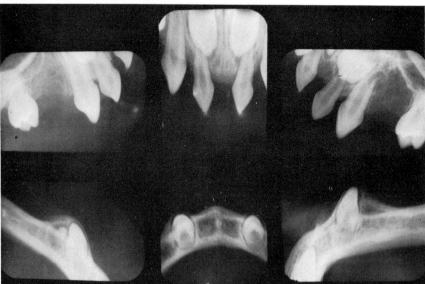

Figure 15-40 Radiographs demonstrate unerupted teeth. There is noticeable lack of alveolar bone because of the absence of teeth.

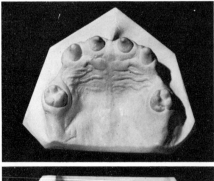

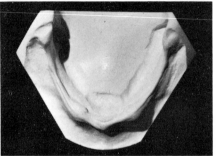

Figure 15-41 Study models. Note lack of ridge development in the mandibular arch.

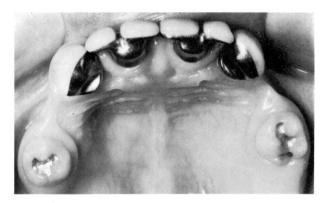

Figure 15-42 Cantilevered crowns (porcelain bonded to gold) on two maxillary conical incisors. This was done to render the typical appearance of four primary incisors. The conical cuspids were also crowned. Note lingual rest areas on these crowns for support of the partial denture.

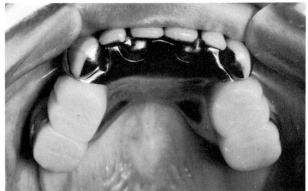

Figure 15-43 Cast cobalt-chromium alloy partial denture seated in maxillary arch. The wide flat teeth were necessary because of the discrepancy in width between the two arches.

Figure 15-44 Lateral view showing the clasps on the primary cuspid and molar. The molar is covered by the partial in order to build up adequate vertical dimension.

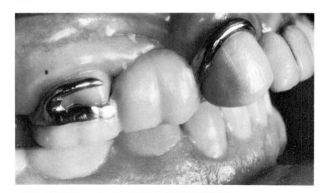

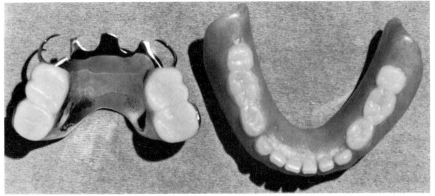

Figure 15-45 Upper partial and lower full denture. Note distal extension of mandibular denture flanges to gain stability.

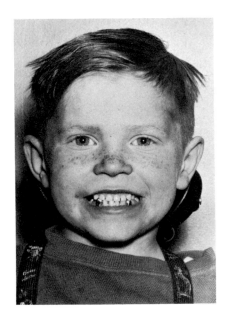

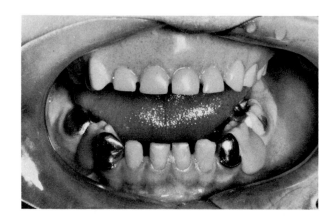

Figure 15-46 A 5-year-old boy with a full maxillary denture and mandibular partial. Teeth were extracted because of rampant caries.

Figure 15-47 Same boy as seen in Figure 15-46. Solder was made to flow on the gingival area of the steel crowns on the cuspids. This was done to provide better retention for the wire clasps.

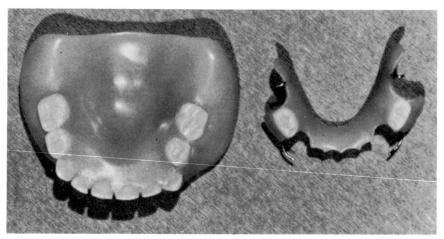

Figure 15-48 View of maxillary denture and mandibular partial of patient shown in Figure 15-47. Note extension of maxillary denture. Mandibular partial has rests on the second primary molars.

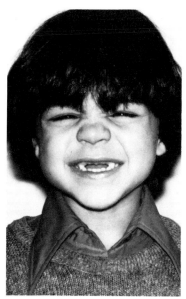

Figure 15-49 A 4¼-year-old boy lost the maxillary central and lateral primary incisors in a traumatic injury.

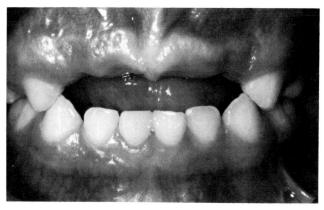

Figure 15-50 Intraoral view of 4½-year-old boy from Figure 15-49. A tongue thrusting habit may result from multiple missing teeth. See Figures 15-51 to 15-53 for appliance designed to prevent initiation of tongue thrusting habit and restore esthetics in this area.

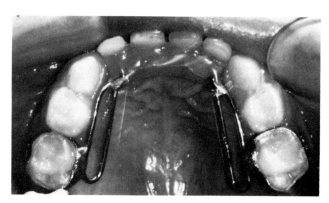

Figure 15–51 Maxillary occlusal view of appliance cemented on the maxillary second primary molar.

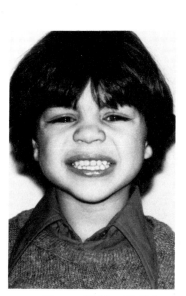

Figure 15-52 Full face view of patient from Figures 15-49 to 15-51.

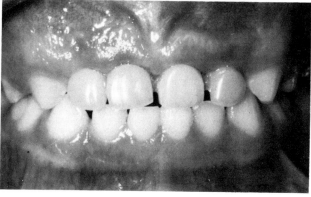

Figure 15-53 Replacement of lost maxillary primary incisors.

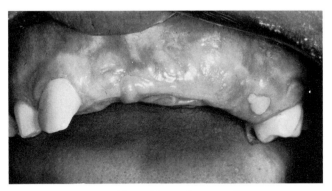

Figure 15-54   A 10-year-old girl lost the maxillary permanent right and left central incisors, left lateral incisor, and the primary left cuspid in an automobile accident. A temporary partial denture was made to restore esthetics and function in the area as well as to prevent mesial drifting of the teeth into the edentulous area. (See Figures 15-55 to 15-58.)

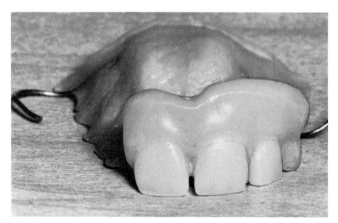

Figure 15-55   Acrylic temporary partial denture with stainless steel wire clasps, in case illustrated in Figure 15-54. Note the slight diastema between the central incisors to make the partial appear more realistic for the age of the patient.

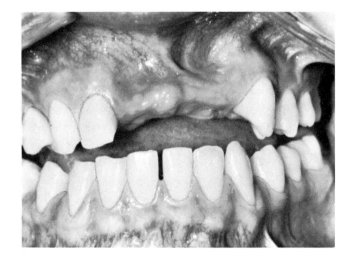

Figure 15-56 Edentulous area following eruption of the permanent cuspid. (Patient from Figure 15-54.)

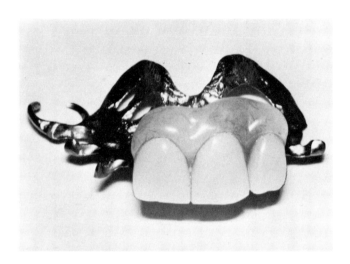

Figure 15-57 Chrome-cobalt partial denture made for the patient described in Figures 15-54 to 15-56, following complete eruption of the permanent teeth. A fixed bridge may be constructed when teeth have reached full maturity.

Figure 15-58 Full face view of patient with partial denture in place

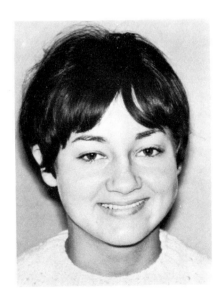

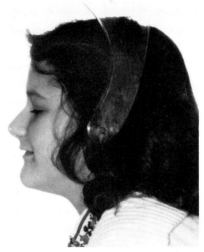

Figure 15-59 Pretreatment photograph of patient at age 10 years, 11 months. Note patient's short lower face height. For treatment of this patient with overdentures, see Figures 15-60 to 15-68. (Figures 15-60 to 15-68 courtesy of Drs. Ken Glover, Michael Spektor, and Ed Johnston, University of Washington, School of Dentistry.)

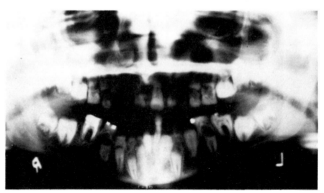

Figure 15-60 Panoramic radiograph reveals the presence of all permanent teeth with delayed resorption of the primary dentition.

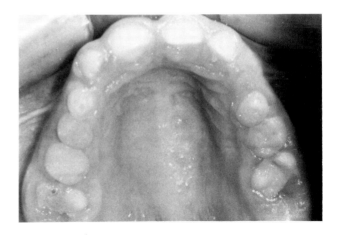

Figure 15-61 Intraoral pretreatment view of the maxillary arch. Note that none of the permanent molars are visible except for the mesiobuccal cusp of the right first molar.

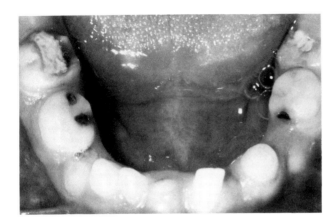

Figure 15-62 Intraoral pretreatment view of mandibular arch. Note the submerged right primary first molar and the delayed eruption of the permanent dentition.

Figure 15-63 Intraoral anterior view exhibiting the anterior and lateral open bite. The patient occludes on the hyperplastic gingival tissue distal to the erupted teeth. This can also be seen on the panoramic radiograph.

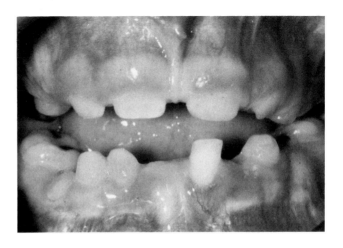

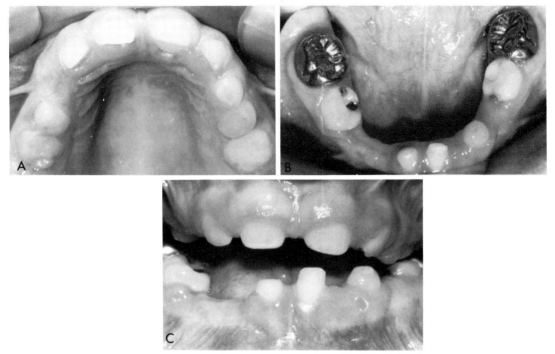

Figure 15-64   Restorative phase at 11 years, 5 months. *A,* Intraoral maxillary arch. Procedures included a median labial frenectomy, surgery of the posterior hypertrophied tissue, and uncovering of the first permanent molars, plus an acid-etch restoration of the occlusal surface of the right permanent molar. *B,* Intraoral mandibular arch. Procedures included surgery of the hypertrophied tissue distal and lateral to the first permanent molars, placement of stainless steel crowns on the first permanent molars, and extraction of some primary teeth. *C,* Intraoral anterior view after restorative, periodontal, and surgical procedures were accomplished with patient under intravenous sedation.

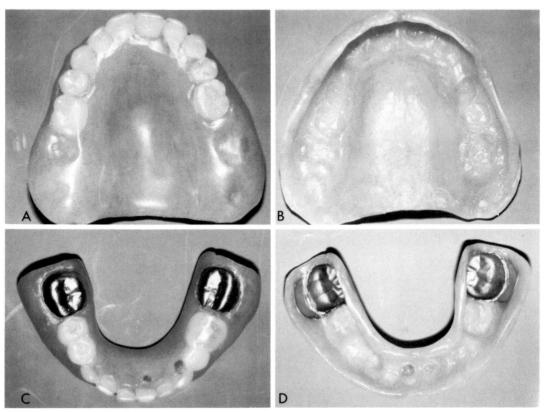

Figure 15-65 Prosthetic phase — overdenture fabrication — at age 11 years and 9 months. *A*, Maxillary overdenture (occlusal view). *B*, Maxillary overdenture (palatal view). Note the indentations for the erupted teeth. *C*, Mandibular overdenture (occlusal view). Note the use of a large stainless steel crown to increase retention and strength in the posterior region. *D*, Mandibular overdenture (inferior view). Note the indentations for the erupted teeth and the use of a soldered loop of wire from the buccogingival surface of the stainless steel crown to accentuate retention in the denture acrylic.

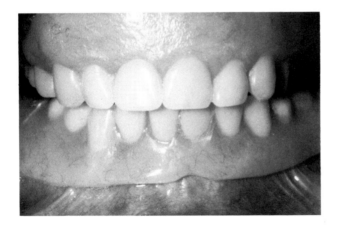

Figure 15-66 Intraoral anterior view with overdentures in place.

Figure 15-67 Extraoral view of the maxillary overdenture and the esthetic result.

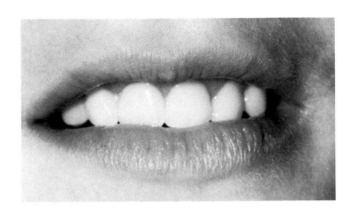

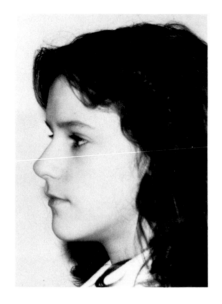

Figure 15-68 Posttreatment view showing the facial balance achieved by the overdentures.

TRAUMA TO THE PRIMARY DENTITION

Chapter 16

Accidents to the primary dentition are extremely common; however, many accident cases are never seen by the dentist, since they are of a very minor nature. In a clinical study[1] of 500 5-year-old children, it was found that 28 per cent evidenced some kind of injury to their anterior teeth. The most common type of trauma was caused by a fall and resulted in small enamel and dentin fractures of the incisors. These accidents accounted for 82 per cent of the total injuries observed. Of the entire group of children, only 4 per cent had experienced complete avulsion or displacement of teeth — a surprisingly low percentage. This probably accounts for the low incidence of observed hypoplasia on permanent incisors, since this is the type of injury that is most likely to damage underlying permanent teeth. Schrieber[2] followed 42 cases of intrusion or displacement of primary teeth and found that more than 20 per cent of these children later evidenced hypoplastic areas on the permanent incisors. He also found that the most common age at which injuries occur to primary teeth is between 1½ and 2½ years. This is the stage of learning to walk, when the small child is relatively uncoordinated.

If the dentist is called in for any emergency involving traumatic injuries to small children, he or she should make every effort to see the patient as soon as possible. It is never advisable to rely on the parent's assessment of the extent of damage. Frequently the child is not very cooperative at this age level, and it may be necessary to postpone radiographic examination and definitive treatment until soft tissue bruises have healed and the child has calmed down. It is very important to carefully examine the dentition for loose or cracked fragments of teeth, for trauma to opposing teeth, and for pulpal exposure. Displaced teeth can be repositioned and even splinted if necessary. Intrusions are usually left alone, and the teeth are allowed to re-erupt. In all such cases, periodic recalls with radiographic evaluation are absolutely necessary. Radiographic coverage must be adequate and should include the areas adjacent to the traumatized tooth as well as the opposing teeth. Discolored and traumatized primary teeth are always a potential hazard, since infection can develop and involve the underlying permanent teeth. If there is any question concerning the pathologic condition around a suspected nonvital incisor, the tooth should be observed closely or else extracted. The parent's concern is an important consideration whenever a young child damages his primary teeth. If the injury is limited to enamel and dentin fracture, it can be predicted in most instances that there will be no effect on the permanent successor. However, if there is intrusion or displacement,

393

especially at ages 1½ to 2½ years, there is the distinct possibility that there will be hypoplastic defects on the underlying tooth when it erupts. This must be considered when questions of medicolegal liability are involved.

In any severe traumatic injury to the primary teeth, jaw fracture should be considered as a possibility. A blow to the chin, for example, may result in fracture of the condyle. It should also be pointed out that whenever soft tissues are bruised and teeth are damaged in injuries that occur outdoors, the child should be referred to his physician for possible tetanus booster injections.

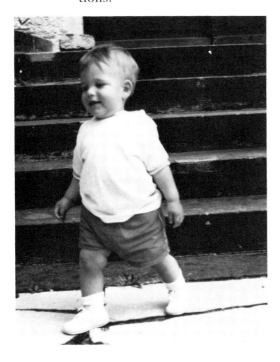

Figure 16–1 Children at this age are highly susceptible to traumatic falls (see Figure 16–2).

Figure 16–2 Accidents to primary teeth are most common at 1½ to 2½ years of age. This is the stage of learning to walk and is a period of underdeveloped motor coordination. (From Schreiber, C. K.: The effect of trauma on the anterior deciduous teeth. Brit. Dent. J. *106*:340–343, 1959).

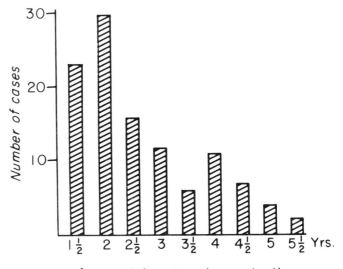

Age at injury to primary teeth

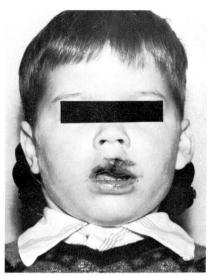

Figure 16–3 Typical appearance of a preschool child following an injury to the lips and teeth. In many of these cases the physician is consulted first. If possible, elective treatment should be deferred until the soft tissue bruising has subsided.

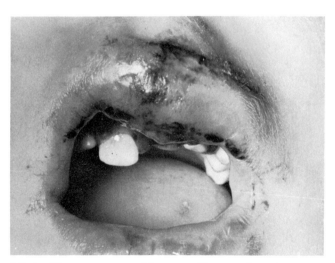

Figure 16–4 Close-up view of the case illustrated in Figure 16–3. One incisor has been avulsed or intruded; the other is quite mobile. Treatment consists of carefully removing loose fragments, taking radiographs to ascertain root condition, and closely observing the dentition over a 6-month period. The opposing arch should always be checked for possible damage. No positive statement can be made at this time concerning possible effects on the underlying permanent teeth.

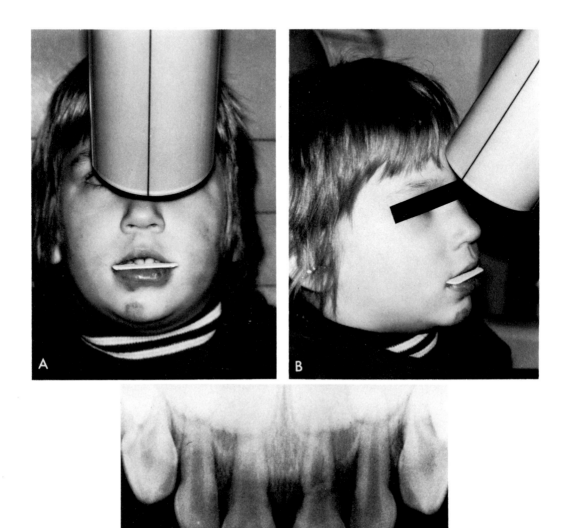

Figure 16–5 Most young children tolerate a maxillary occlusal radiograph much better than a periapical exposure after a traumatic injury. An adult-sized film is used rather than a large occlusal packet (see Chapter 4, Radiography). *A*, Anterior view of film and x-ray head in position for occlusal exposure. *B*, Lateral view of film and x-ray head in position for occlusal exposure. *C*, Radiographic view of occlusal exposure.

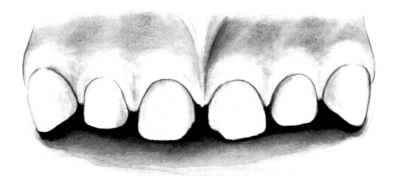

Figure 16–6   Enamel fracture of a maxillary primary incisor.

Treatment

1. Take radiographs to determine the full extent of the injury. Save films for future reference.
2. Smooth the fractured enamel if there are any sharp edges.
3. Schedule periodic check-ups at 6-month intervals.
4. Tooth may become necrotic at a later date and require endodontic therapy or extraction.
5. Tooth may undergo internal resorption and necessitate extraction.

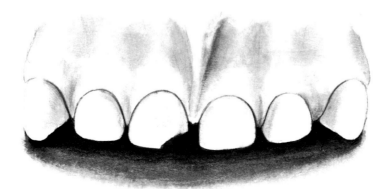

Figure 16–7   Dentin fracture of a maxillary primary incisor.

Treatment

1. Take radiographs to determine the full extent of the injury and save films for reference at future examinations.
2. Depending upon the extent of the exposed dentin, the fractured area may be smoothed over with discs, or, if necessary, a protective base of calcium hydroxide may be placed and covered with an esthetic composite restoration.
3. Schedule periodic check-ups at 6-month intervals. If the tooth becomes necrotic, extraction or endodontic therapy will be required.

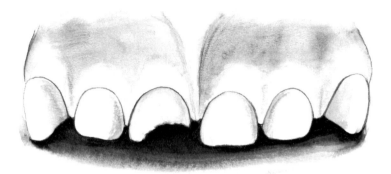

Figure 16–8   Fracture involving the pulp in a maxillary primary incisor.

Treatment

1. Take radiographs and save films for reference at future examinations.
2. If the size of pulpal exposure is pinpoint and the patient is seen immediately after the accident, cap the pulp with calcium hydroxide and place an esthetic composite restoration.
3. If pulpal exposure is large, perform a formocresol pulpotomy and place an esthetic composite restoration.
4. Schedule periodic check-ups at 6-month intervals. If tooth becomes necrotic, extraction or endodontic therapy will be required.

Figure 16–9 Intrusion of the maxillary primary central incisors. Careful clinical examination for pulpal exposures is always indicated. Radiographs should be taken to ascertain root damage. Usually these teeth should be left alone and allowed to re-erupt. Careful follow-up observation is necessary, since they are frequently devitalized by the injury. When this occurs, they should be either treated endodontically or extracted to prevent infection around the developing permanent teeth.

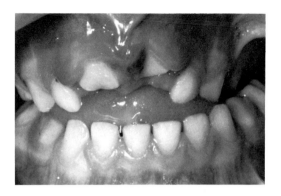

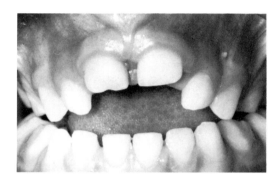

Figure 16–10 Patient seen in Figure 16–9, 6 months after injury. Note slight improvement in position as teeth are starting to re-erupt.

Figure 16–11 Patient seen in Figures 16–9 and 16–10, one year after injury. Note improved position of incisors at this time.

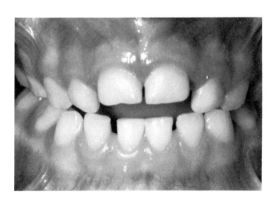

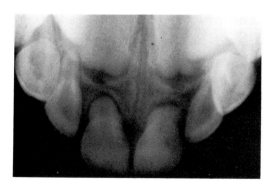

Figure 16–12 Radiograph of patient from Figure 16–11 one year after injury. Note the obliteration of pulp chamber of one incisor as a result of injury. These teeth should be checked every 6 months during the routine recall appointment for any sign of pulpal or periapical degeneration.

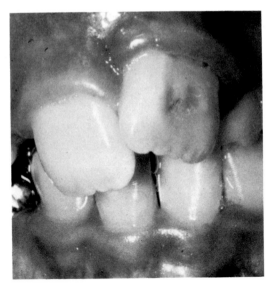

Figure 16–13 Hypocalcification and slight hypoplasia of the maxillary left permanent central incisor. There was a history of traumatic intrusion of the primary central incisor in this area. It is speculated that injuries to permanent incisors from intrusion of primary incisors are dependent upon (1) how deep the primary incisor is intruded, and (2) the amount of calcification completed at time of injury.

An injury of this nature is not likely to affect the underlying tooth if it occurs when the child is 4 to 5 years of age.

Figure 16–14 Hypoplasia of the maxillary right permanent central incisor, with a history of a traumatic intrusion of the primary incisor at age 2½ years. These sequelae are impossible to predict with certainty at the time of the accident.

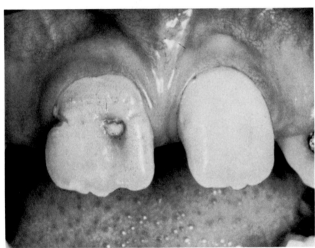

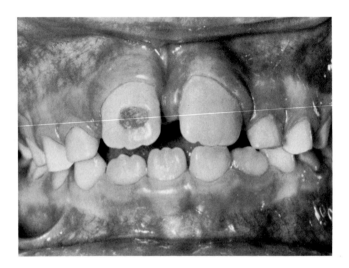

Figure 16–15 Hypoplasia of the maxillary right permanent central incisor. History of trauma similar to that of patient shown in Figure 15–14.

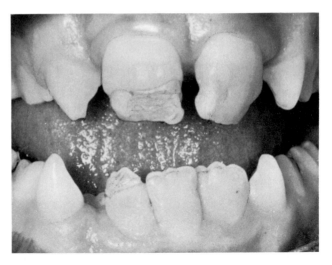

Figure 16–16 Severe hypoplastic defects in maxillary and mandibular permanent incisors. There was a history of facial injury during infancy as a result of an automobile accident. Frequently the dentist is called on to assist in insurance settlements in such cases. Consideration should always be given to the possibility of coronal restorations at some future date.

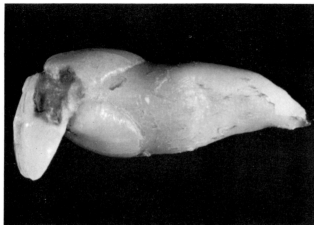

Figure 16–17 Dilaceration of a maxillary permanent central incisor. This is an extreme manifestation of injury to a permanent incisor as a result of a severe intrusion of a primary incisor. (Courtesy Dr. Fredrick Schoenbrodt.)

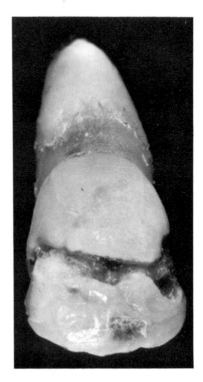

Figure 16–18 Labial view of tooth from Figure 16–17. (Courtesy Dr. Fredrick Schoenbrodt.)

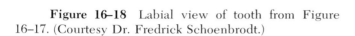

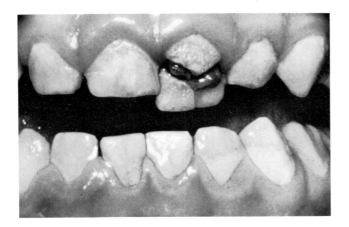

Figure 16-19 A horizontal and vertical fracture of the crown of a maxillary primary central incisor. When a primary tooth is so severely mutilated, extraction is usually the treatment of choice.

Figure 16-20 An 18-month-old child with a mutilated maxillary right primary central incisor—an injury similar to that seen in Figure 16-19. It was necessary to extract this tooth (see Figure 16-21).

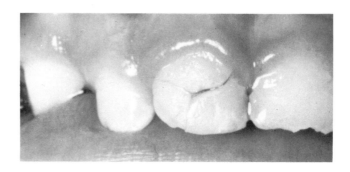

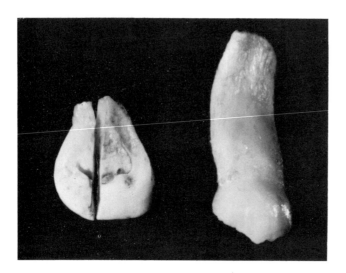

Figure 16-21 View of maxillary primary incisor extracted from patient in Figure 16-20.

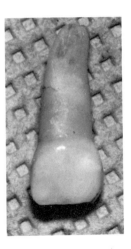

Figure 16–22 Labial view of extracted primary central incisor after traumatic injury. Note that this view gives little hint of why extraction was necessary (see Figure 16–23).

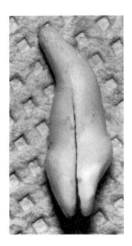

Figure 16–23 Lateral view of same tooth as in Figure 16–22. Note fracture in this view.

Figure 16–24 Fractured tooth from Figures 16–22 and 16–23. Extraction was clearly the treatment of choice in this case.

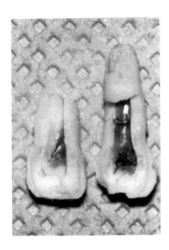

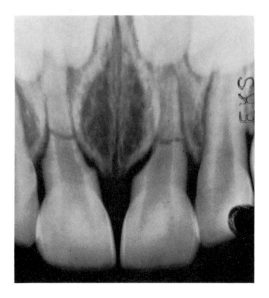

Figure 16–25 Radiograph showing fractured roots of the maxillary primary incisors following a fall. In this case, stabilization of the injured teeth is not indicated, and extraction is the treatment of choice.

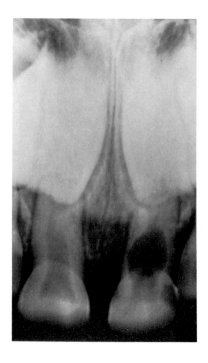

Figure 16–26 Internal resorption in a maxillary primary incisor after a traumatic injury. Note that there is no fracture of tooth structure in this case. Extraction is the treatment of choice.

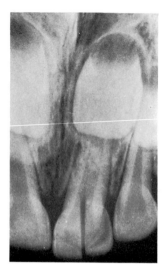

Figure 16–27 Radiograph of a longitudinal fracture extending into the root. Successful restorative treatment of these conditions is unlikely. Extraction is usually the treatment of choice.

Figure 16–28 A 2-year-old child with a displaced mandibular left primary lateral incisor. After the tooth was repositioned, a quick-cure acrylic splint was made that covered the occlusal surface of all primary teeth and opened the bite slightly (approximately 1 to 1½ mm.). The splint was extended just to the gingivae on the buccal and lingual surfaces and secured with zinc phosphate cement. It was left in place for two weeks and well tolerated by the child.

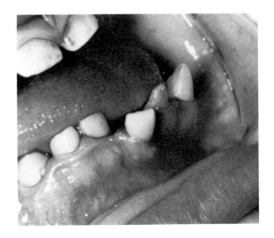

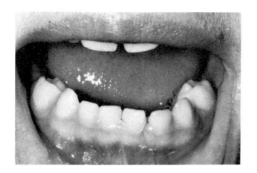

Figure 16–29 Patient seen in Figure 16–28, 2 weeks after the injury with the splint removed. The tooth was in good alignment and was stable.

Figure 16–30 A 3½-year-old child with a displaced maxillary right primary central incisor. The tooth was repositioned, etched with phosphoric acid, rinsed, and dried. The resin and composite splint was then placed.

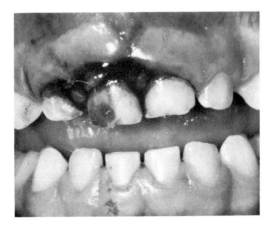

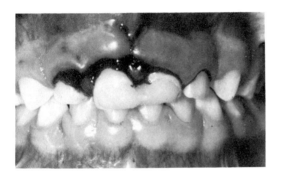

Figure 16–31 Splint placed for patient in Figure 16–30. The splint would have been more durable if it had extended to the right lateral incisor.

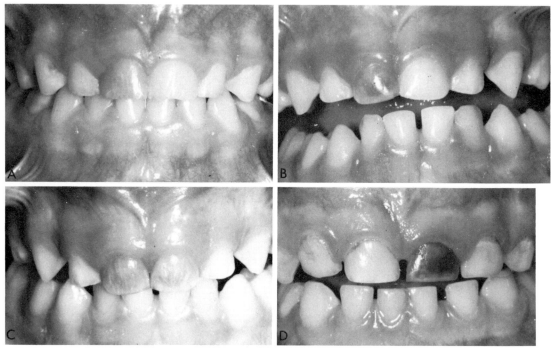

Figure 16–32   Discoloration of maxillary primary central incisors caused by trauma. The darkened appearance occurred as a result of the escape of hemosiderin pigments into the dentinal tubules. These teeth may become lighter or darker and should be checked every 6 months during the routine recall appointment for any sign of pulpal or periapical degeneration. If the tooth becomes necrotic, extraction or endodontic therapy will be required.

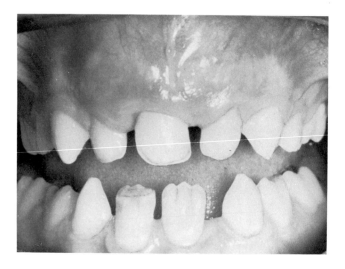

Figure 16–33   Drifting of maxillary primary incisors following the loss of one central incisor. When a primary incisor is lost past the age of 3 to 3½ years, intercanine space usually remains the same. However, some shifting of the remaining incisors may occur. Construction of a bridge or removable appliance is ordinarily not necessary, but may be indicated in some cases when improved esthetics is desired or unusual conditions prevail, such as crowding. (See Chapter 15. Prosthodontics.)

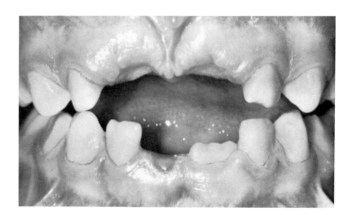

Figure 16–34 At 3½ years of age this child lost both maxillary primary central incisors in an accident. A partial denture was fabricated to restore esthetics.

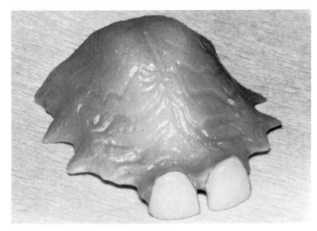

Figure 16–35 Partial denture for child shown in Figure 16–34. Note that no clasps are used. Although retention in this case is excellent without clasps, the clasps should be used when problems of retention are anticipated.

Figure 16–36 Partial denture in place. Note size and spacing of teeth to achieve natural dental appearance for a child of this age.

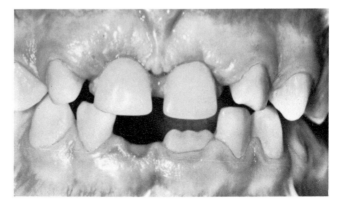

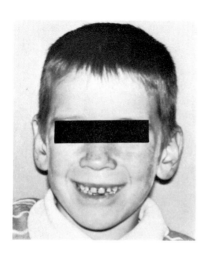

Figure 16–37 Full-face view of child with partial denture in place. Partial is no longer used once the permanent maxillary incisors start to erupt.

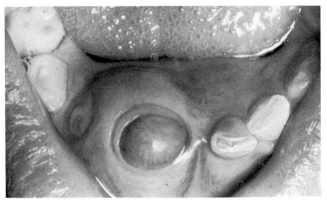

Figure 16–38 Large acute abscess occurring 1 year following a traumatic accident to the mandibular primary incisors. One discolored and nonvital incisor was allowed to remain in the arch because it was asymptomatic. The case was not observed closely and the resultant infection caused gross displacement of the underlying permanent central incisor.

Figure 16–39 Radiograph of teeth shown in Figure 16–38. Note the extensive bone loss and the extreme malposition of the permanent central incisor. This case clearly shows the need for constant observation of traumatized primary teeth and prompt treatment for them if they become nonvital and undergo periapical change.

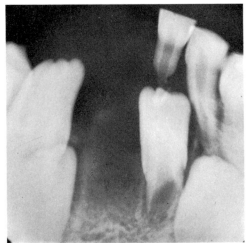

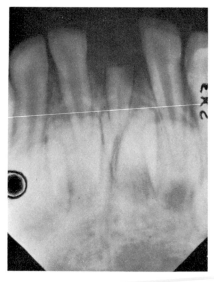

Figure 16–40 Mandibular primary incisor is missing; parents mistakenly considered it to have been completely "knocked out" after a fall.

Figure 16–41 Radiograph of teeth shown in Figure 16–40. A retained root is present as a result of the traumatic accident in which only the crown was broken off. A thorough examination by a dentist, including radiographs, is always desirable in any case of trauma.

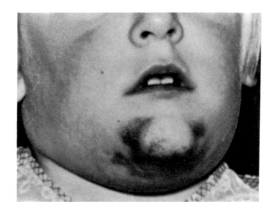

Figure 16–42 Chin of a child who fell over the handlebars of a tricycle. These injuries may cause trauma to the posterior teeth and possibly the condyle of the mandible. A panoramic radiograph is indicated if trauma to the condyle is suspected.

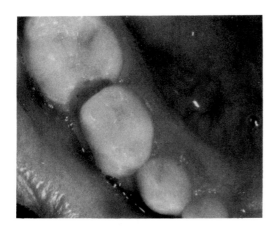

Figure 16–43 Fractured mandibular right second primary molar, resulting from a blow under the chin. There was no condylar fracture in this case. Examination of any patient after an accident should always include gross clinical inspection of all the teeth. Fractured posterior teeth should be treated and followed the same as fractured anterior teeth. Although this is a mesial fracture, mandibular teeth usually fracture on the buccal surfaces — and maxillary teeth on the lingual surfaces — as a result of this type of injury.

REFERENCES

1. Hunton, R. T., and Lust, W. B.: Injuries as found in the anterior primary dentition. Senior thesis. University of Washington, June, 1961.
2. Schreiber, C. K.: The effect of trauma on the anterior deciduous teeth. Brit. Dent. J. *106*:340–343, 1959.

TRAUMA TO THE PERMANENT DENTITION

Chapter 17 _____

The management of injuries to the newly erupted permanent anterior teeth constitutes a recurring problem to the practicing dentist. Studies of these injuries indicate that over 75 per cent occur in children between the ages of 8 and 11 years — the elementary school period. This is a period of growth and development characterized by unrestrained physical activity; the dentition is vulnerable because of the prominence of the permanent anterior teeth during the development of the facial complex. Many minor injuries to these teeth are never seen by the dentist, consequently his experience is likely to be associated with the more traumatic incidents involving gross dentin fracture, pulpal exposure, and occasionally complete avulsion. Davis[3] reported from a study of 2237 students between 7 and 17 years of age that 22.8 per cent had experienced some type of traumatic accident to the anterior teeth. In fractures of the incisors, 74.2 per cent involved the enamel, 24.7 per cent were in the dentin, and only 1.1 per cent involved the pulp. The pulpal fractures are extremely important, however, since these cases are usually the ones that require emergency dental treatment. A report from the Eastman Institute[7] indicates that only 2 per cent of fractured incisors involve root fracture. Little or no information is available concerning the incidence of complete avulsion, but it is comparatively rare.

The causative factors in dental injuries during the childhood years have been documented by Law[4] and are presented in Table 17–1. A wide variety of factors are responsible for these injuries.

411

TABLE 17-1 CAUSES OF FRACTURES AND ENVIRONMENT IN WHICH THEY
OCCURRED IN 1643 ELEMENTARY SCHOOL CHILDREN

Fall	6	Kicked	1
Gold club	2	Door handle	1
Swimming pool	3	Ice	3
Car	6	Roller skating	1
Sidewalk	4	Bathroom	1
Eating candy	1	Telephone	1
Fall from tree	2	Push-ups	1
Beads	1	Trapeze	1
Bike	15	Go-Kart	1
Sink	2	School bus	1
Truck	1	Playground	2
Summer camp	1	Baseball	3
Fight	5	Basketball	1
Sled	4	Boxing	1
Pop bottle	3	Jump rope	1
Pole vaulting	1	Baton	1
Sling shot	1	Merry-go-round	1
Rock	1	Fire escape	1
Marble	1	Train	1

Boys are reported to have twice as many injuries as girls at comparable age levels, which is probably attributable to their participation in more active games and sports.

Prevention is an important consideration, and the only truly preventive measure the dentist can suggest during the elementary school years is early orthodontic correction of markedly protruding maxillary incisors. The child with pronounced labioversion of maxillary teeth is more susceptible to injury than the child with a flat profile with good soft tissue coverage. Lewis[5] and Davis[3] reported a significantly higher incidence of fractured permanent incisors among children with maxillary protrusions in excess of 4 mm. Early referral to the orthodontist is particularly desirable if the child is known to be "accident prone."

The use of mouthguards is especially helpful in preventing accidents to anterior teeth during participation in organized athletics. This is most helpful during the teenage years. Cohen[2] reported excellent results in prevention of dental injuries to Philadelphia high school football players with the mandatory use of individually fitted mouthguards. Most high schools and colleges now require that these appliances be worn in all types of contact sports.

In all cases of accidental injuries to young permanent incisors there are two considerations of prime importance to the dentist: (1) conservation of the pulp, and (2) restoration of the crown. Appropriate treatment of the fractured incisor for pulpal conservation depends upon the nature and severity of the injury. As previously stated, most fractures of the immature permanent tooth do not directly involve the pulp. Many fractures do, however, involve the dentin, and irritants can pass via the dentinal tubules to the pulp. Therefore, the treatment of choice is a sedative dressing held in place by a composite restoration after etching enamel with phosphoric acid. If there is actual exposure of the pulp, immediate treatment is indicated, consisting of a pulpotomy with calcium hydroxide or, if conditions warrant, endodontic treatment. Significant psychological effects can be anticipated if severely fractured anterior teeth are not esthetically restored, particularly in the young teenager.

Complete avulsion of one or more permanent incisors is an uncommon accident, but when it occurs it necessitates immediate, definitive treatment. Studies by Andreasen and Hjorting-Hansen[1] indicate that the length of time the avulsed tooth is out of the mouth before replantation determines the likelihood of success of the treatment. They studied 110 replanted teeth and found that when the extraoral period did not exceed 30 minutes, replantation was successful in 90 per cent of the cases based on absence of root resorption or other pathology. When the extraoral period was 30 to 90 minutes, replantation was successful in 43 per cent of the cases. When teeth were replanted after a 90-minute extraoral period, success was achieved in only 7 per cent of the cases. It would seem advisable in most instances to wash the root of the avulsed tooth and immediately replant and splint, postponing the endodontic treatment for several weeks.

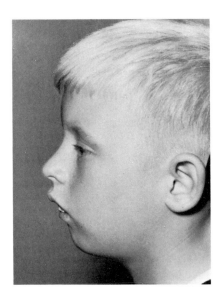

Figure 17–1 Profile of a 10-year-old boy with protruding maxillary central incisors. Children with this type of malocclusion are more susceptible to dental injuries. To help reduce this high rate of dental accidents, children with protruding anterior teeth should receive some orthodontic correction as soon as possible.

Figure 17–2 Same child as shown in Figure 17–1, exhibiting fractured wrist. The "accident prone" child frequently experiences trauma to the teeth. Note the protruding and elongated central incisors with very little lip coverage.

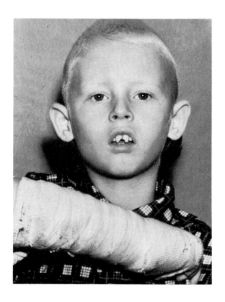

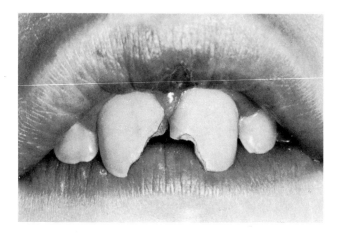

Figure 17–3 Close-up from Figure 17–2, showing diagonal fractures of the enamel and dentin with slight lip involvement. Any fracture involving the dentin requires immediate treatment (see Figures 17–11 through 17–14).

Figure 17–4 Traumatic injury to the maxillary central incisors as a result of a bicycle accident. Although no coronal fracture is visible on intraoral evaluation, it is still necessary to rule out the possibility of a root fracture (see Figure 17–5). Note the absence of a sign of root fractures in Figure 17–5. In cases of concussion such as this, it is necessary to have a radiograph for future reference, since it is possible the severe blow may ultimately cause pulpal degeneration and necrosis. Note slight gingival hemorrhage around maxillary right central incisor; this is why the parent thought the teeth should be evaluated by a dentist.

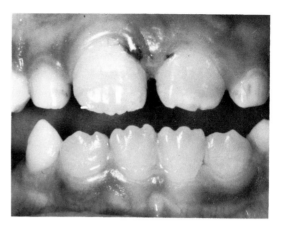

Figure 17–5 Radiograph of maxillary central incisor of patient in Figure 17–4. Note wide open apices. For future reference, this radiograph should be compared with one taken in 6, 12, and 18 months. If root formation continues, it is a good indication that the teeth have survived the original trauma. However, if formation does not continue, as seen in Figure 17–6, it is a sign of pulpal degeneration. The involved tooth must be further tested (electric pulp tester, hot and cold) and endodontics must be considered.

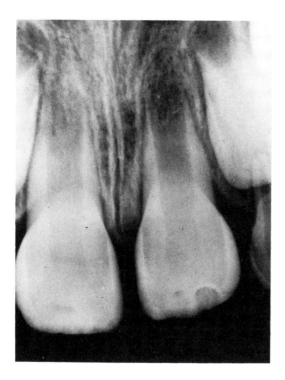

Figure 17–6 Radiograph of maxillary central incisors 18 months after traumatic injury (this is not the same patient as in Figures 17–4 and 17–5). Note the incomplete root formation of left central incisor when compared with root development of right central incisor after traumatic injury. This tooth sustained concussion from the original trauma and, subsequently, pulpal degeneration. When tested, the tooth was found to be nonvital to hot and cold and the vitalometer. It was then treated with the root end closure procedure (see Chapter 9, Pulp Therapy).

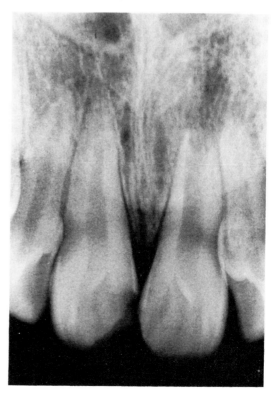

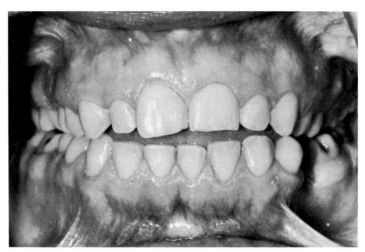

Figure 17–7 Enamel fractures of the maxillary permanent central incisors. The following treatment is recommended:

1. Obtain a history of the accident.
2. Do a thorough oral examination to determine the extent of the injury including any tooth mobility.
3. Take necessary radiographs of involved area to determine extent of injury.
4. Gently smooth the rough edges of fractured enamel.
5. It is wise to check the teeth 6 months following the accident. They may have sustained a severe blow and yet have only slight enamel fractures. In this case, the effect of the concussion may have been great enough to cause the loss of vitality of the involved teeth. Therefore, a vitality test may be made. Such a test taken less than one month following the accident may be unreliable because the pulp may be in a temporary state of shock.
6. These teeth may be reshaped to make them more esthetically acceptable, or a small acid etch restoration may be placed.

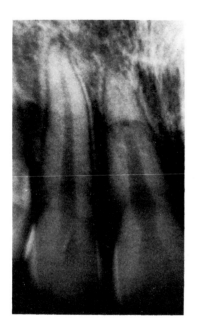

Figure 17–8 Radiograph of patient with a small enamel chip — note root fracture. Since there was no mobility, a splint was not placed. The value of a radiograph for future reference is obvious.

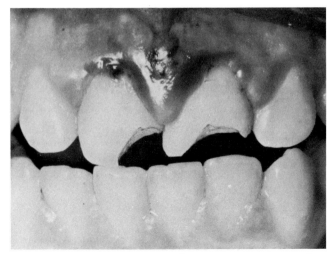

Figure 17–9 Dentin fractures of the maxillary permanent central incisors. The following treatment is recommended:

1. Obtain a history of the accident.
2. Do a thorough oral examination to determine the extent of the injury including mobility.
3. Take necessary radiographs of involved area to determine extent of injury.
4. Treatment options are (A) A sedative dressing and a composite (bandage) placed over fractured tooth structure (see Figures 17–11 through 17–14 for a complete description of this procedure). (B) A composite build-up using acid etching after sedative dressing is placed over the exposed dentin (see Figures 17–17 through 17–20 for a complete description of this procedure). (C) A stainless steel crown with labial composite is placed if the fracture is so severe that neither of the preceding procedures can be used because of a lack of existing tooth structure for retention of the restoration. These are usually severe horizontal fractures involving the pulp, rather than a large dentin fracture (see Figures 17–33 through 17–36 for a complete description of this procedure).
5. The patient should be checked at 6-month intervals, at which time a vitality test can be performed.
6. Permanent restorations may be considered once the fractured teeth have sufficiently erupted and the pulp has receded so that a crown preparation can be made without involving the pulp.

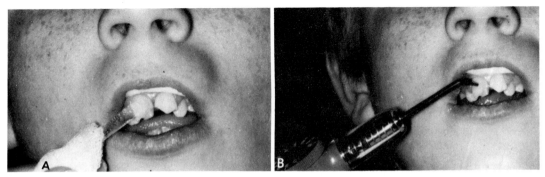

Figure 17–10 Ice or a pulp tester may be used to determine vitally of tooth 6 months after injury. A radiograph taken at this time is also valuable in determining continued root development and associated pulpal vitality.

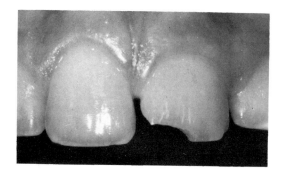

Figure 17–11 Emergency treatment for a sensitive dentin fracture of the maxillary left central incisor. When time does not allow the placement of an esthetic *composite build-up*, a *composite bandage* is suggested to protect the pulp and reduce the patient's discomfort from the exposed dentin (see Figures 17–12 through 17–14 for this procedure).

Figure 17–12 The fracture is gently dried, and a sedative dressing is place over the dentin. Anesthetizing the tooth is usually not necessary, however this decision is left to the judgment of the clinician based on the comfort of the patient during the procedure. A thin layer of resin is placed over the sedative dressing and allowed to dry. The fractured enamel surrounding the sedative dressing is then etched with phosphoric acid for 1 minute, rinsed with water, and air dried. The resin is then placed over the etched area as seen in Figure 17–13.

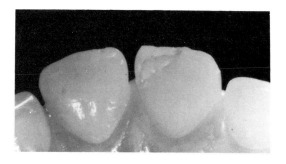

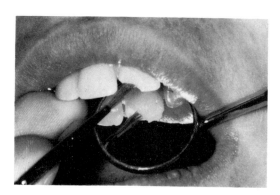

Figure 17–13 Resin placed over etched area.

Figure 17–14 The *composite bandage* is placed over the resin. Note that the contour was not restored at this time. Instead, quick placement of the material and smoothing with a disc was accomplished. If time had permitted, a complete esthetic build-up would have been considered. The patient is now rescheduled for a time that is convenient to both patient and dentist for completion of the composite restoration. During the next appointment, the *bandage* may or may not be left on depending on the preference of the clinician. If it is left on it will be necessary to reduce it slightly. The enamel must then be etched, rinsed, and dried, and composite placed in this area.

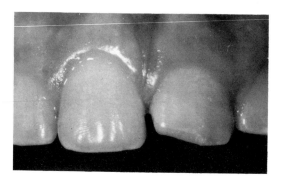

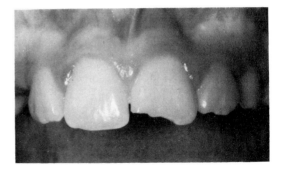

Figure 17–15 Sensitive dentin fracture of the maxillary left central incisor. Whenever possible, the preferred treatment is a *composite build-up* that restores the tooth to its natural esthetic contour, rather than the *composite bandage* as described in Figures 17–11 through 17–14).

Figure 17–16 The fracture is gently dried, and a sedative dressing is placed over the dentin. Anesthetizing the tooth is usually not necessary; however, this decision is left to the judgment of the clinician based on the comfort of the patient during the procedure. A thin layer of resin is placed over the sedative dressing and allowed to dry. The enamel surrounding the sedative dressing is etched with phosphoric acid for 1 minute. It is then rinsed with water and air dried. The resin is applied over the etched enamel, which is carried to the tooth with a modified crown form (see Figure 17–17).

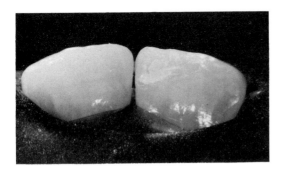

Figure 17–17 Composite placed with a modified crown form. A perforation is made in the incisal angle of the crown to prevent bubbles from forming in this area. Note extrusion of composite through perforation.

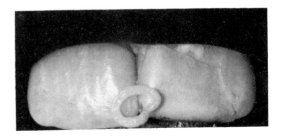

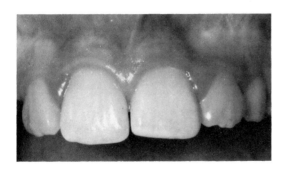

Figure 17–18 Finished *composite build-up*. Note that too much composite was removed from the incisal angle. This type of restoration may start to discolor in several years and may have to be replaced at a later date. In order to prevent dislodgment, patients are warned not to chew hard foods with these restorations.

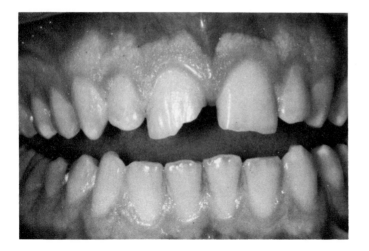

Figure 17–19   A 17-year-old patient with large fractures of the maxillary central incisor. This patient preferred *composite build-ups* to anterior crowns.

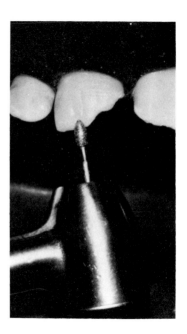

Figure 17–20   After teeth have been cleaned with a nonglycerin-containing prophylaxis paste, their shade is taken to determine color match with the restorative material to be used. Anesthesia should be considered in preparing a labial and lingual chamfer. The rubber dam is then placed and the chamfer is made with burs or diamonds depending upon the preference of the clinician (see Figures 17–27 and 17–28 for suggested chamfers).

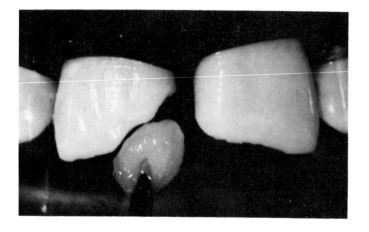

Figure 17–21   The phosphoric acid is placed for 1 minute, then rinsed with water and dried. A thin layer of resin is placed, and the composite is carried to the tooth in a pretrimmed crown form.

Figure 17–22 Contoured composite build-ups immediately after rubber dam removal. Diamonds, burs, and fine discs work well in achieving contour and final finish of the composite. A resin glaze is placed over the finished composite and allowed to dry just before rubber dam removal (many consider this step optional).

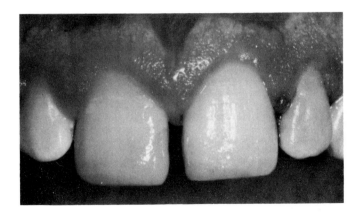

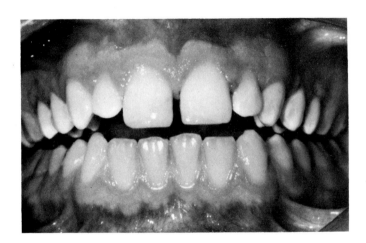

Figure 17–23 Labial view of composite build-ups shown in Figures 17–19 through 17–22. Note that composite appears slightly darker than the rest of tooth. Since tooth structure has dehydrated under the rubber dam, it is natural that it appears slightly lighter. Within hours, moisture will return to these areas, and the color match should be excellent (see Figure 17–24).

Figure 17–24 Composite restorations several days after treatment — note color match. The dehydrated areas have now returned to their normal shade. These restorations may start to discolor in several years and may have to be replaced or reveneered at a later date.

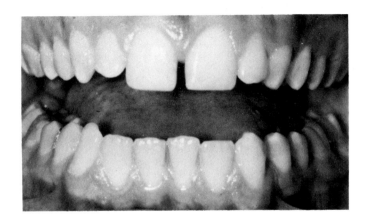

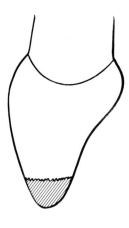

Figure 17–25 Drawing of butt-joint composite restoration after acid etching fractured enamel. This is usually reserved for small fractures (see Figures 17–26 through 17–28).

Figure 17–26 Drawing of overlapping composite restoration *without* chamfer after acid etching enamel. The disadvantage of this technique is that a greater bulk of composite must be placed on the labial surface to achieve the desired esthetic appearance as compared with the chamfer described in Figures 17–27 and 17–28. Another disadvantage of this technique is the fragile feather edge of composite at the union of composite and enamel. This gradually fractures away, leaving a roughened area that results in poor esthetics.

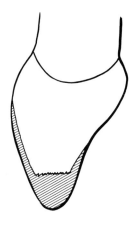

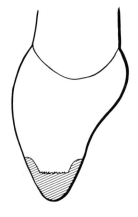

Figure 17–27 Drawing of chamfer and overlapping of composite restoration after acid etching enamel. This technique is frequently used with large dentin fractures (see Figure 17–28).

Figure 17–28 Drawing of more extensive chamfer than in shown in 17–27. It is sometimes desirable for esthetics to overlap more of the labial surface than is displayed in Figure 17–27.

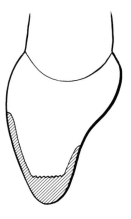

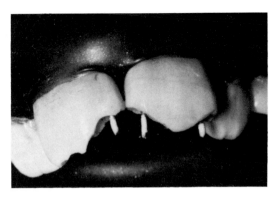

Figure 17–29 Prior to the perfection of acid etching procedures, pins were frequently used with large composite restorations.

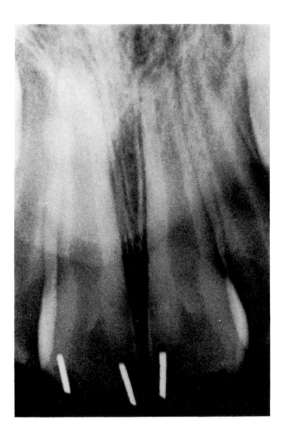

Figure 17–30 Radiograph of patient seen in Figure 17–29. Note proximity of pins to large coronal pulp chambers. Pins are not used as frequently since acid etching procedures have been perfected.

Figure 17–31 Adult with fractured maxillary right central incisor. Rather than having a full esthetic crown placed, this patient preferred a composite build-up after acid etching.

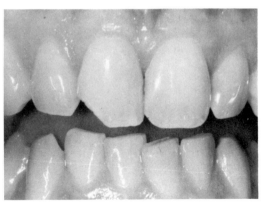

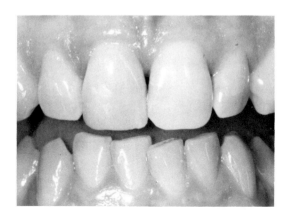

Figure 17–32 Composite build-up after acid etching. This patient was extremely happy with this procedure rather than having to undergo a full crown preparation.

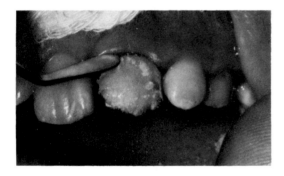

Figure 17–33 Placement of composite in labial window of stainless steel crown.

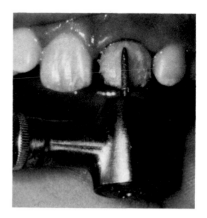

Figure 17–34 Diamonds, multibladed finishing burs, and discs work well to finish composite restorations.

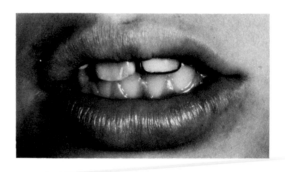

Figure 17–35 Finished restoration.

Figure 17–36 Extraoral view of finished restoration. This is a temporary procedure until a permanent restoration may be placed. The stainless steel crown does not extend more than 1 mm. beneath the tissue. This area is meticulously polished in order to cause as little tissue irritation as possible.

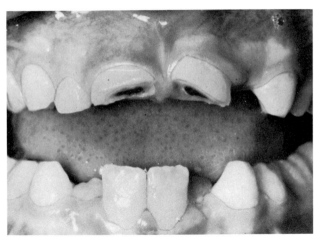

Figure 17–37 Large pulpal exposures of the maxillary permanent central incisors. The following treatment is recommended:

1. Obtain a history of the accident.
2. Do a thorough oral examination to determine the extent of the injury including any tooth mobility.
3. Take necessary radiographs of involved area to determine extent of injury.
4. A pulpotomy should be performed if the following conditions exist: (A) The dental pulp is exposed. (B) The pulp is vital and shows moderate hemorrhage. (C) The apex of the root is not fully developed.
5. Pulpotomy technique is as follows: (A) Isolate the tooth with a rubber dam. (B) Amputate the coronal pulp. (C) Place a paste of calcium hydroxide over the amputated pulp (approximately 1 mm. thick). (D) Fill the chamber with zinc oxide–eugenol or zinc phosphate cement. (E) Place a temporary esthetic restoration such as an acid etch with composite build-up. (F) In two to three months there should be a bridging of dentin over the amputation site. (G) A permanent restoration is placed after the incisors have recovered from the injury.
6. If a pulpotomy is not indicated, endodontic treatment should be initiated to save the tooth.

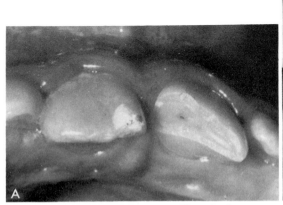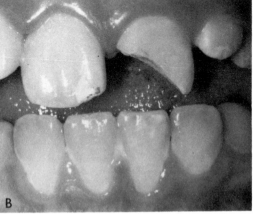

Figure 17–38 Note small pulpal exposure of the maxillary left central incisor. Some individuals prefer pulp capping in an injury of this nature if (1) It is no larger than a pinpoint exposure. (2) The exposure is of short duration—no longer than several hours. (3) The apex of the root is not fully developed. (4) The pulp is vital and shows moderate hemorrhage. *A.* Incisal view. *B.* Labial view.

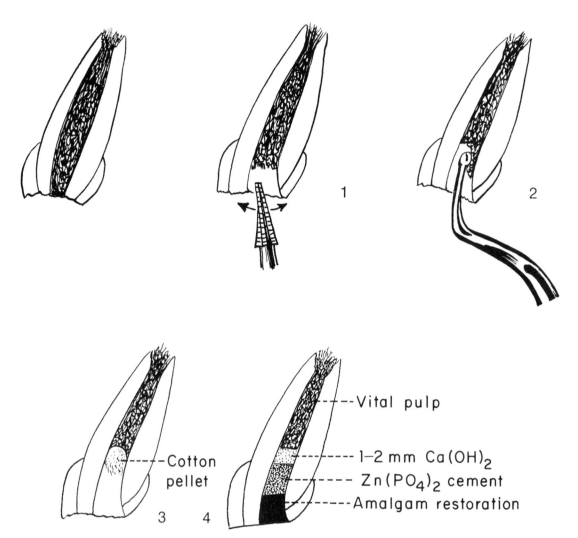

Figure 17–39. Pulpotomy on young permanent incisor when the exposure is caused by traumatic injury in a young tooth with incomplete apical development (upper left-hand figure). Procedure:

1. Access is gained with a tapered fissure bur.
2. Pulp is amputated at cementoenamel junction with sharp spoon excavator.
3. A sterile cotton pellet is used to control hemorrhage.
4. A layer of calcium hydroxide (approximately 1 to 2 mn. thick) is placed against the amputated pulp followed by a base and amalgam restoration. A *composite build-up* using acid etching may now be performed to restore the esthetic appearance of these injured teeth. If there is not enough tooth structure remaining to adequately do a composite build-up with acid etching, a stainless steel crown with an esthetic labial window may be placed (see Figures 17–33 through 17–36).

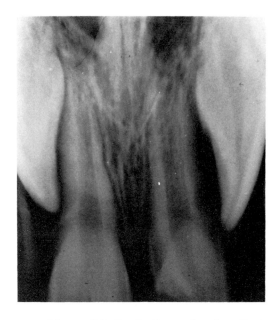

Figure 17-40 Preoperative radiograph of patients seen in Figure 17–37. Note wide open apices. Calcium hydroxide pulpotomies are indicated for these teeth (see Figure 17–41).

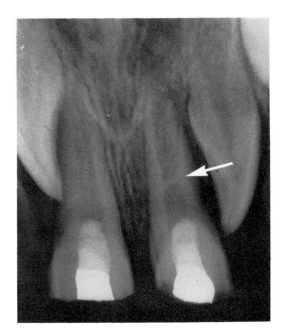

Figure 17–41 Radiograph of patient seen in Figures 17–37 and 17–40, 1½ months after calcium hydroxide pulpotomies were performed on both maxillary central incisors. Note location of dentin bridge formation. In this case pulpal tissue was amputated too far apically with resultant bridging in this location. For preferred location of dentin bridging, see Figure 17–42.

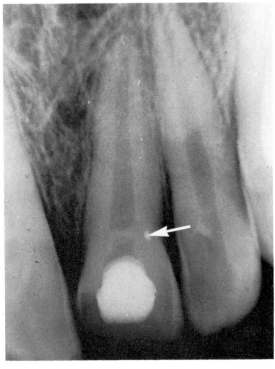

Figure 17–42 Radiograph of preferred location of dentin bridging following a calcium hydroxide pulpotomy. In this case the coronal pulpal tissue was amputated just short of the cementoenamel junction.

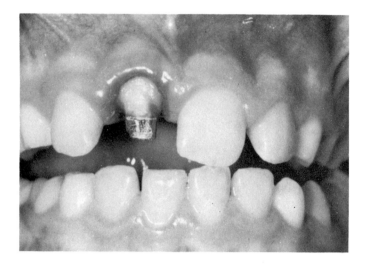

Figure 17-43 Maxillary right permanent central incisor with dowel and crown build-up (see Figures 17-44 through 17-45).

Figure 17-44 Crown cemented in place over dowel and gold build-up. Note gingival irritation around the crown. Everything possible should be done to minimize this when placing any restoration under the gingiva.

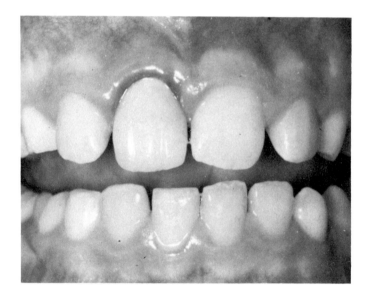

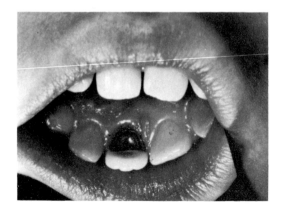

Figure 17-45 Lingual view of patient seen in Figure 17-43 and 17-44.

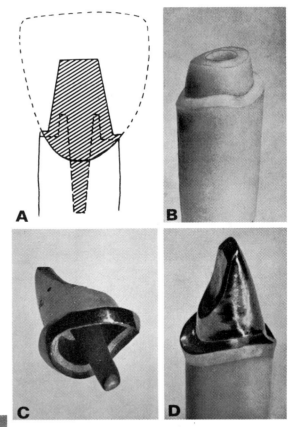

Figure 17–46 Full coping with collar and dowel. Preparation for restoration with a jacket crown. (From Ingle, J. I.: *Endodontics*, 1st ed., Lea & Febiger, Philadelphia, 1965, p. 621.)

A, Schematic drawing of the preparation and casting. *B*, Preparation that emphasizes subgingival shoulder. *C*, Internal surface of the casting. Note the shoulder and collar and the bulk and length of dowel. *D*, Casting cemented in place. Restoration with a jacket crown will complete the case.

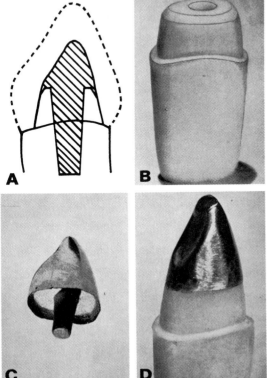

Figure 17–47 Dowel and extension for increasing the length of preparation of a fractured crown. (From Ingle, J. I.: *Endodontics*, 1st ed., Lea & Febiger, Philadelphia, 1965, p. 623.)

A, Schematic drawing. *B*, Preparation for coping to extend length of remaining tooth. *C*, Internal surface of the casting. Note the collar and the bulk and length of the dowel. *D*, Casting cemented in place ready for impression for jacket coverage.

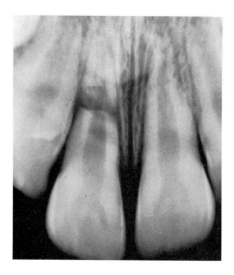

Figure 17–48 Root fracture of a maxillary right central incisor. The following treatment is suggested:

1. Stabilize the tooth with a splint, leaving it on for 6 to 8 weeks.
2. Eliminate trauma to the occlusion.
3. Allow the root to heal (see Figures 17–49 and 17–50).
4. If the pulp becomes devitalized, endodontic treatment should be initiated.

Figure 17–49 Root fracture following a traumatic injury. Tooth was stabilized with an acrylic splint for 6 weeks. (Courtesy Dr. David C. Dilts.)

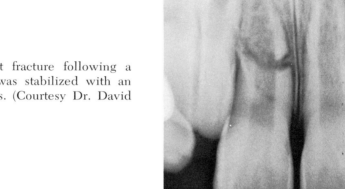

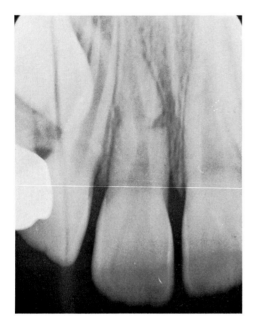

Figure 17–50 Same tooth as shown in Figure 17–49, after 1 year. Note extensive repair. The pulp of the tooth is vital. (Courtesy Dr. David C. Dilts.)

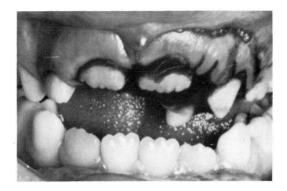

Figure 17–51 Intruded maxillary right and left permanent central incisors with incomplete root formation. Intruded permanent incisors with incomplete root formation are left alone to re-erupt.

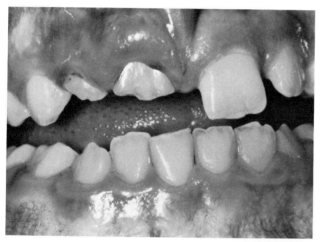

Figure 17–52 Intruded maxillary right central and lateral incisors. Since the roots of these intruded permanent incisors were completely developed, they were repositioned and stabilized with a splint.

Figure 17–53 Mutilated crown. Lack of sufficient coronal tooth structure and extension of the fracture below the gingival margin complicates treatment of this tooth.

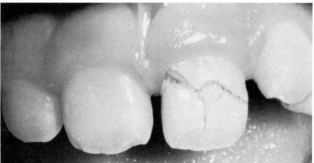

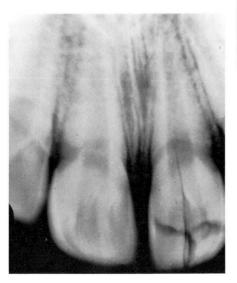

Figure 17–54 Radiograph of the tooth shown in Figure 17–53. Note the longitudinal fracture that penetrates the root. Successful endodontic treatment of this case would be questionable. Extraction may be necessary.

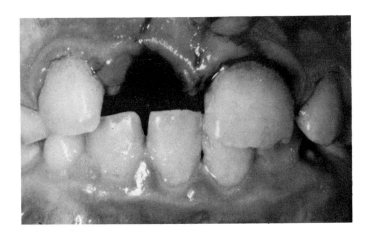

Figure 17–55 Appearance of patient immediately after injury who has avulsed the maxillary right permanent central incisor. Provided the tooth is knocked out in one piece, the parent or patient should rinse it off in water and, if possible, reposition it as seen in Figures 17–56 and 17–57. The patient should then see the dentist immediately so that the replanted tooth may be evaluated, stabilized, and followed in the future.

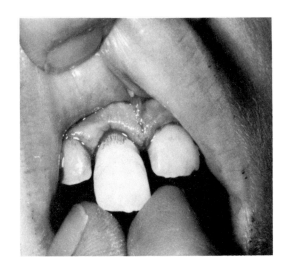

Figure 17–56 Tooth being repositioned by parent after it was rinsed off with water (see Figure 17–57).

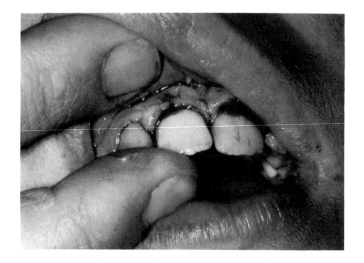

Figure 17–57 Parent repositioning tooth and holding for a moment immediately after it was rinsed in water. A tetanus booster is necessary if patient is not up to date with the last injection. Current status of tetanus immunity is the dentist's responsibility, along with the parent and physician.

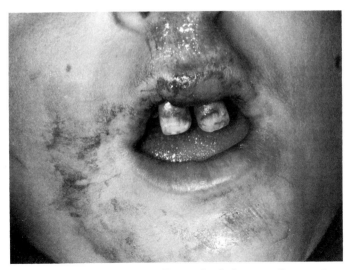

Figure 17-58 This patient traumatically avulsed the maxillary right and left permanent central incisors. Within 20 minutes the dentist was contacted by telephone, at which time he advised the parent to do the following:

1. Rinse teeth with water.
2. Reposition teeth back in their respective sockets.
3. Hold in place and go immediately to the dental office for further treatment.
4. If not able to reposition, have patient place tooth in buccal sulcus while being transported to the dentist.

Note that teeth were repositioned but placed in the wrong sockets. This should present no problem, as they can quickly be repositioned once in the dental office (see Figures 17–59 through 17–62).

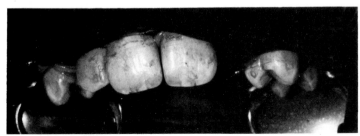

Figure 17–59 Same patient seen in Figure 17–58. After the anesthetic was infiltrated over the apices of the maxillary central incisor sockets, the teeth were repositioned and the rubber dam was placed for ease of placing the splint (see Figures 17–60 and 17–61).

Figure 17–60 Placement of acid etch splint in patient illustrated in Figures 17–58 and 17–59. After rubber dam was placed, the teeth were thoroughly cleaned, etched for 1 minute, rinsed and dried, and a passive labial arch wire was imbedded in the resin and composite (see Figure 17–62).

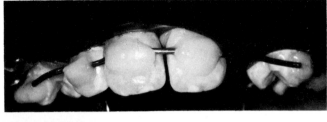

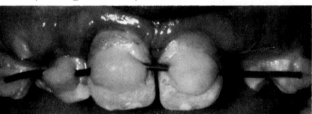

Figure 17–61 Appearance of splint immediately after rubber dam was removed. Patient returned in 3 days, at which time endodontic therapy was started. These splints are usually removed in 2 to 4 weeks after the injury.

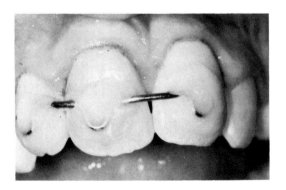

Figure 17–62 Acid etch and wire splint with composite placed after the maxillary right permanent central incisor sustained a severe root fracture. Note loops placed in wire for added retention. This is optional.

Figure 7–63 Acid etch and composite splint placed after the maxillary right and left central incisors were traumatized with resulting mobility. Although this splint is effective, it is more difficult to remove than the wire and composite type.

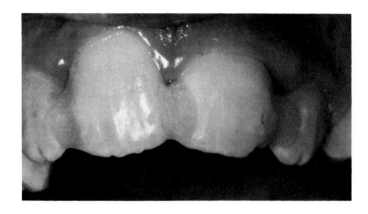

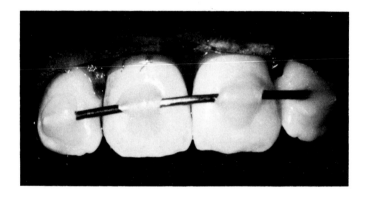

Figure 17–64 Acid etch and wire splint with composite after maxillary right and left permanent central incisors were traumatically retruded. The splint was removed after 4 weeks. The wire was cut interproximally, and each segment of composite was removed. multibladed finishing burs and finishing discs work well for removing this type of splint.

Figure 17–65 Tooth in position 1 month after replantation. Ankylosis, followed by resorption of the root, often occurs in these cases. However, if the tooth remains in position until all the permanent teeth have erupted, the replantation should be considered a success.

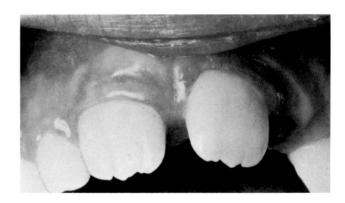

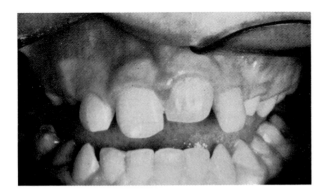

Figure 17–66 Ankylosis of a maxillary left central incisor after replantation. The adjacent teeth continued to erupt, leaving the replanted incisor at the former incisal level. When this occurs the replanted tooth may be restored to the new incisal level with a full crown or porcelain jacket. (From Ingle, J. I.: *Endodontics* 1st ed., Lea & Febiger, Philadelphia, 1965, p. 601.)

Figure 17–67 Resorption of the root of a maxillary left central incisor following replantation.

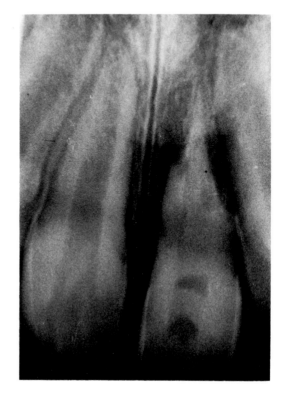

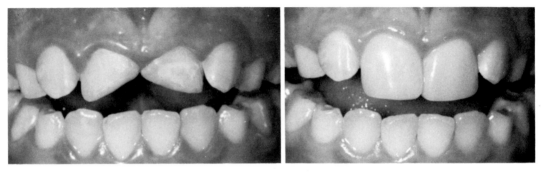

Figure 17–68   Treatment of two fractured permanent incisors with veneers.* This procedure is best accomplished in two appointments. The first appointment is spent discussing the procedure with the patient and obtaining an impression of the involved area. Precise grinding of the veneer is necessary until it fits the exact gingival contour on the model (see Figure 17–69A).

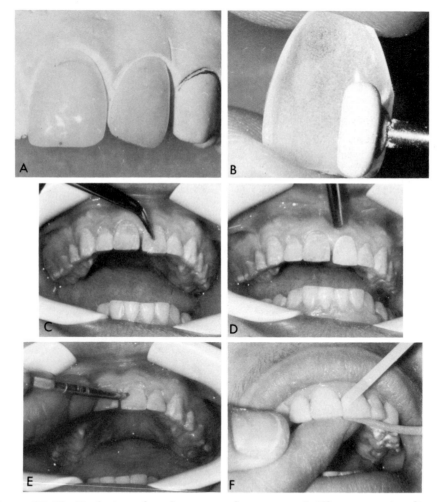

Figure 17–69   Technique for placement of veneers.* A. The veneer is adjusted to the model by meticulous grinding. B. Final step is pressure adaptation of veneer to model. C. Tooth is etched for one minute with phosphoric acid. D. Tooth is rinsed and dried. E. A thin layer of resin is applied to tooth. F. After veneer has been conditioned the lingual surface is filled with composite and placed on the tooth. To prevent bonding to adjacent teeth a celluloid matrix strip is placed interproximally. All excess composite is removed, the interproximal area is finished with strips as demonstrated here, and the incisal area is completed with discs.

*Mastique—L. D. Caulk Co.

436

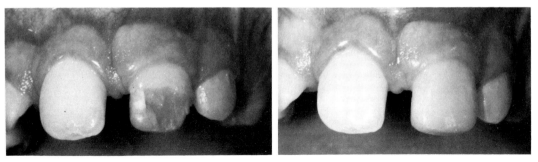

Figure 17-70 This tooth was damaged as a result of a traumatic intrusion of the primary incisor at an early age. A veneer* was placed on the hypoplastic permanent central incisor.

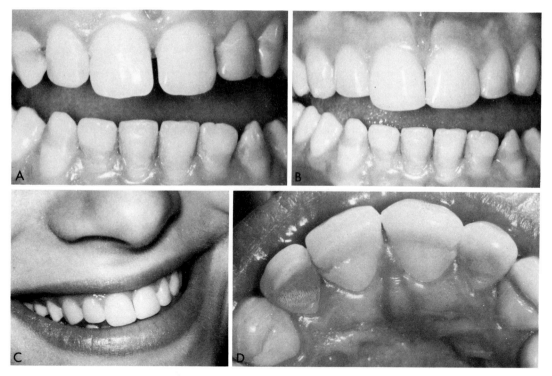

Figure 17-71 Veneers* were placed on this 16-year-old girl's teeth to eliminate the diastema and cover the band of hypoplastic enamel which appears in the middle of several incisors. The hypoplastic area had previously been restored by acid etching and placement of a composite which had discolored. A. Pretreatment view. B. Post-treatment view. C. Facial view after placement of veneers. D. Incisal post-treatment view (note that the labio-lingual dimension is slightly increased).

*Mastique—L. D. Caulk Co.

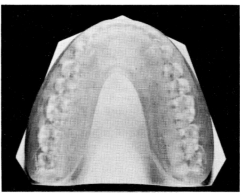

Figure 17-72   Mouth protector on model. Mouth protectors should be worn by all individuals participating in contact sports to prevent or decrease the severity of dental accidents. According to Stevens[6] the custom-made variety (fabricated from impressions and models by dentists using a durable firm material such as vinyl plastic or resilient acrylic) is the superior protector, and athletes should secure this type whenever possible. The studies of Stevens also indicate that mouth protectors should have an even occlusal imprint of the teeth from the opposing arch, or at least be graduated in thickness on the occlusal surface (thinner in the molar areas and thicker in the incisor areas). The imprints of the mandibular teeth in the protector serve to prevent posterior displacement of the mandible when impact is received.

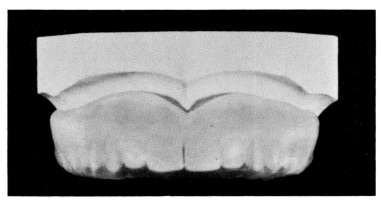

Figure 17-73   Anterior view of mouth protector. The mouth protector must not impinge on the frenum areas.

REFERENCES

1. Andreasen, J. O., and Hjorting-Hansen, E.: Replantation of teeth. I. Radiographic and clinical study of 110 human teeth replanted after accidental loss. Acta Odont. Scand. 24:263–286, 1966.
2. Cohen, A.: Improvements in mouthguards. Dental Digest 71:68–70, 1965.
3. Davis, J. M.: The relationship of overjet to the incidence of subjects with fractured young permanent anterior teeth. Master's thesis. University of Washington, June, 1967.
4. Law, D. B.: Prevention and treatment of traumatized anterior teeth. Dent. Clin. North Am., 1961, pp. 616.
5. Lewis, T. E.: Incidence of fractured anterior teeth as related to their protrusion. Angle Orthodont. 29:128–131, 1959.
6. Stevens, O. O.: Mouth protectors: evaluation of twelve types — second year. J. Dent. Child. 32:137–143, 1965.
7. Sundvall-Hagland, I.: Olyeksfallsskador paa Tänder och Parodontium under Barna-aaren. In Nord. Klin. Odont., Vol. II, 1960.

MANAGEMENT OF THE CHILD PATIENT

Chapter 18 _____

> *"We approach all problems of children with affection.*
> *Theirs is the province of joy and good humor.*
> *They are the most wholesome part of the race for they*
> *are the freshest from the hands of God."**

The Preschool Child

Successful management of the preschool patient is not only essential to accomplishment of treatment procedures, but it is even more important in laying a foundation for future acceptance of dentistry as a health service. The child who is comfortable in the dental environment during his or her early years will also usually be a good patient in the school-age and teenage period. Although some persons have intuitive skill in understanding and directing the behavior of small children, any dentist who has a sincere desire to treat them can be very successful by following known guidelines and principles of behavior modification.

In order to obtain rapport with the preschool child and carry out dental operations, it is necessary to have some idea of his or her language and motor and social development. Utilizing this knowledge, step by step procedural acquaintance, accompanied by constant reinforcement of good behavior, will result in positive conditioning.

Fear and anxiety are probably the most important emotional blocks with which the dentist contends. Small children may acquire fear of the dentist from conversations overheard at home and also from discussions with playmates. In some cases they may actually have been exposed to a traumatic

_____

*From Herbert Hoover's White House Conference on Children, 1930.

situation in the hospital or the physician's office. First visits to the dentist, therefore, should be structured so that the child will have a pleasant and interesting experience. Definitive treatment should not be attempted on the first appointment. Time must be spent in getting acquainted with the child and in carrying out routine diagnostic procedures: examination, prophylaxis, and radiographic survey. Small children need to know and have confidence in their dentist. For this reason the first appointment should not be delegated to auxiliary personnel.

Making the preschooler feel comfortable and confident in the dental office requires that all personnel in the dental office reflect an aura of friendliness and personal interest. The dentist should be pleased to see the child patient and should express this feeling in voice and demeanor. Positive statements such as, "It's nice to see you today," or "What a lovely dress," are preferable to thoughtless questions or remarks directed primarily to parent figures. Voice inflection, too, can be a factor in gaining rapport and cooperation. Certainly there is much to be gained by courteous remarks such as "Thank you for opening your mouth so widely," and use of the word "Please." At all times lavish praise is effective with preschool children and helps to build their confidence in the dentist. At this age level it is advisable to use some verbal distraction by conversation about topics appropriate to the child's interests. This could include clothes, pets, favorite foods, or reference to birthdays or similar events. Avoid discussion of school, athletics, or other subjects beyond the child's experience.

The dentist who sees small children also needs to establish friendly physical contact, since his eventual treatment will certainly involve intimate physical contact. This can be achieved by such devices as taking the child's hand when entering the operatory, helping him into the chair, and giving him a gentle hug when the appointment is over. It should be pointed out, however, that at the time of the initial contact with the preschool child the dentist should maintain a distance and avoid too precipitous physical advances.

Whether the parent should be in or out of the dental operatory has been a controversial subject among pedodontists. Certainly with a very young child — two or three years of age — it is advisable to have the parent present for the first two or three appointments. The decision to allow the parent of an older child in the operatory is up to the dentist. Most successful pedodontists, however, do prefer to exclude the parent if the child is uncooperative. Management of the uncooperative child involves firmness on the part of the dentist and positive communication of the behavioral limits acceptable while treatment is being carried out. In this regard, the use of drugs to modify child behavior is largely a matter of individual preference. The experienced operator, who structures appointments carefully and gains the confidence and trust of patients, will encounter few behavior problems serious enough to interfere with the accomplishment of dental treatment. The very young child who has a complex dental problem, or the preschooler who is seriously disturbed and does not respond to the usual approach, constitutes a group that should be considered for treatment under a general anesthetic in the hospital operatory.

Giving the preschooler a small gift or token after each dental appointment is a sound procedure from a psychological standpoint, as long as there is no implication of its being a bribe or reward for good behavior. The young child cannot be expected to appreciate the long-term benefits of oral health and, therefore, the prospect of dental appointments is not especially appealing. The anticipation of receiving a small gift changes this attitude, however, and in many instances results in the child eagerly looking forward to seeing his or her dentist.

Much has been written concerning the physical arrangement of offices in which children are treated. Although this is largely a matter of personal taste, there should be some attention given to creating an attractive environment in which the child will feel welcome and comfortable. The dentist must be careful not to allow the decorating theme to be exclusively devoted to the interest level of the preschooler, however, or older children will feel out of place. The reception room should be cheerfully furnished with the possible inclusion of a corner with a child-sized chair and table. Books appropriate for various age levels should be available and in good condition. The operating areas should be uncluttered and free of visible instruments that may create unnecessary anxiety. Highly antiseptic odors are undesirable as are medicinal soaps and hand creams. A pleasantly flavored mouthwash can be beneficial to patient and dentist alike.

In conclusion, it should be emphasized that although the physical aspects of the reception room and operatory should be carefully structured to create a favorable atmosphere, no amount of unusual decor will take the place of a sympathetic and friendly operator who has secured the trust and confidence of his small patient.

The School-Age Child

Children in the mixed dentition period, between the ages of 6 and 12, are usually more amenable to reason than their younger counterparts; consequently, less problems are encountered in their behavior management. As in dealing with the preschool child, however, it is equally important to establish rapport and to follow the principles of procedural acquaintance with the school-age child, although necessarily on a more sophisticated level.

Reinforcement of acceptable behavior is still a desirable approach, especially if complicated procedures are anticipated. Verbalization can be effected on a more adult basis with children this age, and school is a favorite topic of discussion. Comments on dress are quite appropriate for girls, whereas boys enjoy talking about sports or hobbies. A noncooperative school-age child may be more difficult to manage than a preschooler because the emotional problem has had more years to develop. It is extremely important in these cases to allow more time for getting acquainted and gaining the confidence and respect of the patient. It is possible to explain long-term objectives of treatment at this age and to point out the consequences of negligence.

Tranquilizers are frequently of benefit if these children are unduly apprehensive. In some instances, when fear of injection is the chief hurdle to be surmounted, alternative procedures can be suggested. With some children an agreement can be reached to proceed with treatment without local anesthesia. In others, nitrous oxide–oxygen analgesia may be an acceptable alternative. The use of a pressure anesthetic device is another approach that may be helpful. Rarely is it necessary to resort to general anesthesia and the hospital operating room in order to complete the required dentistry for this age group of patients. Exceptions to this would include the very disturbed child with urgent dental needs and the mentally retarded or otherwise handicapped child.

The Adolescent Patient

Management problems with the adolescent dental patient are likely to be in the nature of noncooperation in home care recommendations and failure to keep appointments, rather than an outright refusal of treatment or overt expressions of anxiety such as temper tantrums. However, since children in this age group often manifest severe dental problems associated with a high caries rate, they represent an extremely important area of concern for the dentist.

Some guidelines for the practitioner who treats this age group are necessary, as there is a clear need during the patient's adolescent period for the dentist to change certain aspects of his or her approach.

The adolescent is characterized by a desire for personal independence and an aversion to adult authority. Recognizing these facts, the dentist can structure management of the adolescent patient to avoid unnecessary problems. For instance, the parental role should be minimized, and the adolescent patient, as much as possible, should be involved in the dental office procedures. Thus, appointments should be made directly with the patient; the opportunity for an adolescent to work out his or her own schedule is a pleasurable and confidence-building activity. Such thoughtfulness on the part of the dental staff will result in the patient feeling mature and important. There should be no criticism or unsympathetic remarks concerning dress, hair styles, or teenage fads. Instructions on oral hygiene should be carried out on an adult level without assuming an authoritarian attitude. If the adolescent equates the dentist with a reprimanding or critical adult figure (perhaps a parent or teacher), the patient will not accept treatment readily and may fail to cooperate at all. A supportive, understanding approach will be far more successful with the teenage patient, and every effort should be made by all members of the dental office team to work toward this end.

It is axiomatic, however, that the fundamental principles of behavior modification successful with young children should be utilized with the adolescent as well. Reinforcement of good behavior, step-by-step procedural acquaintance, and courtesy all help in creating a favorable dentist-patient relationship.

SEDATION

Chapter 19

MARC W. ANDERSON

Fear, pain, and anxiety in the dental patient can be controlled through the appropriate application of various psychological, physical, and pharmacological techniques. When selecting any of these methods, it is important to remember that:

Pain is a localized sensation of discomfort that is highly subjective in nature. The patient's feeling of pain must be accepted as a valid perception.

Fear is the patient's response to a known external danger.

Anxiety is the patient's response to a threat or to an unknown.

The young child's first dental visit can involve pleasant curiosity and minimal apprehension or extreme fear and anxiety. In most cases, simple unthreatening introductory techniques are effective. In some instances, however, there is a need for premedication to be used if treatment is to be successful. The need for medication also may be considered for the child who has undergone one or more negative dental experiences.

When medications are used, the practitioner's selection of a specific agent should be guided by a standard of desirable characteristics. These are:

1. Patient acceptance
2. Wide safety margin
3. Short duration of onset
4. Rapid recovery
5. Titratability
6. Reversibility
7. Predictability
8. Ease of administration
9. Reasonable cost

Pharmacological methods are never a substitute for understanding a patient's needs and anxiety. Psychological aspects of good patient management must not be forgotten. Medications given in an attempt to override this aspect of patient management are contraindicated. Psychological manage-

444

ment, however, can be complemented with medication, each having specific purposes and indications. Clinical situations vary greatly and therefore no one technique will be effective in all cases.

It is important to clearly distinguish between conscious sedation and general anesthesia. Sedation is conceptually and physiologically distinct from general anesthesia — and from analgesia.

General anesthesia is the elimination of all sensations and is accompanied by a state of unconsciousness.

Sedation is the calming of a nervous, apprehensive individual by the use of systemic drugs without inducing loss of consciousness.

Analgesia is the diminution or elimination of pain in the conscious patient.

A sedated patient should:

1. Always be arousable and at no point so sedated that he or she cannot respond to commands and/or carry on an intelligible conversation.

2. Have maintenance of all protective mechanisms, especially the laryngeal reflex.

3. Experience no more depression of the cardiovascular and pulmonary system than would a relaxed, unapprehensive patient.

Even when the patient's medications are carefully selected and individualized, failures do occur. Parents must be told before medications are tried that a few visits may be necessary in order for the most effective drug to be properly selected. In addition, the possibility of general anesthesia in the hospital should be discussed. When a prescribed medication has been given to the child and sedation is inadequate (i.e., the needed service cannot be performed), no additional medication is to be given at that appointment. The addition of medications can lead to overlap in peak concentrations of drugs. The result can be an over-sedated child. The patient who is inadequately sedated at one appointment must come in for another appointment, at which time the same drug at a higher dose might be given, a different medication may be tried, or a decision to utilize general anesthesia may be made.

It is not the intent of this chapter to evaluate all of the available methods of sedation. Rather, the methods illustrated represent techniques that have been popular, safe, and effective in clinical practice.

Oral Medications

The oral medications described in this section are those that are safe, easily administered, well-accepted by the child, inexpensive, and clinically successful. The onset and effect of any oral medication will vary from individual to individual. There may be different effects on the same individual on different occasions depending on the stomach contents, the time of the day the medication is given, and the anxiety of the child on that particular day. Maximum absorption occurs when oral medications are given with water or clear juice to a patient with an empty stomach. Sedatives given in oral medications can have effects that last for several hours. Of course, with sedative medications, a decrease in dosage as appropriate should be attempted over the course of the child's appointments to encourage the realization in the child that he or she is capable of compliant behavior. The child's recognition that it is possible to cope with the dental situation will build self-esteem and may make the child a "model patient," eliminating the need for further medication.

Oral medications are usually available in tablets or capsules or in liquid forms. Most children prefer the liquid forms, which are uniformly acceptable in taste. However, a liquid medication may be resisted by the stubborn child despite a pleasant taste. One must ask the parent if the child has refused oral medications in the past.

Some oral medications can be used in conjunction with nitrous oxide–oxygen sedation. However, when varying drugs and differing routes of administration are combined, the predictability of action decreases while the possibility of over-sedation or light anesthesia increases.

DIAZEPAM

The sedative diazepam is an anti-anxiety agent that has muscle relaxant and amnestic effects. It should induce sleepiness, slight ataxia, and decreased anxiety in the child who is initially uneasy in the dental environment. The child may still be "fussy" upon sitting in the dental chair, but kind reassurance usually ameliorates this behavior. Since diazepam is a known amnestic, the child may not remember the successful dental treatment just completed. Therefore, at the completion of treatment (and in the presence of the parent), the child should be complimented for "great" behavior and compliance.

Diazepam is *usually* given in one dose *one hour* before the dental appointment. However, for those children who have difficulties sleeping in anticipation of the next morning's dental appointment, diazepam may be given in two doses: the first dose the night before the morning appointment, and the next dose *one hour* before the appointment.

Diazepam tablets are only about one-third the size of aspirin and therefore are easily swallowed. They have a very bland taste if swallowed whole. When chewed, however, they have an objectionable bitter taste. If the child will not swallow pills, it would be advisable to have the parent thoroughly crush the tablet between two teaspoons and mix with sugar and water or a sweet juice. The total powder and liquid volume should be approximately one teaspoon. The child is encouraged to follow the dose with a small glass of water.

Diazepam should begin to work within twenty to thirty minutes and be fully effective in one hour. Peak duration of action is approximately two hours. However, due to diazepam's absorption, deposition, and metabolism, full recovery can take up to 24 hours in the individual patient.

Valium

Diazepam is sold under the name Valium.

Availability:
Tablets	2 mg white
	5 mg yellow
	10 mg light blue
Liquid	None available for use orally.

Dose Suggestions:
1. Valium is not to be used if the child weighs less than 25 pounds.
2. For children aged:
   2 to 3 years—2 mg to 6 mg per dose
   4 to 5 years—5 mg to 10 mg per dose
   6 to 9 years—5 mg to 12 mg per dose
   10 to 12 years—5 mg to 15 mg per dose
3. Doses larger than 15 mg are not recommended.

Note: Diazepam is useful in controlling unwanted muscle movements such as those seen in patients with cerebral palsy. However, intravenous medication is much more effective in controlling these movements than is oral diazepam.

HYDROXYZINE

Hydroxyzine is an ataractic drug that will have a profound calming effect on the child. It will provide peace of mind and emotional indifference or stability. Therefore, the child will react in a more balanced manner (and should not be atactic). Hydroxyzine's effects last for two to four hours; full recovery can take several hours. Its use is indicated in the shy, timid, and/or anxious child. Frequently, the practitioner will encounter a child whose anxiety level is so high that the usual environmental introduction and the show-tell-do techniques cannot be accomplished. Hydroxyzine would be the ideal drug in such a patient. It would have enough of a calming effect to allow for the usual office routine and would permit some rapport between dentist and patient. Depending on the reaction of the child, the dentist could then elect to use the medication as needed (in an increased dose or a decreased dose) at the next visit (of course, no medication at all may be required).

Hydroxyzine is *usually* given in one dose *two hours* before the dental appointment. However, for those children who have difficulty sleeping in anticipation of the next morning's dental appointment, hydroxyzine may be given in two doses: the first dose the night before the morning appointment, the next dose one hour before the appointment itself. The peak effect of hydroxyzine given orally occurs in one to two hours and lasts for some two to four hours.

Like diazepam, hydroxyzine is frequently used as a co-medication with nitrous oxide. That is, hydroxyzine is used to reduce the child's anxiety level to such a degree that the nose piece can be introduced and nitrous oxide then used to achieve the desired sedation level.

Atarax and Vistaril

Hydroxyzine hydrochloride is sold under the name Atarax; hydroxyzine pamoate is sold under the name Vistaril.

Availability:

Atarax tablets	10 mg orange
	25 mg green
	50 mg yellow
Atarax liquid	10 mg/5 ml. This syrup has a pleasant minty taste.
Vistaril capsules	25 mg two-tone green
	50 mg green and white
Vistaril liquid	25 mg/5 ml. This oral suspension has a pleasant lemon taste. One must remember to shake the bottle prior to administration to ensure homogeneity.

Dose Suggestions:

1. Neither Atarax nor Vistaril is to be used if the child weighs less than 25 pounds.
2. For children aged:
   2 to 3 years and mildly anxious—1 mg per pound (2 mg/kg) of body weight
   2 to 3 years and very anxious—1 to 2 mg per pound (2–4 mg/kg) of body weight
   4 to 6 years—2 mg per pound (4 mg/kg) of body weight
3. No dose should exceed 75 mg.

HYDROXYZINE AND CHLORAL HYDRATE

Drug combinations are utilized in order to obtain effects that are not achievable with the use of a single agent. With the combination of hydroxyzine and chloral hydrate, an anti-anxiety calming effect (from the hydroxyzine) and a sedative hypnotic effect (from the chloral hydrate) may be obtained. This combination has been helpful in the preschool child. Too often, though, the dentist selects this combination inappropriately. If hydroxyzine alone is not effective with the "stubborn" or "spoiled" child, one might think that the addition of chloral hydrate will add enough sedation to produce a calm sleepiness in the child. However, the reaction that often occurs is an undesirable one — the patient is sleepy but combative. The chloral hydrate and hydroxyzine combination is best reserved for the child who needs the anti-anxiety effect of hydroxyzine to help accept the dental environment and the chloral hydrate sedative effect to aid in sleepiness while undergoing a dental procedure. The child might, at the start of a procedure, show some resistance in the form of crying, but more physical activity is uncommon; often, in time, the child will go to sleep (this sleep is one from which the child is easily aroused). Peak effects occur 45 minutes to 2 hours after administration. (Thus the child waiting in the dental office for any length of time between administration and the actual appointment may become ataxic and sleepy, and should not be allowed to wander around the office unattended.)

Hydroxyzine and Noctec

Commercial preparations of hydroxyzine (Atarax and Vistaril) have already been described; Noctec is the name under which chloral hydrate is sold.

Availability:

Hydroxyzine   as previously described (see p. 448)
Noctec syrup   500 mg/5 ml

Dose Suggestions:

1. Hydroxyzine—⅔ the normal dose previously cited (p. 448)
2. Noctec syrup — 12 mg per pound (25 mg/kg) of body weight
3. Dosage for sedative effect in 30-lb child:
   20 mg of hydroxyzine and 360 mg of Noctec

NITROUS OXIDE–OXYGEN SEDATION

The popularity of nitrous oxide–oxygen sedation is easily understandable: recovery from such sedation is rapid, and the effects of the sedative — nitrous oxide — are predictable (in terms of onset and duration of action) and are reversible, thus allowing for a wide margin of safety. However, equipment for sedating patients with nitrous oxide and oxygen is expensive, and special training in its use is required. Technical and safety problems with the installation and maintenance of equipment (and the risk of potentially catastrophic accidents) have prompted several agencies to issue guidelines on nitrous oxide–oxygen sedation. Various recommendations now cover maintenance and installation requirements, monitoring of occupational chronic low-dosage exposure to nitrous oxide, and the proper training of persons who administer N_2O—O_2 sedation.

The American Dental Association's Council on Dental Materials and Devices has guidelines on acceptable nitrous oxide–oxygen sedation machines and devices, nitrous oxide–oxygen scavenging equipment, and nitrous oxide–oxygen waste gas monitoring equipment. In addition, the National Fire Protection Association has published standards for the use of nitrous–oxide oxygen. These standards deal primarily with installation of equipment and with fire safety. Most local fire departments have standards that are derived from the national ones, with supplemental guidelines appropriate to the local community. Finally, technical information on the control of occupational exposure to nitrous oxide–oxygen in the dental operatory — specifically the control of expired waste gas and equipment leakage — is available in government publications.

The nature of the *volume* and the *concentration* of nitrous oxide delivered to the patient is often misunderstood. The patient requires a specific volume of gas per unit of time. An average adult needs a volume of approximately 7.5 liters per minute. In a child, the requirement is about 3 to 6 liters per minute, depending on the child's size. The total volume of gas required must be continuously administered.

Concentration is usually expressed in terms of percentage. Two liters per minute of nitrous oxide and two liters per minute of oxygen equals four liters per minute total gas flow. The nitrous oxide concentration at this rate is fifty per cent. The volume of gas delivered usually remains constant, but the concentration of nitrous oxide and oxygen can be varied.

It is important to describe to the patient the effects of nitrous oxide, from the initial signs and symptoms to the desired state of sedation and analgesia. This description prepares the child for the known effects of the drug and makes the experience a pleasurable one. When the initial effects are well described and the child then feels them, he or she will readily accept the mild euphoria, sedation, and analgesia that will soon follow. The dentist can offer suggestions of a pleasant warm feeling, of a floating sensation, or of being on a boat. In this way, the child is allowed to take advantage of the known dissociation in a fun way. Thus, the effects of the drug are greatly enhanced by the power of suggestion. The child prefers to be in his or her own world rather than concentrating on the dental environment and the procedures that are about to be undertaken. Table 19–1 lists the signs and symptoms the patient may experience and at what concentration of nitrous oxide they can be expected.

TABLE 19–1   EFFECTS OF NITROUS OXIDE

NITROUS OXIDE CONCENTRATION	SIGN OR SYMPTOM
10%	Usually none
20%	Muscle relaxation (usually felt first in legs)
	Body warmth
	Slight sleepiness
	Slight euphoria
	Tingling of hands and feet
	Ringing in ears (usually not reported)
30%	Circumoral and tongue tingling
	Giddiness
	Exaggerated hearing
	Mild dissociation
	Mild euphoria
	Analgesia
	Mild sleepiness
	Amnesia
	Sweating
40%	Dissociation
	Euphoria
	Dysphoria
	Nausea
	Increased sleepiness
	Uncoordinated muscle movements

Note that while desirable effects are achieved with concentrations of nitrous oxide in the 20–40% range, individual response to nitrous oxide can be variable.

Figure 19–1 The arrows in this drawing represent most of the points from which waste gases can contaminate the dental operatory. When equipment is well maintained and properly installed, only the gas not inhaled by the patient should escape, and if the room is adequately ventilated and scavenging is utilized, there should be no contamination by this gas. (Illustration from Whitcher, C. E., Zimmerman, D. C., Tonn, E. M., and Piziali, R. L.: Control of occupational exposure to nitrous oxide in the dental operatory. J.A.D.A. 95(4): 766, October, 1977.)

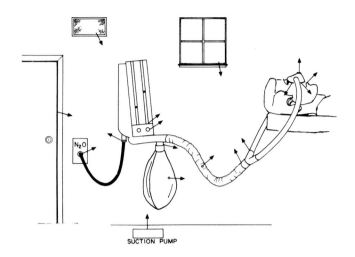

N₂O

SUCTION PUMP

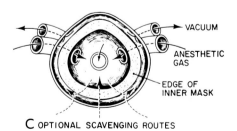

A — HOLE FOR VACUUM RELIEF

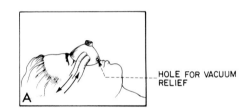

---ROOM AIR INLET
----ADJUSTABLE VALVE
-----EXHALED GASES

VACUUM
ANESTHETIC GASES

B OPTIONAL SCAVENGING ROUTES

Figure 19–2 Waste gas escape into the operatory can be significant unless a scavenging mask is utilized. Drawing A shows a scavenging mask in place; B and C show the functional details of the mask. (Illustration from Whitcher, C. E., Zimmerman, D. C., Tonn, E. M., and Piziali, R. L.: Control of occupational exposure to nitrous oxide in the dental operatory. J.A.D.A. 95(4): 771, October, 1977.)

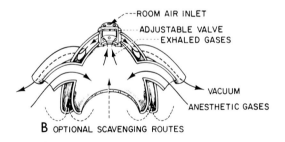

VACUUM

ANESTHETIC GAS

EDGE OF INNER MASK

C OPTIONAL SCAVENGING ROUTES

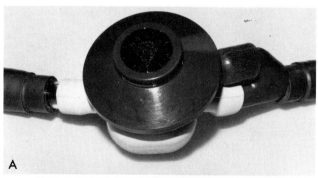

A

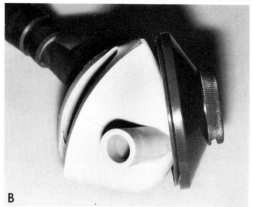

B

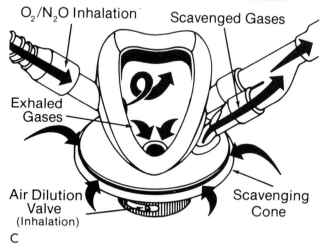

O$_2$/N$_2$O Inhalation

Scavenged Gases

Exhaled
Gases

Air Dilution
Valve
(Inhalation)

Scavenging
Cone

C

Figure 19–3 A nitrous oxide scavenging nose piece. (A) Front view. (B) Side view. (C) The drawing shows how the scavenging device functions with a vacuum. The use of a rubber dam encourages nose breathing, which improves the effectiveness of the scavenging system. (Illustration courtesy Fraser Sweatman, Inc.)

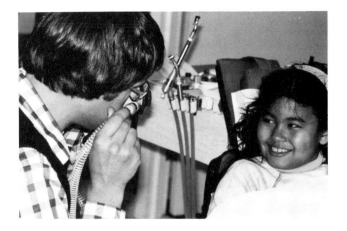

Figure 19–4 Oxygen flow is started and the child is shown how the mask looks and fits on the nose. A very small amount of fragrant liquid swabbed inside the nose piece can be used to conceal the odor of the rubber.

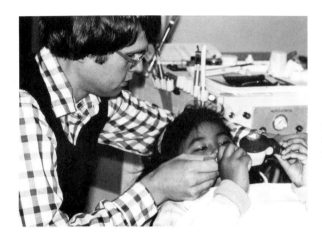

Figure 19–5 The nose piece should not be placed abruptly on the child. Instead, it should be handed to the child for investigation and placement.

Figure 19–6 While the nose piece is being adjusted by the child, one should repeat the description of the initial effects of nitrous oxide. The nitrous oxide can then be started.

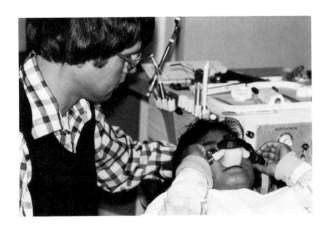

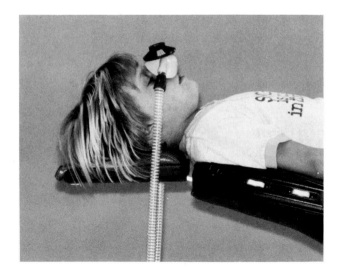

Figure 19–7 The conducting tubing should be adjusted loosely behind the patient to allow freedom of movement by the child.

Figure 19–8 Even when operating on maxillary anterior teeth, the dentist will find that the nose piece is not a significant physical obstacle.

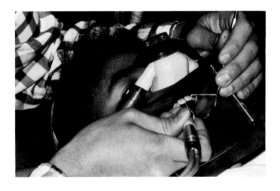

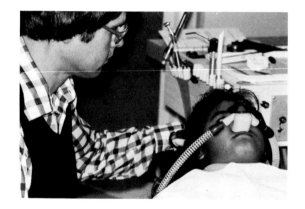

Figure 19–9 The final result is a relaxed, happy patient. At the completion of the procedure, the patient is given 100% oxygen for five minutes in order to "flush" the nitrous oxide from the body.

THE HANDICAPPED CHILD

Chapter 20 _____

by MICHAEL R. FEY
and
PATRICK K. TURLEY

Treatment of the handicapped child requires more time, energy, preparation, and thought than does treatment of the normal child. However, the dentist who includes the handicapped child among his patients will be rewarded far beyond monetary considerations. The total number of handicapped children is relatively small, and even those persons limiting their practices to children are called upon to treat relatively few. Fortunately, there is increased emphasis today on the need for adequate dental service for this segment of the population. Progress in dental education, along with new concepts of normalization and deinstitutionalization, is enlarging the role of the dentist in providing oral health care.

The words "handicapped child" denote an exceedingly wide range of conditions. It should be recognized that the handicapped condition can be physical, mental, or social. The actual dental problems associated with these children are usually the same as those affecting normal children. However, they are often more severe because of neglect, and almost always more difficult to correct, especially from a management standpoint.

455

Except in institutions where the children's total health is supervised by administrative personnel, the dental care of the handicapped is frequently neglected. Causative factors in this neglect seem to be ignorance of the dental problems that can and will develop and an aversion on the part of the parents to subject their child to additional treatment procedures not related to the main problem. In many cases the family, feeling sorry for the child, attempts to overcompensate by giving him cookies, candies, and other cariogenic foods. In addition, oral hygiene is frequently very difficult to carry out and may be totally neglected. The end-result, as might be expected, is a child who is in the most desperate need of help. To compound all this, the family with a handicapped child oftentimes will have other associated problems, such as insurmountable medical expenses, emotional problems with other children as a result of overattention to the affected child, and even dissension between parents as to the proper care of the affected child.

Paramount to good dental care for the handicapped is the dentist's attitude toward these children and their parents. The operator must learn to accept the unusual sights, sounds, and actions that he observes and hears upon meeting these children. Some of them cannot control their physical actions (as in cerebral palsy); consequently, treatment can be very frustrating. Others who need the careful intimate attention of the dentist may not be esthetically pleasing patients. Some, such as the mentally retarded, make sounds and movements that may be quite different from those of the usual child patient. Conversely, the hemophiliac may appear perfectly normal, but his tissue response is exaggerated and requires special consideration. The child with cystic fibrosis may have paroxysms of coughing in the middle of treatment. The dentist, therefore, must develop an attitude of concern for treating the dental problems and avoid being personally affected by the child's physical condition.

Whether treatment is performed in the dental office or in the hospital under general anesthesia, it is wise to consult with the family physician and obtain as much information as possible concerning the nature of the condition and precautions that should be observed. The goal in treating the handicapped child is to render the same dental care as that afforded the more normal child.

Deafness

Dental treatment for the deaf child requires that the operator be able to communicate the procedures through visual demonstration, touch, taste, and smell. Knowledgeable parents can assist the dentist in many cases, relaying the necessary information in an understandable fashion. If lip reading is a capability of the child, explanations should be given simply and with reasonable speed. The operator must remember that his lips must be visible to the patient to effect communication. Adequate time to establish rapport is essential when treating the deaf child.

I. DEAFNESS

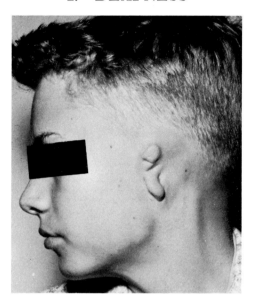

Figure 20–1 The deaf child requires extra attention for demonstration of the treatment which will be carried out. Time spent at this will be repaid in a more cooperative patient. It is most important to reduce apprehension in handicapped children to the minimum.

Blindness

It is necessary to spend considerable time explaining all aspects of dental treatment when dealing with a blind person. The person must never be moved without being told what is going on. Demonstration using touch (including letting the patient feel instruments), smell, and taste can be helpful in acquainting the blind patient with dental procedures. The need for thorough education in oral hygiene and other preventive procedures is especially important. The parent especially needs to be involved in the basics of preventive dentistry so that proper guidance can be maintained in the home environment.

II. BLINDNESS

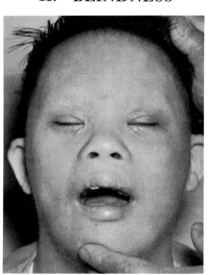

Figure 20–2 Blindness in a child requires that the dentist explain all procedures in great detail, particularly those involving noises, e.g., suction and drill. Constant physical contact is important. Patience, firmness, and kindness are key prerequisites for the successful treatment of these children.

Mental Retardation

The mentally retarded probably represent the largest percentage of handicapped children. Fortunately, the majority of those who fall into this classification are affected to a very mild degree and can be managed by careful adherence to the recognized principles of child management overlaid with a willingness to spend extra time and effort compared with other children. Each child is an individual, and there will be cases requiring drug therapy and in a few instances treatment in a hospital or institution. *The dentist who treats the mentally handicapped should be willing to make the effort to treat these patients in the office environment, and with an understanding approach he will succeed in the majority of instances.* Those who are not amenable to treatment in the private office should be referred to a children's hospital or pedodontist.

III.   MENTAL RETARDATION

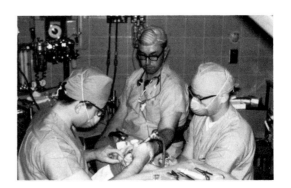

Figure 20–3   Although office treatment is usually possible, the more severely handicapped patient may require hospitalization and treatment under a general anesthetic.

Hemophilia

INTRODUCTION

Hemophilia is a hereditary disorder of the blood clotting mechanism that occurs in approximately 1 in 10,000 individuals. The basic types of hemophilia are as follows:

1. Hemophilia A — (Factor VIII deficiency) classic hemophilia, most common type, limited to male sex.

2. Hemophilia B — (Factor IX deficiency) clinically indistinguishable from hemophilia A but has thromboplastin component deficiency.

3. Factor XI deficiency — Plasma thromboplastin deficiency.

4. Von Willebrand's disease — (Factor VIII deficiency and impaired platelet plug formation).

CLINICAL FEATURES

1. Severe hemophilia, 0 to 2 per cent of deficient factor — spontaneous bleeding, mainly in joints.

2. Moderate hemophilia, 2 to 5 per cent of deficient factor — bruise easily, persistent bleeding if exposed to trauma.

3. Mild hemophilia, 5 to 30 per cent of deficient factor — prolonged bleeding only after severe trauma or surgery.

The two basic screening tests used for hemophilia are the partial thromboplastin time and bleeding time. The bleeding time is normal in the hemophilias but abnormal in von Willebrand's disease because of the platelet disorder. Partial thromboplastin time is usually prolonged in the hemophilias, although it is sometimes normal in hemophilia A and von Willebrand's disease. Specific clotting factor assays determine the nature of the clotting defect.

ORAL FINDINGS

Hemorrhage, which can result from trauma or normal tooth exfoliation and eruption, may be prolonged in the patient suffering from severe hemophilia. Gingival bleeding as the result of tooth brushing is not a problem in healthy tissue.

TREATMENT AND PROGNOSIS

There is no cure for the hereditary disorder of hemophilia. Prevention of bleeding episodes is of utmost importance. In the case of a bleeding episode, hemophilia A and von Willebrand's disease are treated with cyroprecipitate, whereas hemophilia B is treated with fresh frozen plasma or factor IX complex — human (Konyne). In the event of a surgical procedure, factor levels should be increased to levels above 25 per cent. For patients with severe hemophilia who suffer from frequent spontaneous bleeding, home transfusion of cyroprecipitate is the treatment of choice. The use of cyroprecipitate and fresh frozen plasma with epsilon aminocaproic acid has proved effective in controlling oral bleeding and has had the additional benefit of reducing the amount of replacement therapy and the length of hospitalization needed (numerous episodes of blood product replacement greatly increase the patient's risk of hepatitis and also create a risk for the practitioner treating the patient).

The course of the disease is variable depending on the severity of the factor deficiency. Patients with severe hemophilia can develop chronic synovitis and arthritis from repeated hemarthrosis. Muscle weakness and atrophy can also result. The introduction of factor replacement therapy has made the treatment of bleeding from trauma or planned surgery a controllable procedure. The introduction of home replacement therapy for patients with severe hemophilia should help to decrease the long-term effects of spontaneous bleeding that have been seen previously.

FACTORS AFFECTING DENTAL TREATMENT

To reduce the necessity of restorative dental procedures, prevention of dental disease is of the utmost importance. Usually, rubber cup prophylaxis can be performed without factor replacement therapy, which must be used for restorative dental procedures or oral surgical procedures. The rubber dam should be used in all operative procedures, because it offers protection from accidental trauma to the oral soft tissues. The improvement of orthodontic appliances and techniques such as direct-bonding orthodontic brackets has made orthodontic treatment possible even for patients suffering from the most severe hemophilia.

IV. HEMOPHILIA

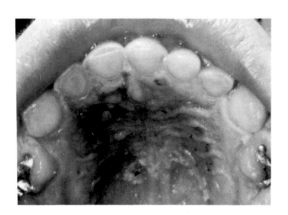

Figure 20–4 A small gingival laceration resulted in continued oozing in this 5-year-old hemophiliac with an inhibitor to Factor VIII. A small percentage of hemophiliacs produce antibodies in response to Factor VIII replacement therapy, making this form of hemorrhage control difficult.

Figure 20–5 An acrylic splint that covered the palate and extended into the vestibule was cemented in place with periodontal packing for a period of 10 days, after which the bleeding stopped.

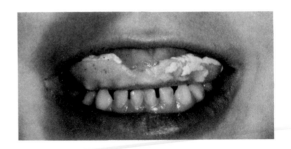

IV.   HEMOPHILIA *Continued*

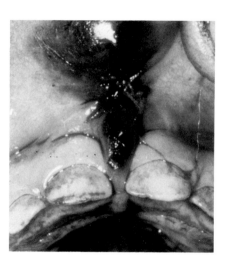

Figure 20–6   Lacerated frenum in a 19-month-old hemophiliac who has an inhibitor to Factor VIII. The area was sutured and the patient was given aminocaproic acid (Amicar) for 13 days to prevent lysis of the clot.

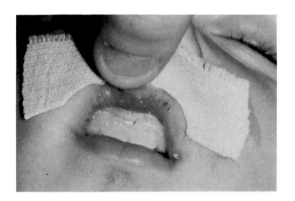

Figure 20–7   When frenum started oozing 48 hours after suturing, acrylic splint was cemented in place to hold gauze packing over frenum. An extraoral bandage was placed to apply slight pressure to the lip and to minimize facial movement of injured area.

Figure 20–8   Healing frenum approximately 4 weeks following initial injury.

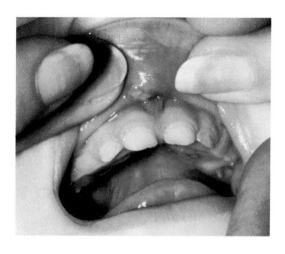
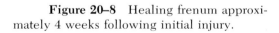

IV. HEMOPHILIA *Continued*

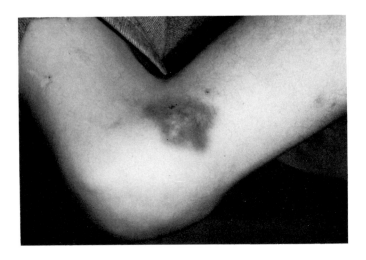

Figure 20–9 Common clinical findings in severe hemophilia are ecchymosis and hemarthrosis. Both of these findings are present in the right elbow of a 9-year-old boy with 1 per cent Factor VIII.

Figure 20–10 Extrusion of resorbed central incisors following a blow to the face in a 7-year-old male with 10 per cent Factor VIII.

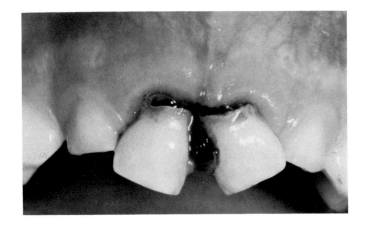

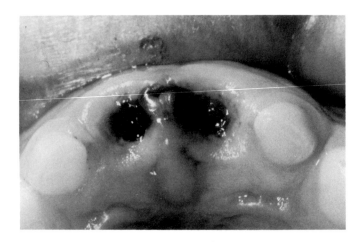

Figure 20–11 Patients with mild hemophilia experience prolonged bleeding only after severe trauma or surgery. Removal of crowns resulted in immediate hemostasis following a few minutes of steady pressure (same patient as in Figure 20–10).

Down's Syndrome

INTRODUCTION

Down's syndrome is one of the most common disorders associated with mental retardation. The first adequate description of the condition was made by Langdon Down (1866) who attempted to classify mental deficiency according to racial or ethnic origins. From this historic paper the term "mongol" originated. It has subsequently been replaced by most clinicians with the term "Down's syndrome" or trisomy 21.

The overall incidence of this condition in newborn white infants is approximately 1 in 600 or 700 births. Differences in incidence between various races or ethnic groups have not been reliably established.

ETIOLOGY

Down's syndrome was the first human condition to be recognized as being the result of a chromosomal aberration. In a majority of cases, the presence of an extra chromosome results from maternal primary nondisjunction that seems to be related to the age of the mother. There is a higher incidence of Down's syndrome with increased maternal age.

CLINICAL FEATURES

Characteristics of a general nature include small stature, short extremities, short and broad hands with transverse palmar creases, clinodactyly of the fifth finger with only one flexion crease, hyperflexibility and generalized hypotonia in young children that becomes less pronounced with increasing age. Probably the most prominent characteristic is mental retardation. Increased susceptibility to upper respiratory infections and a higher incidence of congenital heart disorders are medical problems that may complicate treatment.

OROFACIAL FEATURES

Many of the physical diagnostic features are located in the head area. Those of importance include a short and broad neck, ear deformity, a flat and broad nasal bridge, oblique palpebral fissures, prominent epicanthal folds, a fissured tongue, a low incidence of dental caries, a marked susceptibility to periodontal disease, delayed eruption of both primary and permanent dentitions, congenitally missing teeth, tooth anomalies including size and shape, and relative mandibular prognathism as a result of midface deficiency.

TREATMENT AND PROGNOSIS

The mortality rate in Down's syndrome is higher than that of the general population. The causes of early mortality are primarily related to congenital heart and gastrointestinal abnormalities and pneumonia.

Although patients with Down's syndrome have a lower-than-normal susceptibility to dental caries, there is an increased incidence of periodontal disease. Loss of periodontal support can be found as early as the preteenage years.

A posterior cross bite or anterior open bite can be observed in many patients. An underdevelopment of the midface accounts for the prognathic appearance and abnormal dental relationships. The etiology of an anterior open bite is primarily attributed to the physiological forward positioning of the tongue.

A special factor to take into consideration when planning dental treatment for patients with Down's syndrome is the high incidence of congenital heart defects in these patients. Obviously, protecting affected patients against complications is critical, and prophylactic antibiotic coverage to prevent bacteremia should, in particular, be included in treatment planning.

These children usually respond well to tender loving care. Sedation may be necessary to manage behavior for routine dental procedures, depending on the degree of mental retardation.

V. DOWN'S SYNDROME

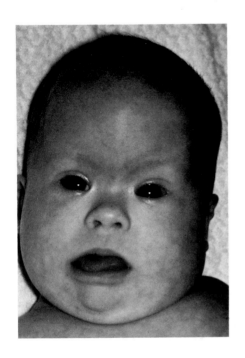

Figure 20–12 Infant with Down's syndrome. Note small head circumference, epicanthic folds, upslanting palpebral fissures, low nasal bridge, small nose, open mouth with protruding tongue, and cutis marmorata (skin mottling). (Courtesy M. Michael Cohen, Jr., Seattle, Washington.)

V. DOWN'S SYNDROME *Continued*

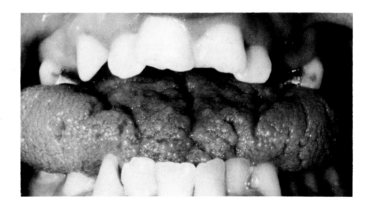

Figure 20–13 Although true macroglossia is uncommon, the tongue appears relatively large because of a small oral cavity.

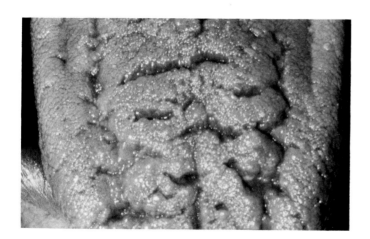

Figure 20–14 Deep fissures of the tongue are commonly present.

Figure 20–15 A 14-year-old female with Down's syndrome exhibiting severe chronic gingival inflammation with loss of alveolar support. Early periodontal disease is a prominent oral feature with Down's syndrome. Although local factors from poor oral hygiene seem to play a large part in early bone destruction, these individuals appear to be more susceptible to periodontal disease than individuals without Down's syndrome.

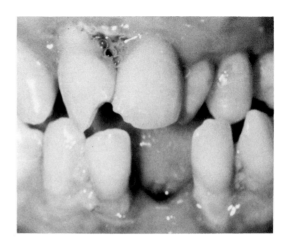

V. DOWN'S SYNDROME *Continued*

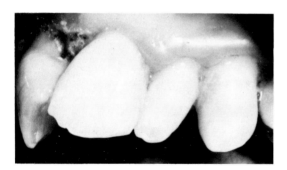

Figure 20–16 Note the abnormal shape of the lateral incisor and cuspid in this patient. Microdontia and abnormal morphology are common in Down's syndrome.

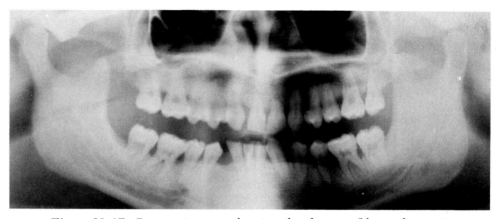

Figure 20–17 Panoramic x-ray showing the degree of bone destruction in a 17-year-old male with Down's syndrome.

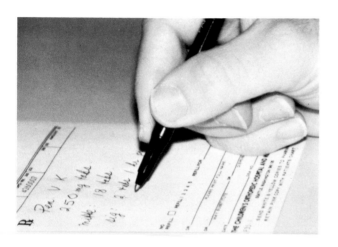

Figure 20–18 Prophylactic antibiotic coverage must be considered because of the high incidence of congenital heart defects in Down's syndrome. Consequently, the health history should always be reviewed prior to treating these patients.

V. DOWN'S SYNDROME *Continued*

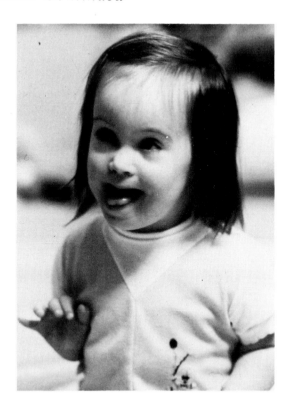

Figure 20–19 A 4-year-old child with Down's syndrome. These youngsters respond well to tender loving care. (Courtesy Dr. Richard R. Rolla, Child Development and Mental Retardation Center, University of Washington, Seattle.)

Cerebral Palsy

INTRODUCTION

Cerebral palsy is a motor disorder of the brain resulting from congenital or acquired factors. It is one of the most frequently occurring syndromes associated with physical handicapping conditions in children.

ETIOLOGY

Congenital disorders comprise about 85 per cent of all cases of cerebral palsy, with the most common being cerebral anoxia, trauma, premature birth, toxemia of pregnancy, Rh incompatibility, and congenital malformations of the brain. Postnatal trauma, meningitis, or vascular phenomena occurring in the early developmental years account for the remaining cases of cerebral palsy.

CLINICAL FEATURES

The major motor disorders of congenital cerebral palsy emerge as a result of the maturation of an abnormal nervous system. Clinical classification of cerebral palsy can be made according to the nature of the motor disturbance:

1. Spasticity — the most common type, reflex hyperexcitability, abnormal posture of limbs, limitation in extension of forearms, swallowing difficulties, and excessive drooling.

2. Athetosis — uncontrollable and involuntary muscular activity, facial muscle distortions and drooling usually present.

3. Rigidity — contraction of most muscles, diminished movement.

4. Ataxia — disturbance of postural balance and coordination of muscle activity.

5. Atonia — diminished muscle tone with flabby, weak muscles.

Mental retardation is often associated with this major motor handicap and can be found in 50 per cent of cases. Seizure disorders are found in approximately 30 per cent of cases. Visual problems as well as hearing, speech, and learning disabilities that are related to visual-motor-perceptual abnormalities are also frequently seen.

ORAL MANIFESTATIONS

Abnormal oral manifestations are generally attributed to the neuromuscular disorder. Bruxism is a common phenomenon, found especially in the spastic and athetoid type of motor disturbances. An increased incidence of dental protrusion is exhibited in these individuals, which is more than likely related to the presence of a strong tongue and perioral musculature. Gingival inflammation is commonly present because of mouth breathing and poor oral hygiene. The use of phenytoin (Dilantin) for seizure control may cause gingival hyperplasia. The incidence of dental caries is reportedly higher than average in persons with cerebral palsy; however, the cause is probably secondary to poor oral hygiene rather than an inherent susceptibility.

TREATMENT AND PROGNOSIS

Prognosis of this nonfatal and uncurable condition is dependent largely upon the presence and severity of associated mental handicaps. Physical therapy is employed to enhance control of motor activities. Surgical procedures may be required to relieve joint deformities caused by excessive muscle stresses or for tendon lengthening to aid in walking. Occupational therapy is designed to develop self-help skills. Other adjuncts in treatment include the management of severe behavior disorders and control of seizures with appropriate medications.

FACTORS AFFECTING DENTAL TREATMENT

The control of abnormal muscle activity and the management of mental retardation are major concerns in providing dental care. Parents or guardians are enlisted to provide much of the oral hygiene care. Difficulties in mastication and swallowing often result in a diet consisting of soft foods that are usually high in carbohydrates. This diet, combined with the prolonged retention of food particles in the mouth resulting from abnormal oral muscular activity, enhances the difficulty of oral hygiene. Consequently, the use of stainless steel crowns is frequently preferable compared with large amalgam restorations.

VI.   CEREBRAL PALSY

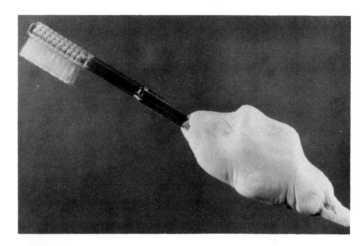

Figure 20–20 Aids for the home care of disabled individuals. Addition of acrylic to the handle helps in the grasp of a toothbrush by the patient. Electric toothbrushes and floss holders are also recommended.

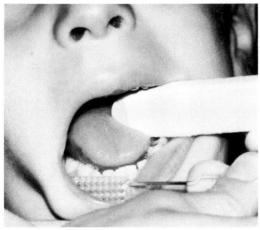

Figure 20–21 A simple mouth prop made from several tongue depressors taped together greatly aids the parent and dentist in cleaning the teeth of a child with cerebral palsy or a mental handicap.

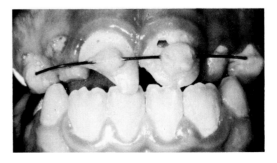

Figure 20–22 Maxillary protrusion combined with a neurological disorder leads to frequent episodes of dental trauma. Note wire and acrylic stabilization.

VI.   CEREBRAL PALSY *Continued*

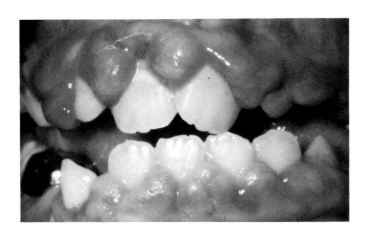

Figure 20–23   Development of gingival hyperplasia with the use of phenytoin (Dilantin) for seizure control. Although poor oral hygiene is thought to initiate the hyperplasia in many cases, other factors such as allergic or autoimmune reactions may be involved. Use of a medium bristle toothbrush for daily gingival massage in addition to tooth brushing may be helpful in reducing tissue hyperplasia. Surgical removal of the tissue is indicated for esthetics or if occlusal function is hindered.

Figure 20–24   Attrition of the dentition may result from bruxism associated with the neuromuscular disorder.

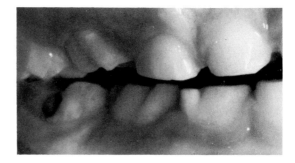

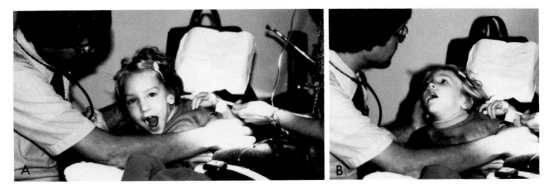

Figure 20–25   Control of body movements is a major factor in treating individuals with cerebral palsy. Use of sedation can be beneficial in the dental office.

Juvenile Rheumatoid Arthritis

INTRODUCTION

Juvenile rheumatoid arthritis (JRA) is one of the most crippling diseases affecting children. There are approximately 200,000 children in the United States less than 15 years of age suffering from JRA. Females are affected more frequently than males in a ratio of 3:1.

ETIOLOGY

Exact causes of the disease are unknown, although infection and autoimmune factors have been suspected.

CLINICAL FEATURES

Clinical features include swollen and stiff joints, with loss of motion and pain upon movement. Synovitis is chronic and can last anywhere from several weeks to several years. If the inflammation persists, permanent joint damage can result. The proximity of the osteogenic growth center to the inflamed synovium has been thought to cause growth disturbances in the involved bones. Premature closure of epiphyses may occur, resulting in markedly hypoplastic bones at maturity. Cephalometric radiographs may show a decreased height of the ramus, a decreased length in the body of the mandible, and a posterior rotation of the mandible. The presence of antegonial notching is shown in Figure 20–27.

ORAL FINDINGS

The reported incidence of temporomandibular joint (TMJ) involvement in juvenile rheumatoid arthritis varies from 18 to 86 per cent. TMJ involvement is found in only the systemic polyarticular and polyarticular types of JRA. Micrognathia is often seen when the growth disturbance in the condyle is severe. Other common findings include decreased lower face height, tendency for open bite, protrusion of incisors, and Class II, Division I malocclusion. Ankylosis of TMJ with its associated growth deformities has been reported.

TREATMENT AND PROGNOSIS

Treatment of the disease is symptomatic and is aimed at maintaining comfort and function. Salicylates are the safest anti-inflammatory drugs and are most widely used. Physical therapy is important in maintaining range of motion and muscle strength. At least 75 per cent of children with JRA do not suffer from permanent disabilities. The latter include permanent joint damage, loss of vision from iridocyclitis, and emotional trauma from chronic illness.

FACTORS AFFECTING DENTAL TREATMENT

Tenderness in the temporomandibular joint and limitation in opening are often encountered in the JRA patient. These factors can increase the difficulty of providing routine dental care. Many JRA patients are on salicylates to decrease the inflammatory aspect of their disease, and this factor should be considered in the anticipation of any oral surgical procedures, since intensive salicylate therapy may produce decreased blood prothrombin (delayed clotting). Since abnormal mandibular growth is inevitable in many of these patients, orthodontic referral should be made early to enable better planning of orthodontic and orthognathic treatment.

Orthodontic treatment can greatly improve the status of the malocclusion often found in the JRA patient. In the case of the severe mandibular dysplasias, orthognathic surgery combined with orthodontic therapy provides the best treatment for the occlusal and facial esthetic problems encountered. Some clinicians recommend that such treatment be performed early to avoid the development of the poor self-image associated with the facial deformity. Owing to the inadequate mandibular body length and the resulting high incidence of impactions, the early removal of third molars is recommended in those patients displaying retarded growth of the mandible in the presence of healthy first and second molars.

VII. JUVENILE RHEUMATOID ARTHRITIS

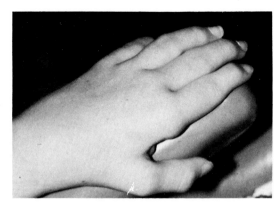

Figure 20–26 Joint swelling in the fingers of a 12-year-old female with polyarticular arthritis.

VII. JUVENILE RHEUMATOID ARTHRITIS *Continued*

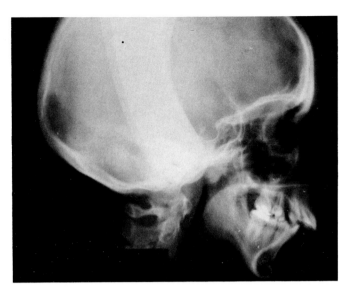

Figure 20–27 Cephalometric radiograph of a 14-year-old female with polyarticular arthritis. These patients often present with Class II, Division I malocclusion and open bite. Note the decreased height of the ramus and marked antegonial notching. The patient required extraction of mandibular (and maxillary) second molars because of inadequate length in the body.

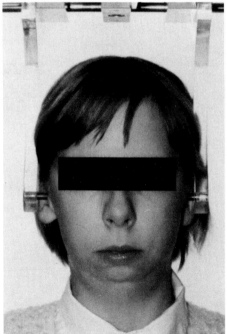

Figure 20–28 Frontal photograph of a 12-year-old female with polyarticular arthritis, showing retruded mandible and obvious short lower face height.

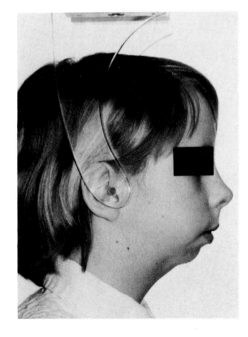

Figure 20–29 Lateral photograph of same patient showing convex profile and obvious micrognathia. Because of the poor self-image that develops in many of these patients, orthodontic referral should be made early to enable better planning of orthodontic and orthognatic treatment.

Leukemia

INTRODUCTION

Leukemia is the most common malignant disease affecting prepubertal children. The incidence in the United States is approximately 3.5 per 100,000, with 40 per cent occurring between the ages of 3 and 5 years.

Chronic leukemia occurs in only 1 to 4 per cent of all childhood leukemias. Acute forms account for 96 to 99 per cent (acute lymphoblastic leukemia, 65 to 85 per cent; acute monocytic, 1 to 5 per cent; and acute undifferentiated the remainder).

ETIOLOGY

The etiology of leukemia is unknown, although it appears to be related to both genetic and environmental factors.

CLINICAL FEATURES

The presenting symptoms of the various types of acute leukemias are similar. Lethargy, fever, pallor, purpura, and pain initially bring the child to the physician. The basic clinical features involve bone marrow failure caused by the displacement of normal blood elements by leukemic cells and infiltration of other tissues by leukemic cells. The consequences of bone marrow failure include anemia, infection resulting from inadequate neutrophils and lymphocytes, and bleeding caused by depressed platelet counts. Diagnosis is confirmed by examination of the bone marrow, which is hypercellular with 60 to 100 per cent blast (immature) cells.

ORAL FINDINGS

The orofacial manifestations can occur early in the disease and may lead to the initial diagnosis. Although the clinical picture is highly variable, petechiae and ecchymoses are often the most common findings in acute lymphoblastic leukemia, followed by pallor, ulcers, and bleeding. Gingival hypertrophy, which is uncommon in the lymphoblastic type, is often the most common finding in the myelogenous or monocytic forms. Lymphadenopathy has been reported as the most common finding in head and neck examinations, and positive findings have been reported as visible on panoremic radiographs. Leukemic infiltration can occur in most areas of the oral cavity, including the buccal mucosa, tongue, gingiva, jaws, and pulp of teeth. *Candida albicans* infection, resulting from antibiotic therapy and the resultant alteration in microflora, is a common finding in acute leukemia.

TREATMENT AND PROGNOSIS

Less than 50 years ago leukemic children could be expected to live no longer than 9 months. Today, however, more than 50 per cent of the children diagnosed with acute lymphoblastic leukemia will have complete remission and discontinuation of therapy in 5 years. Although the other forms of leukemia have higher mortality rates, the number of long-term survivors continues to increase with advances in treatment.

The treatment of leukemia can be divided into three phases:

1. Induction of remission: Multiagent chemotherapy is employed to decrease the blast cell population in order to permit regeneration of normal marrow elements.

2. Central nervous system prophylaxis: The normal administration of chemotherapy does not reach certain areas of the body, such as the CNS, and hence these areas must be treated separately to prevent the development of "extramedullary" leukemia.

3. Maintenance of remission: Once remission has been achieved, maintenance chemotherapy must be continued or the patient will relapse in 2 to 4 months.

FACTORS AFFECTING DENTAL TREATMENT

The major factors influencing dental treatment in leukemia are the complications of the disease, i.e., neutropenia (inadequate neutrophils) and thrombocytopenia (inadequate platelets). Because of these complications, the management of the oral pathologic condition is dependent on the nature of the problem.

1. Management of acute infections: All acute pathology should be treated prior to initiating remission induction chemotherapy, which will further suppress bone marrow elements. Blood counts should be known in order to provide the necessary supportive care (antibiotics and blood component therapy). The following conditions are considered acute: deeply carious, necrotic, or abscessed teeth; other orofacial abscesses; dental or bony fractures; and oral hemorrhage.

2. Management of caries: Treatment of routine caries should be postponed until the child is in remission and then only after the attending hematologist has been consulted.

3. Management of soft tissue: Chemotherapy can cause severe oral ulcers and mucositis. Gingival hypertrophy and hemorrhage may reflect complications of the disease (leukemic infiltration of tissue and thrombocytopenia) but commonly represent an exaggerated response to local factors. Aggressive oral hygiene, including brushing, flossing, and frequent rinsing, can prevent or minimize such problems. Oral Candida infections can be treated with nystatin rinses.

VIII.   LEUKEMIA

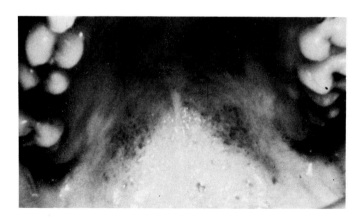

Figure 20–30 One of the most common intraoral manifestations of leukemia is petecchiae. Although they can occur on the lips or buccal mucosa, they are often seen at the junction of the hard and soft palate and may lead to the initial diagnosis. (Courtesy Dr. A. Morgan, Seattle.)

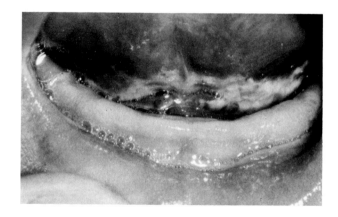

Figure 20–31 Leukemic patients receiving antibiotics or chemotherapy have a high incidence of *Candida albicans* infections. Note area of moniliasis beneath the tongue of this young infant with leukemia. To prevent such infections, nystatin mouth rinses should be used prophylactically every 2 hours.

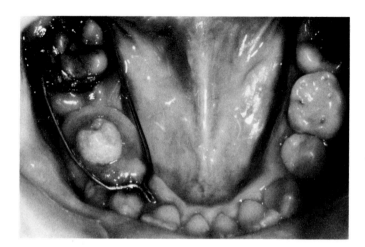

Figure 20–32 Intraoral photograph of a 12-year-old male who presented with a chief complaint of soreness in the area of his space maintainer. (Note enlarged tissue in this area.) Blood studies 2 days later revealed relapse of acute myelogenous leukemia.

VIII. LEUKEMIA *Continued*

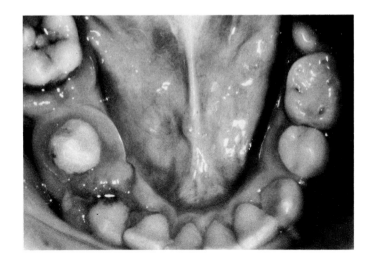

Figure 20–33 After removal of the appliance it was noted that the gingival hypertrophy was apparent only on the side of the appliance, and not on the side devoid of local irritating factors.

Sickle Cell Anemia

INTRODUCTION

Sickle cell anemia is a chronic hereditary hemolytic anemia predominantly affecting the black population.

ETIOLOGY

Inheritance is autosomal recessive. Carriers of the heterozygous gene for sickling are identified as having sickle cell trait. True sickle cell anemia is present when the individual has a homozygous gene for sickling. The basic defect occurs in the hemoglobin molecule of the erythrocyte. Deoxygenation results in distortion of the erythrocyte into a sickle-shaped cell. The clinical manifestations of the disease occur when small vessels are occluded by increased numbers of the less soluble sickled red blood cells.

CLINICAL FEATURES

The chief clinical manifestation of the disease is the acute exacerbation or crisis. These periodic acute forms of sickle cell anemia are associated most commonly with severe pain in the abdomen, muscles, and joints. The acute vaso-occlusive crises may be initiated by infections, dehydration, hypoxia, acidosis, or a combination of these. Infarctions within small bones of the extremities may produce painful swellings of the hands and feet in early childhood.

Other types of crises involve pooling of large volumes of blood in the liver and spleen, with resulting circulatory collapse. Various radiological changes can be seen in skeletal bones, resulting from areas of thrombosis and infarction or loss of trabeculation due to bone marrow hyperplasia.

CRANIOFACIAL FEATURES

The most noted features are the changes seen within the mandibular alveolar bone. These include decreases in radiodensity of bone, larger marrow spaces, bony infarctions, loss of definitive cortical plates, and interdental cuffing of the interproximal bone.

TREATMENT AND PROGNOSIS

Therapy for the individual with sickle cell anemia is mainly supportive, since there is presently no cure. Avoidance of crisis producing factors such as infections and hypoxia is stressed. Treatment of acute episodes includes analgesics for pain relief, correction of any dehydration and acidosis, and appropriate antibiotic therapy for infections.

FACTORS AFFECTING DENTAL TREATMENT

The potential problems posed by any infection points out the necessity for preventive dental measures. Early signs or symptoms of infection require aggressive treatment. Administration of prophylactic antibiotics prior to dental surgical procedures should be considered to minimize the chance of postoperative infection.

Although conditions of hypoxia are to be avoided, use of nitrous oxide–oxygen analgesia is generally not contraindicated.

IX. SICKLE CELL ANEMIA

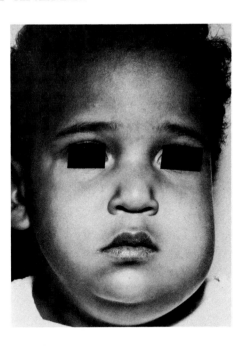

Figure 20–34   The most significant feature in the treatment of individuals with sickle cell anemia is the prevention of infections that might trigger an acute exacerbation of the disease.

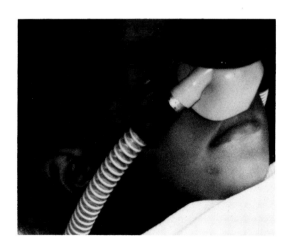

Figure 20–35   If nitrous oxide is used, hypoxia *must* be avoided. (See Chapter 19.)

X. DIABETES MELLITUS

Diabetes Mellitus

INTRODUCTION

Diabetes mellitus is a disorder of carbohydrate metabolism resulting from absolute or functional insulin deficiency. The prevalence in children less than 15 years of age is approximately 1 in 2500. However, the percentage of known diabetics in the adult age group is much higher, being somewhere in the range of 1 in 100.

ETIOLOGY

Diabetes is considered hereditary and is probably a recessive trait.

CLINICAL FEATURES

The onset of diabetes mellitus in children can be sudden with the classic symptoms of polyuria, thirst, itching, hunger, weakness, and weight loss. The excretion of excessive amounts of urine during the day and night leads to increased thirst and dryness of the skin. The juvenile form of diabetes, if untreated, is characterized by ketosis, acidosis, and hyperglycemia. In contrast, its occurrence in adults, sometimes called maturity onset diabetes, generally presents hyperglycemia without ketosis.

Vascular complications that are commonly associated with diabetes include coronary arteriosclerosis and retinopathy. Generally, impairment of vascular flow slows the healing of injuries and increases the incidence and severity of infections. The decreased life expectancy for patients with diabetes is attributed to the associated vascular disease. Myocardial infarctions account for a majority of deaths among diabetics.

ORAL FINDINGS

Patients with diabetes that goes untreated show a significant increase in caries and periodontal disease. However, patients with properly controlled diabetes show no significant differences in caries and periodontal disease when compared with the normal population. If anything, a lower caries rate may be seen because of the controlled diet. Other oral symptoms may include a dry and burning sensation, especially in the tongue.

TREATMENT AND PROGNOSIS

Restoring normal metabolic conditions in juvenile diabetics involves the administration of insulin. Daily insulin injections are tailored to the individual needs of the patient. The type and amount of insulin required depends on time of injection, diet, exercise or daily activity, presence of infection, fever, other medical conditions, and the size of the patient.

Insulin shock or hypoglycemia may occur with an overdose of insulin or when too little food is taken after the injection. Signs of insulin-induced shock include restlessness, pallor, reduction in temperature, and sweating. If untreated, it may lead to confulsions and coma. Administration of oral or intravenous glucose rapidly corrects the condition.

FACTORS AFFECTING DENTAL TREATMENT

In uncontrolled diabetes, medical advice should be sought before instituting any treatment. Dental appointments for patients with controlled diabetes should be scheduled at a time that does not interfere with the administration of medication or meals. Adjustments in medication are generally not needed for routine dental care. However, the physician may elect to modify the insulin dosage for a surgical procedure.

XI.   EPILEPSY

Epilepsy

INTRODUCTION

Epilepsy is a recurrent convulsive disorder characterized by states of unconsciousness, tonic or clonic muscle spasms, and other abnormal behavior. In the early school years, the prevalence of epilepsy is between 1 and 2 per cent.

ETIOLOGY

Epilepsy may stem from cerebral abnormalities, possibly related to birth injuries, or may be idiopathic in nature.

CLINICAL FEATURES

The dentist should be familiar with the two most common types of epileptic manifestations, gran mal and petit mal seizures. Grand mal seizures are characterized by generalized convulsions with tonic and clonic phases of muscle spasms. There is loss of balance, with an unsupported patient falling to the ground or floor. The pupils dilate and the eyeballs roll upward. Facial distortion occurs, and the head is thrown backward or to one side. As the tonic phase continues, respiratory movements are arrested and cyanosis occurs. This phase lasts about 30 seconds, after which the patient usually sleeps soundly for a brief period. Headaches and a generalized state of confusion may be present on regaining consciousness. Although a number of medications have been utilized for controlling the seizure activity phenytoin (Dilantin) remains the drug of choice for gran mal seizures.

Petit mal seizures are characterized by momentary or transient loss of consciousness. There may be a brief upward rolling of the eyeballs, nodding of the head, or slight quivering of the body. Attacks of this type are usually less than 30 seconds in duration, after which the individual resumes normal activity. Seizure medication therapy may be necessary in some cases of extensive petit mal activity.

ORAL FINDINGS

Overgrowth of gingival tissues is characteristic of patients on phenytoin therapy. No significant oral changes occur from the disease itself. Tooth fractures are common from falls.

FACTORS AFFECTING DENTAL TREATMENT

If a grand mal seizure occurs during dental treatment, the main concern is the prevention of a self-inflicted injury by the patient. Insertion of a towel or similar object between the teeth may be useful in preventing injury to the teeth. The patient should be positioned so there is the least likelihood of falling or striking nearby objects. If rubber dam clamps are used in a patient who is subject to seizures, it is advisable to have a length of dental floss attached to the clamp to permit retrieval in case of aspiration.

Petit mal seizures usually present no major problem other than delaying treatment until the child returns to a normal state.

Overgrowth of gingival tissues (phenytoin hyperplasia) can be partially controlled by careful oral hygiene. However, in severe cases, surgical removal of the hyperplastic tissue is the treatment of choice. Consultation with the physician is advisable to determine whether alternate drug therapy is possible to avoid phenytoin hyperplasia. In all patients with epilepsy, the dentist should avoid using removable appliances because of the danger of aspiration.

Cleft Lip and Palate

INTRODUCTION

Cleft lip and/or palate occurs in approximately 1 of every 700 live births in the United States. Cleft palate forms in the absence of midline contact and fusion of lateral palatal shelves in the developing maxillary processes. A cleft of the lip and alveolus is a result of the failure to maintain an epithelial fusion between the median nasal process and maxillary processes. These events occur between the eighth and tenth week of embryological development.

ETIOLOGY

In addition to its association with numerous congenital syndromes, maternal use of thalidomide and phenytoin has been identified as causing cleft lip and palate. For those cases with no recognizable genetic pattern, a multifactorial causation has been suggested, one in which there appears a strong familial tendency interacting with a variety of environmental influences to produce the cleft.

CLINICAL FEATURES

The presence of midfacial deformity in a patient with cleft palate is obvious. The development of a concave profile appears to be dependent upon the original severity of the defect as well as the type and timing of surgical repair. Associated disorders include speech defects due to incomplete velopharyngeal closure and frequently loss of normal lip, alveolar ridge, and dental relationships. Anatomical defects within the eustachian tubes and frequent inner ear infections lead to a high incidence of hearing impairment.

ORAL FINDINGS

Dental anomalies associated with cleft palate include congenitally missing teeth, supernumerary teeth, fused teeth, malformed teeth, malposed teeth, and altered dental eruption in the area of the cleft.

FACTORS AFFECTING DENTAL TREATMENT

Rehabilitation of a cleft lip and palate requires a program involving the pediatrician, plastic and oral surgeons, otolaryngologist, dentist, orthodontist, speech therapist, social worker, and child psychologist. Although the timing of surgical correction varies with the degree of involvement, closure of the cleft lip is generally performed as soon as the child is able to withstand the surgical procedures under a general anesthetic. This is usually performed around 12 to 14 weeks after birth. Soft tissue closure of a cleft palate is recommended around 2 years of age to facilitate speech development.

In addition to routine dental care, the dentist may be needed to provide prosthetic replacement of missing teeth or esthetic management of malformed teeth. Maxillary arch collapse is a frequent occurrence; therefore children with a cleft palate and/or lip require early monitoring and treatment by the orthodontist. Palatal expansion is usually required.

XII. CLEFT LIP AND PALATE

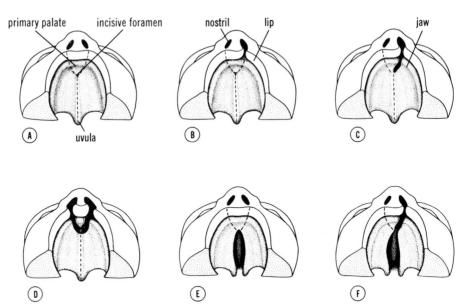

Figure 20–36 Classification of cleft lip and palate. The incisive foramen is commonly used as the landmark to separate isolated cleft lip from cleft palate. *A*, Normal, *B*, Unilateral cleft lip not involving the alveolus, *C*, Cleft lip involving alveolar ridge to incisive foramen, *D*, Bilateral cleft of lip and alveolus, *E*, Isolated cleft palate, *F*, Unilateral cleft lip and palate. (From Langmen, J.: *Medical Embryology*. Baltimore, Williams & Wilkins Co., 1975, p. 345.)

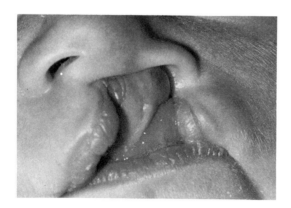

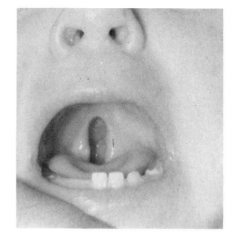

Figure 20–37 Unilateral cleft of lip and alveolar ridge. Presence of unilateral cleft lip appears on the left side twice as often as the right side. (Courtesy M. Michael Cohen, Jr., Seattle.)

Figure 20–38 Isolated cleft of the soft palate. (Courtesy Dr. Oscar Beder, Seattle.)

XII. CLEFT LIP AND PALATE *Continued*

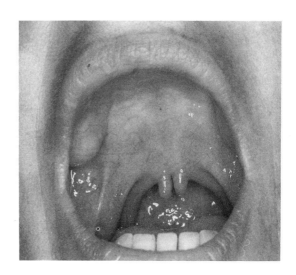

Figure 20–39 A bifid uvula is considered an incomplete expression of a cleft palate. Although this disorder has no dental implications, its presence may be associated with a submucous cleft. (Courtesy Dr. Oscar Beder, Seattle.)

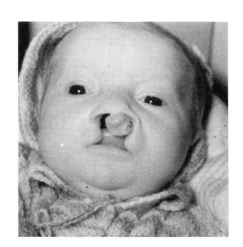

Figure 20–40 Frontal view of intant with bilateral cleft lip and palate. (Courtesy Dr. Oscar Beder, Seattle.)

Figure 20–41 Lateral view of patient in Figure 20–40. (Courtesy Dr. Oscar Beder, Seattle.)

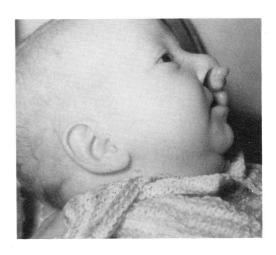

XII. CLEFT LIP AND PALATE *Continued*

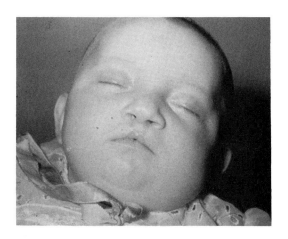

Figure 20–42   Repair of bilateral cleft lip of patient seen in Figures 20–40 and 20–41. Surgical closure of the cleft lip is accomplished as soon as the infant is able to withstand the general anesthesia and surgery. This is usually within 3 to 4 months after birth. Closure of the palate is delayed until initial speech development, in order to afford normal growth of the maxilla. (Courtesy Dr. Oscar Beder, Seattle.)

Figure 20–43   Maxillary arch collapse and associated dental malocclusion necessitates early orthodontic services. (Courtesy Dr. R. William McNeill, Seattle.)

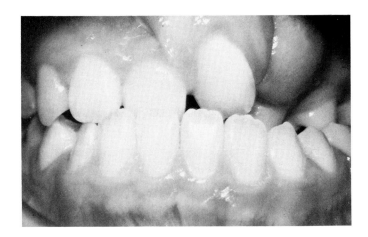

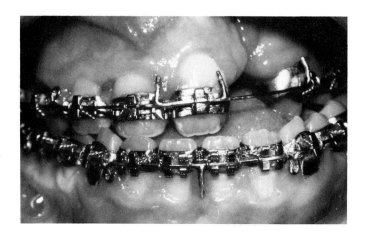

Figure   20–44   Orthodontic treatment generally precedes any definitive prosthetic therapy. (Courtesy Dr. R. William McNeill, Seattle.)

XII.   CLEFT LIP AND PALATE *Continued*

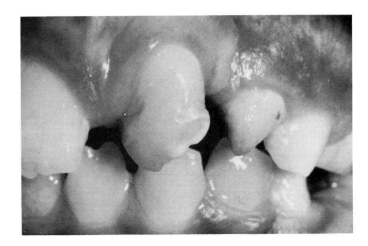

Figure 20–45   Abnormal morphology and hypoplastic enamel on a central incisor adjacent to cleft in alveolar ridge.

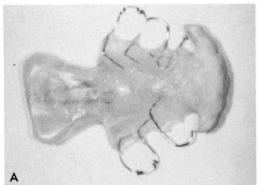
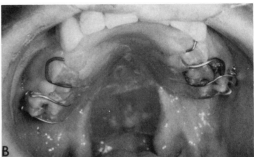

Figure 20–46   Construction of an obturator may be necessary for those clefts in which surgical closure is not possible. The obturator seals off the intraoral cavity from the nasal cavity to aid in speech and mastication. (Courtesy Dr. Oscar Beder, Seattle.)

Congenital Heart Disease

INTRODUCTION

Congenital heart disease occurs in approximately 6 of every 1000 newborn infants. It is important that the dentist recognize the importance of adequate oral health care for these individuals.

Congenital heart lesions can be divided into cyanotic and acyanotic types. The most common of these are as follows:

Acyanotic

Atrial septal defect
Ventricular septal defect
Patent ductus arteriosus
Pulmonic stenosis
Aortic stenosis

Cyanotic

Tetralogy of Fallot
Transposition of great vessels
Tricuspid atresia
Totally anomalous pulmonary venous return

The reader is referred to the Appendix for a schematic representation of the anatomy and physiology of some of these defects.

ETIOLOGY

Maternal diseases such as rubella or viral myocarditis are known to cause abnormalities in the fetal heart. Children born with Down's syndrome (a chromosomal abnormality) have a higher incidence of congenital heart disease. The chances of having an additional offspring with a congenital heart disorder is increased if one offspring or parent is affected. The mode of inheritance is thought to be polygenic.

CLINICAL FEATURES

The clinical findings are highly variable and depend on the type of lesion and the severity of the particular defect. In the acyanotic forms, the patient may be asymptomatic with no positive history, or may present with a history including dyspnea and exercise intolerance or congestive heart failure and cyanosis in the severe forms. The cyanotic forms usually present with a history of cyanosis, dyspnea, exercise intolerance, tachypnea, and spells of hypoxia. Cyanosis with clubbing of the fingers and the presence of systolic murmur also characterize the cyanotic forms.

TREATMENT AND PROGNOSIS

Although approximately 70 per cent of infants born with congenital heart disease can be helped with surgery, 50 per cent of these children will die during the first year of life if there is no surgical intervention. Although the clinical course is highly variable among the different types and within the same type of defect, the prognosis throughout childhood is usually good if the child has survived the first year without major symptoms. Congestive heart failure, subacute bacterial endocarditis, and pulmonary vascular disease are major complications of the acyanotic forms, whereas congestive heart failure, hypoxia, and thrombosis characterize the complications of the cyanotic types of defects.

Following the identification of a cardiac problem, the patient is referred to a cardiologist — the timing dependent on the presence of significant symptoms. Children with severe problems usually limit their own activity. Angina, syncope, or abnormalities in the electrocardiogram may warrant further limitation and possibly the consideration of catheterization and surgery. Decisions concerning surgical intervention are based on the natural history of the defect and the surgical morbidity and mortality. Elective cardiovascular surgery is usually recommended at the preschool age.

FACTORS AFFECTING DENTAL TREATMENT

Bacterial endocarditis, though relatively uncommon in children, may sometimes occur as a result of dental treatment. In order to prevent the occurrence of this serious complication, children with congenital heart defects should receive prophylactic antibiotics prior to dental treatment. Dental abscesses are especially dangerous; hence an aggressive oral hygiene program is a necessity. Daily use of topical fluorides is recommended in those children with high caries susceptibility. Because of varying opinions concerning the preferred regimen of prophylactic antibiotic coverage, it is recommended that the child's pediatrician or cardiologist be consulted prior to performing any dental procedures.

XIII.   CONGENITAL HEART DISEASE

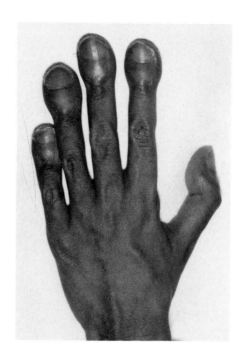

Figure 20–47   An 8-year-old female with inoperable cyanotic heart disease displaying typical clubbing of the fingers.

Figure 20–48   An 8-year-old white female with transposition of the great vessels, atrial septal defect, ventricular septal defect, and, because of her cyanotic heart disease, a hematocrit of 87 (normal is 37). Cyanosis was apparent in the lips and tongue.

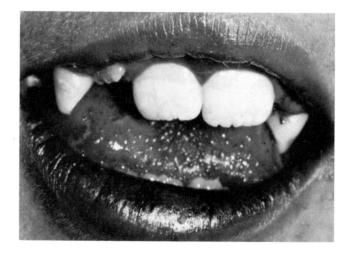

REFERENCES

I. *Deafness*

1. Kopra, M. A.: A brighter future for deaf people. Rehabil. *40*(5):35–38, 1974.
2. Brownstein, M. P.: Dental care for the deaf child. Dent. Clin. North Am., *18*:3, 1974.

II. *Blindness*

1. Lebowitz, E. J., An introduction to dentistry for the blind. Dent. Clin. North. Am. *81*:3, 1974.

III. *Mental Retardation*

1. *Mental Retardation — A Handbook for the Primary Physician*. A Report of the American Medical Association Conference on Mental Retardation, April 9–11, 1964.
2. Krauss, B. S., Clark, G. R., and Okra, S. W.: Mental retardation and abnormalities of the dentition. Am. J. Ment. Defic. 72:905–917, 1968.

IV. *Hemophilia*

1. Nakai, T. R., Peterson, J. C., and Law, D. B.: Current concepts in the management of hemophilic pedodontic patients. J. Dent. Child. 41(5):361–366, 1974.
2. Needleman, H. L., Kaban, L. B., and Kevy, S. V. The use of epsilon-aminocaproic acid for the management of hemophilia in dental and oral surgery patients. J. Am. Dent. Assoc. 93:586–590, 1976.
3. Grossman, R. C.: Orthodontics and dentistry for the hemophiliac patient. Am. J. Orthod. 68:391–403, 1975.

V. *Down's Syndrome (Trisomy 21)*

1. Cohen, M. M., Sr., and Cohen, M. M., Jr.: Oral Manifestations of Trisomy G_1 (Down Syndrome). In *Birth Defects: Original Article Series*, Bergsma, D. (ed.), Vol. VII, No. 7, June 1971, pp. 241–251. White Plains.
2. Gorlin, R. J., Pindborg, J. J., and Cohen, M. M., Jr.: *Syndromes of the Head and Neck*, Chapter 21, McGraw-Hill Book Co., New York, 1977, pp. 96–98.
3. Nowak, A. J. (ed.): *Dentistry for the Handicapped Patient*, The C. V. Mosby Co., St. Louis, 1976.

VI. *Cerebral Palsy*

1. Nowak, A. J. ed.): *Dentistry for the Handicapped Patient*, The C. V. Mosby Co., St. Louis, 1976.
2. McKay, R. J., and Vaughan, V. C. (eds.): *Nelson Textbook of Pediatrics*, W. B. Saunders Co., Philadelphia, 1975, pp. 1423–1425.

VII. *Juvenile Rheumatoid Arthritis*

1. Barriga, B., Lewis, T. M., and Law, D. B.: An investigation of the dental occlusion in children with juvenile rheumatoid arthritis. Angle Orthod. 44(4):329–335, 1974.
2. Martis, C. S., and Karakasis, D. T.: Ankylosis of the temporomandibular joint caused by Still's disease. Oral Surg. 35:462–466, 1973.
3. Smith, D. W., and Marshal, R. E.: *Introduction to Clinical Pediatrics*, Chapter 32, W. B. Saunders Co., Philadelphia, 1972, pp. 220–224.

VIII. *Leukemia*

1. Sutow, W. W., Viehi, T. J., and Fernbach, D. J.: *Clinical Pediatric Oncology*, The C. V. Mosby Co., St. Louis, 1973.

2. Curtis, A. B.: Childhood leukemias: osseous changes in jaws on panoremic dental radiographs. J.A.D.A. 83:844–847, 1971.

IX.   *Sickle Cell Anemia*

1. Powell, E. A., and Januska, J. R.: Sickle cell anemia: chronology, natural history, and implications for dental practice. Quart. Nat. Dent. Assoc. 31:72–81, 1973.
2. McKay, R. J., and Vaughan, V. C., eds.: *Nelson Textbook of Pediatrics*, W. B. Saunders Co., Philadelphia, 1975, pp. 1124–1126.
3. Michelson, R. K., and Whitmore, R. B.: Sickle cell anemia in the dental patient. Oral Surg., Oral Med., and Oral Path. 21:19–24, 1967.

X.   *Diabetes Mellitus*

1. Bernick, S. M., et al.: Dental disease in children with diabetes mellitus. J. Periodont. 46(4):241–245, 1975.
2. Cohen, D. W., et al.: Diabetes mellitus and periodontal disease: two-year longitudinal observations. Part I. J. Periodont. 41:709–712, 1970.
3. Paulsen, E. P., and Colle, E.: Diabetes Mellitus. In *Endocrine and Genetic Diseases of Childhood and Adolescence, Gardner, L. I., ed. W. B. Saunders Co., Philadelphia, 1975.*

XI.   *Epilepsy*

1. Dummett, O. W.: Oral tissue reactions from Dilantin medication in the control of epileptic seizures. J. Periodontol. 25:112, 1954.
2. Gibberd, F. B., Dunne, J. F., Handley, A. J., and Hagleman, B. L.: Supervision of epileptic patients taking phenytoin. Br. Med. J. 1:147–149, 1970.
3. Buchanan, R. A., and Allen, R. J.: Diphenylhydantoin and phenobarbital levels in epileptic children. Neurology (Minneap) 21:866–871, 1971.

XII.   *Cleft Lip and Palate*

1. Georgiade, N. G., and Hagerty, R. F.: *Symposium on Management of Cleft Lip and Palate and Associated Deformities.* The C. V. Mosby Co., St. Louis, 1974.
2. McKay, R. J., and Vaughan, V. C., eds.: *Nelson Textbook of Pediatrics*, W. B. Saunders, Philadelphia, 1975, pp. 1423–1425.
3. Nowak, A. J., ed.: *Dentistry for the Handicapped Patient*, The C. V. Mosby Co., St. Louis, 1976.

XIII.   *Congenital Heart Disease*

1. Morgan, B. C., and Kawabori, I. Cardiovascular Disorders. In Smith, D. W., *Introduction to Clinical Pediatrics*, W. B. Saunders Co., Philadelphia, 1977.
2. American Heart Association. *If Your Child Has A Congenital Heart Defect.* Dallas, 1970.

APPENDIX

It is not unusual for a dentist to have patients with congenital or acquired heart defects (e.g., rheumatic valvular heart disease). It is important for the practitioner to be aware of the dental implications of treating these patients and the anatomical configuration of such defects. Consultation with the child's physician is important in determining type, doses, duration of action, and route of administration of antibiotics to be prescribed. At the time of publication, the most current recommendations on prophylactic antibiotic measures for children with congenital or acquired heart defects appear in a 1977 report by the Committee on Rheumatic Fever and Bacterial Endocarditis, American Heart Association, 7320 Greenville Avenue, Dallas, Texas 75231. This report should be referred to for complete information on which cases require prophylaxis; for the joint recommendations of the American Heart Association and the American Dental Association, the following sources can be consulted: "Prevention of Bacterial Endocarditis" (a brochure published by the American Heart Association); *Circulation*, 56:139A, 1977; and the *Journal of the American Dental Association*, 95:600, 1977.

Recommended antibiotics for protection against bacterial endocarditis in dental patients with an existing heart condition are listed on the next page.

ANTIBIOTIC REGIMEN	DOSAGE INFORMATION
1. For most patients: **PENICILLIN**	*a. Intramuscular plus oral:* ADULTS: 600,000 units of procaine penicillin G mixed with 1,000,000 units of aqueous crystalline penicillin intramuscularly 30–60 minutes prior to dental procedure, followed by 500 mg penicillin V orally every 6 hours for 8 doses. CHILDREN: 30,000 units aqueous penicillin G/kg mixed with 600,000 units of procaine penicillin intramuscularly (not to exceed adult dose). For children less than 27 kg, the dose of penicillin V is 250 mg every 6 hours for 8 doses. *b. Oral only:* ADULTS: 2.0 gm of penicillin V 30–60 minutes prior to dental procedure and then 500 mg every 6 hours for 8 doses. CHILDREN LESS THAN 27 KG: 1.0 gm of penicillin V 30 minutes to one hour prior to dental procedure and then 250 mg every 6 hours for 8 doses.
2. For those allergic to penicillin: **ERYTHROMYCIN**°	ADULTS: 1.0 gm orally an hour and a half to two hours prior to dental procedure and then 500 mg every 6 hours for 8 doses (or Regimen 4). CHILDREN: 20 mg/kg orally an hour and a half to two hours prior to dental procedure and then 10 mg/kg (not to exceed adult dosage) every 6 hours for 8 doses (or Regimen 4).
3. For those at higher risk of infective endocarditis and not allergic to penicillin:† **PENICILLIN** plus **STREPTOMYCIN**	ADULTS: Intramuscular penicillin as outlined above in Regimen 1a, plus streptomycin 1.0 gm intramuscularly, both given 30–60 minutes before dental procedure; then penicillin V 500 mg orally every 6 hours for 8 doses. CHILDREN: Timing of doses is same as for adults. Aqueous penicillin dose is 30,000 units/kg mixed with 600,000 units procaine penicillin. Streptomycin dose is 20 mg/kg (not to exceed adult dosage). For children less than 27 kg, the dose of penicillin V is 250 mg every 6 hours for 8 doses.
4. For higher risk patients allergic to penicillin:† **VANCOMYCIN** (IV) plus **ERYTHROMYCIN** (oral)	ADULTS: Vancomycin 1 gm intravenously over 30–60 minutes, begun 30–60 minutes before dental procedure; then erythromycin 500 mg orally every 6 hours for 8 doses. CHILDREN: Timing of doses is same as for adults. Dose of vancomycin is 20 mg/kg. Dose of erythromycin is 10 mg/kg every 6 hours for 8 doses (not to exceed adult dose).

°Erythromycin may also be selected for those receiving oral penicillin as continuous rheumatic fever prophylaxis.

†This category particularly includes patients with prosthetic heart valves.

494

The illustrations in this Appendix are included as a convenient reference on normal and abnormal anatomy of the heart. (Figures 1 to 10 modified from American Heart Association manual "If Your Child Has a Congenital Heart Defect.")

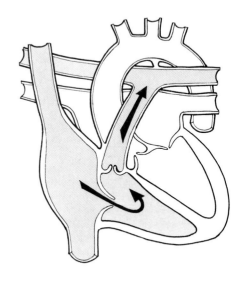

Figure 1 Normal heart function. Venous blood, low in oxygen, returns to the heart through the superior vena cava and enters the right atrium. This low-pressure chamber then empties blood into the right ventricle through the tricuspid valve. Contraction of the right ventricle drives blood under low pressure through the pulmonary valves and artery to the lungs for oxygenation.

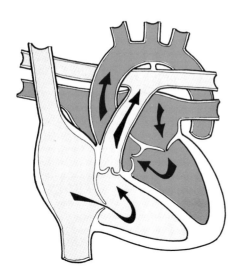

Figure 2 Normal heart function. Bright red blood, which has been oxygenated, returns to the heart through the left atrium. Once the blood passes into the left ventricle, it is pumped out the aortic valve into the body's general circulation. Pressure within the left ventricle is high and equals that of the patient's blood pressure.

Figure 3 Patent ductus arteriosus. During normal fetal development a shunt exists between the pulmonary artery and aorta, allowing blood to bypass the lungs. This open passageway usually closes spontaneously within a few weeks after birth. Failure to close allows continued shunting of blood through this passageway. Because of differences in arterial pressure, however, the aortic blood flows back into the pulmonary circulation. The heart is forced to work harder to supply sufficient blood for general circulation. Correction of this defect usually involves surgical ligation of the passageway or division and suture of the ductus.

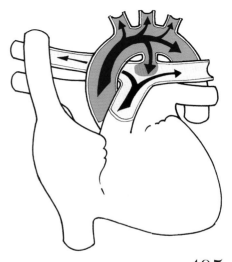

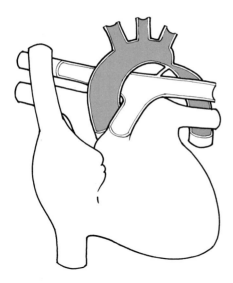

Figure 4 Coarctation of the aorta. Constrictions of the aorta result in a diminished flow blood to those parts of the body served by the aorta distal to the constriction. The majority of such constrictions occur just below the origin of the left subclavian artery. Development of hypertension can lead to congestive heart failure or intracranial hemorrhage. Correction of the disorder generally involves excision of the constricted area with subsequent closure of the ends or grafting.

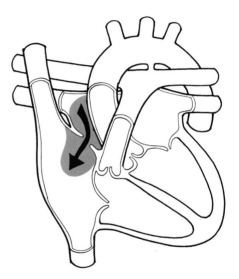

Figure 5 Atrial septal defect. Openings in the septum or wall separating the right and left chambers shunt the blood returning from the pulmonary circulation into the right chambers for a return trip to the lungs. As in ductus arteriosus, a septal defect results in cardiac inefficiency. Loud murmurs can often be detected in patients with septal defects. If surgical closure is necessary, it is usually carried out in childhood.

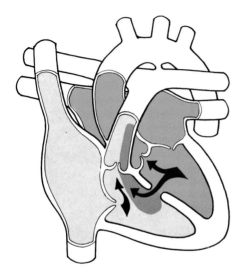

Figure 6 Ventricular septal defect.

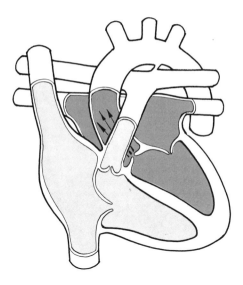

Figure 7 Aortic stenosis. Narrowing or stenosis of the aortic valve decreases the outflow of blood for general body circulation and creates high pressure in the left ventricle. The constriction in most cases is caused by thickening of the leaflets. Most affected children are asymptomatic and have otherwise normal physical development.

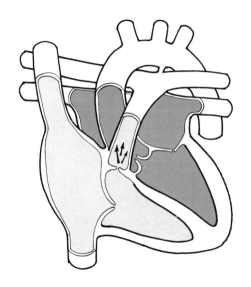

Figure 8 Pulmonic stenosis. Constriction of the pulmonary valve decreases the rate of blood flow through the lungs for oxygenation and increases the right ventricular pressure. Surgery is generally indicated when the pressure is high.

Figure 9 Tetralogy of Fallot. This disorder is the result of several cardiac defects, including a ventricular septal defect, pulmonary stenosis, dextroposition of the aorta, and right ventricular hypertrophy. Insufficient oxygen in the blood results in cyanosis, most notably seen in the mucous membranes of the lips and mouth and in the fingernails. Clubbing of fingers is common. Patients with an uncomplicated tetralogy of Fallot usually undergo total correction of the defect by open heart surgery before adolescence.

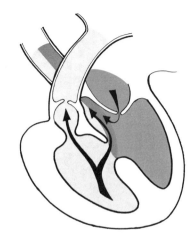

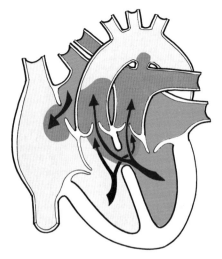

Figure 10   Transposition of the great vessels. Transposition of the great vessels involves a reversal in the normal attachment of the pulmonary artery to the right ventricle and the aorta to the left ventricle. This results in essentially two closed circulatory systems, with the pulmonary flow going through the left chamber of the heart back to the lungs and blood from the general circulatory system going only through the right chamber with no means of reoxygenation. Infants born with this disorder can survive only when there are co-existing cardiac defects that allow oxygenated blood to reach the aorta (e.g., septal defects, patent ductus arteriosus).

INDEX

Note: Page numbers in *italics* refer to illustrations; page numbers followed by "t" refer to tables.